Volume 2

MERRILL'S ATLAS *of*

RADIOGRAPHIC POSITIONING & PROCEDURES

Nicholas Armietti

3/4 / 1

1ˢᵗ volume Ribs On
Wed· ✓

Volume 2

MERRILL'S ATLAS *of*

RADIOGRAPHIC POSITIONING & PROCEDURES

Eugene D. Frank, MA, RT(R), FASRT, FAERS

Bruce W. Long, MS, RT(R)(CV), FASRT

Barbara J. Smith, MS, RT(R)(QM), FASRT

Jeannean Hall Rollins, MRC, BSRT(R)(CV)

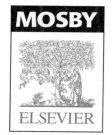

MOSBY

ELSEVIER

MOSBY
ELSEVIER

11830 Westline Industrial Drive
St. Louis, Missouri 63146

WORKBOOK FOR MERRILL'S ATLAS OF RADIOGRAPHIC
POSITIONING & PROCEDURES, VOLUME 2, EDITION 11

Volume 2

Two-volume set

ISBN-13: 978-0-323-04215-4
ISBN-10: 0-323-04215-5
ISBN-13: 978-0-323-04216-1
ISBN-10: 0-323-04216-3

Notice

Neither the Publisher nor the Authors assume any responsibility for any loss or injury and/or damage to persons or property arising out of or related to any use of the material contained in this book. It is the responsibility of the treating practitioner, relying on independent expertise and knowledge of the patient, to determine the best treatment and method of application for the patient.

The Publisher

ISBN-13: 978-0-323-04215-4 (Volume 2)
ISBN-13: 978-0-323-04216-1 (Two-volume set)
ISBN-10: 0-323-04215-5 (Volume 2)
ISBN-10: 0-323-04216-3 (Two-volume set)

Publisher: Andrew Allen
Executive Editor: Jeanne Wilke
Senior Developmental Editor: Linda Woodard
Publishing Services Manager: Patricia Tannian
Project Manager: Kristine Feeherty
Design Direction: Paula Ruckenbrod
Cover Designer: Paula Ruckenbrod

Printed in the United States of America

Last digit is the print number: 9 8 7 6 5 4 3 2

Preface

This two-volume workbook has been developed to accompany *Merrill's Atlas of Radiographic Positioning and Procedures* (commonly referred to as *Merrill's Atlas,* or just *Merrill's*). The chapters in this workbook are presented in the same order as the first 31 chapters of *Merrill's Atlas of Radiographic Positioning and Procedures.* The workbook is also a useful companion to *Mosby's Radiography Online: Anatomy and Positioning for Merrill's Atlas of Radiographic Positioning & Procedures.* However, the material presented in this workbook can function as a useful review for any anatomy and positioning course or as a review for the certification exam. The exercises found in this workbook are designed to give you a thorough review of osteology, anatomy, physiology, arthrology, and radiographic examinations.

FEATURES

All chapters that have essential projections are divided into two sections: an anatomy section and a positioning section.
- The anatomy sections consist of various exercises such as labeling and identification diagrams, short-answer and multiple-choice questions, matching exercises, and crossword puzzles.
- The positioning sections include short-answer and multiple-choice questions, true-false statements, fill-in-the-blank statements, matching exercises, identification exercises, and comparisons of standard radiographic projections.
- At the end of each chapter are multiple-choice questions that review the entire chapter.
- Answers for all exercises are provided at the end of each volume.

NEW TO THIS EDITION

- New Chapter 2, "Compensating Filters," added to review essential information now included in *Merrill's*
- Several new questions and exercises to practice application of abbreviations commonly used in radiography
- New review questions on the axiolateral projection (Coyle method) of the elbow

- New review questions on the AP oblique projection (Grashey method) of the shoulder
- New exercises on the acetabulum and anterior pelvic bone projections included in the eleventh edition of *Merrill's*
- Five new chapters provided to review pediatric, geriatric, mobile, surgical and computed tomography (CT) procedures
- New vascular anatomy images added to Chapter 25, "Circulatory System"
- All new images in Chapter 26, "Sectional Anatomy for Radiographers"
- Previous edition Chapter 23, "Temporal Bone," merged with the anatomy and procedures of Chapter 20, "Skull"

Some of the radiographic projections included and described in *Merrill's Atlas* are for reference purposes only and are no longer routinely performed in radiologic imaging facilities. Therefore we have chosen to focus on essential terminology, anatomy, and positioning information for the projections identified as necessary by the ARRT competencies, the *Merrill's* Advisory Board, and the authors' research.

Some chapters of *Merrill's Atlas* (Volumes 1 and 2) have limited radiographic applications or consist of radiographic procedures rarely performed today because of technological advances in adjunct medical imagery modalities (e.g., CT, magnetic resonance imaging, and sonography). Because those chapters do not include radiographic examinations deemed essential for entry-level competency, this workbook provides only cursory coverage for those chapters.

You will receive the maximum benefits from this workbook by first studying the appropriate corresponding anatomic and radiographic sections from *Merrill's Atlas* and *Mosby's Radiography Online* and then completing the workbook review exercises that relate to the chapter of interest. Finally, the self-test at the end of the chapters is an excellent tool to assess preparedness for your course exam. We hope you enjoy this workbook as a complement to your study of radiography.

Jeannean Hall Rollins

Acknowledgments

I am deeply honored to have the opportunity to contribute to the profession I love and enjoy. There are no words sufficient to express my appreciation to everyone who supported me through the revision of this workbook. First and foremost, I want to recognize my husband, Jon, who took on many extra family responsibilities so that I would have time to work on publishing outside of my teaching responsibilities. I cannot possibly say "thank you" enough for all of the love, support, and encouragement. You are an amazing husband, father, and friend. My children, Jonathan, Hannah, Wesley, and Taylor, also helped out in a million little ways that added up to a major contribution. I want to thank each of you for your positive attitudes, patience, and understanding. I love all of you with all of my heart.

The radiologic sciences faculty at Arkansas State University has been very helpful and supportive. Ray Winters, Melanie Burnette, Donna Caldwell, Jennifer DeClerk, Lyn Hubbard, and Tracy White are the best colleagues imaginable. Thank you all for the professional advice and personal shoulders. I would be remiss if I didn't recognize the unwavering support of the Dean of the College of Nursing and Health Professions, Dr. Susan Hanrahan. She has no idea how much she means to the entire RS program.

I would not have had this opportunity were it not for the recommendation of Eugene Frank. I am very grateful for his confidence in me, not to mention his advice and support throughout the process. He has been and continues to be a wonderful mentor. I have also learned a great deal from Bruce Long and Barbara Smith, the coauthors of *Merrill's*. I have thoroughly enjoyed working with the team, and I appreciate the quick responses to (too) many questions. The spirit of teamwork demonstrated has made this project an unforgettable experience.

To Jeanne Wilke and Linda Woodard, the editors at Elsevier: Thanks for putting up with me! Linda's sense of humor and patience have eased my anxiety too many times to count. Jeanne is truly an amazing person in every possible way. She has cared enough to listen to more than work-related issues. Her confidence and support mean so much, and I have truly enjoyed getting to know and work with her throughout this project.

Finally, this workbook is for the radiography students. I sincerely hope you find it useful in your study of our profession. You are embarking on a very challenging yet rewarding career path. I am honored to have been a part in helping you obtain your goal of becoming a radiographer. Welcome to the profession!

Jeannean Hall Rollins

Contents

Answers to Exercises

13 Trauma Radiography

The condition of some trauma patients sometimes requires a radiographer to alter procedures associated with routine radiographic examinations. All radiographers must be competent in performing trauma radiography. This exercise pertains to trauma radiography. Provide a short answer for each of the following questions.

1. Define *trauma*.

   A sudden unexpected, dramatic or, forceful or violent event

2. How does a level I trauma center differ from a level IV trauma center?

   Level 1 - T.C. provide the most comprehensive, wheras Level 4 provide stabilization of pt.'s and basic injury care

3. Within how many feet from the x-ray tube should appropriate shielding be provided to patients on nearby stretchers when performing mobile radiography?

   6 feet.

4. List five symptoms of shock that can be readily observed by a radiographer.

   cool, clamy skin, excessive sweating or drowsiness, thirst & loss of conciousness

5. Concerning providing information to key personnel, what procedure should a radiographer perform if it is necessary to deviate from the routine projections?

   Document any alterations for the referring physician & notify the Radiologist

6. What should be the first projection performed for a trauma patient with a cervical injury?

   Lateral projection, dorsal decubitus position

7. When is it necessary to perform the lateral projection for the cervicothoracic region?

   When the entire C7-T1 interspace is not well demonstrated with the lateral projection.

1

8. What condition must be met before attempting to move the patient's arms for the lateral projection of the cervicothoracic region, dorsal decubitus position?

permission is granted from the attending physician after review of the lateral projection.

9. When performing the lateral projection for the cervicothoracic region, dorsal decubitus position, when may the central ray be caudally angled?

when the pt can not depress the tube side shoulder.

10. When performing the lateral projection of the cervicothoracic region, dorsal decubitus position, what is the purpose for using a long exposure time with the patient breathing normally?

To blur rib shadows

11. When performing the anteroposterior (AP) axial projection on a patient who is not on a backboard or x-ray table, who should lift the patient's head and neck so that a radiographer can position the image receptor (IR) under the patient?

The attending physician

12. When performing the AP axial oblique projection for cervical vertebrae, why should you *not* use a grid IR?

The compound central ray angle will cause grid cut-off

13. When performing the AP axial oblique projection for cervical vertebrae on a supine trauma patient, how should the central ray be directed with a nongrid IR?

15°-20° cephalad as well as 45° mediolaterally.

(compound angle)

14. When performing the AP axial oblique projection for cervical vertebrae on a supine trauma patient, where should the central ray enter the patient?

Slightly lateral to the MSP at the level of the thyroid cartilage, and passing through C-4

15. When demonstrating lumbar vertebrae on a trauma patient who is supine on a backboard, what should be the first projection performed?

Lateral Projection Dorsal Decubitus position.

16. When performing the lateral projection for thoracic vertebrae on a trauma patient who is supine on a backboard, how should the central ray be directed?

horizontal and perpendicular to the center of IR.

17. When performing the AP projection of the abdomen on a trauma patient, what should be obtained before moving the patient to the radiographic table?

permission from the attending physician to transfer the pt to the exam table.

18. When performing the AP projection of the abdomen on a trauma patient, what procedure should the radiographer do if the patient's abdomen becomes increasingly distended and firm to the touch?

Immediateley notify the attending physician.

19. When performing the AP projection of the abdomen on a trauma patient on a gurney, why must the grid IR be perfectly horizontal and the central ray directed perpendicularly to the IR?

To prevent grid-cut-off and image distortion.

20. When performing the AP projection of the abdomen, left lateral decubitus position, why should the patient be placed in the left lateral recumbent position for at least 5 minutes before making the exposure?

To allow any free air that may be present to rise & be visualized.

21. What emergency medical conditions are of primary concern with pelvic fractures?

Internal hemmorhaging and hemmhorhagic shock.

22. What action should a radiographer initiate if a head trauma patient has unequal pupils or experiences a decrease in the level of consciousness?

Immediately alert the attending physician.

23. When performing the acanthioparietal projection, reverse Waters method, for facial bones on a supine trauma patient, how should the infraorbitomeatal line (IOML) be positioned with reference to the IR?

approximately perpendicular.

24. What is the general rule concerning demonstrating adjacent joints when radiographing long bones on trauma patients?

Always include both joints

25. What is the general rule concerning immobilization devices when radiographing upper and lower limbs on trauma patients?

Do not remove unless directed by the attending physician.

Define the following abbreviations:

26. CPR: cardio-pulmonary resuscitation

27. MVA: motor vehicle accident

28. GSW: gun shot wound

29. CVA: cerebro vascular accident

30. ED: emergency dept.

31. OML: orbital meatal line

32. IOML: infra orbital meatal line

33. MML: mentomeatal line

34. IVU: intravenous urography

35. EAM: external acoustic meatus

SELF-TEST: TRAUMA RADIOGRAPHY

Answer the following questions by selecting the best choice.

1. Which of the following is an example of blunt trauma?

   a. Frostbite
   b. Gunshot wound
   c. Impalement injury
   d. Motor vehicle accident

2. Which procedure should be performed when taking radiographs to localize a penetrating foreign object?

   a. Reduce kVp to produce short-scale contrast.
   b. Mark entrance and/or exit wounds with a radiopaque marker.
   c. Provide a written description of the location of the entrance wound.
   d. Use twice the usual source-to-image distance to increase detail of structures.

3. Which procedure should a radiographer perform if a trauma patient begins to experience a seizure?

   a. Provide a drink of water.
   b. Roll the patient onto the side.
   c. Inform the attending physician.
   d. Cover the patient with a blanket.

4. Which of the following symptoms is associated with stroke injuries?

   a. Slurred speech
   b. Cool, clammy skin
   c. Excessive sweating
   d. Increased drowsiness

5. Which of the following statements is not an appropriate rule for trauma radiographers?

   a. Always make at least three radiographs for each area of injury.
   b. Never leave a trauma patient unattended during imaging procedures.
   c. Never remove any immobilization device without physician's orders.
   d. Always ask the attending physician before giving a trauma patient anything to eat or drink.

6. Which of the following projections should be the first one performed for a multiple-trauma patient?

   a. AP lumbar spine
   b. Lateral lumbar spine, dorsal decubitus position
   c. AP cervical spine
   d. Lateral cervical spine, dorsal decubitus position

7. When performing the AP axial oblique projection for cervical vertebrae on a supine trauma patient, how should the central ray be directed if only one angle is used?

   a. 15 degrees cephalad
   b. 45 degrees cephalad
   c. 15 degrees lateromedially
   d. 45 degrees lateromedially

8. When performing the AP projection of the abdomen on a trauma patient, what should be obtained before moving the patient to the radiographic table?

   a. Vital signs
   b. Written consent from the patient
   c. Permission from the attending physician
   d. Lateral C-spine projection in dorsal decubitus position

9. Which of the following procedures should the radiographer perform if a trauma patient has bleeding wounds?

   a. Protect the IR with plastic.
   b. Enclose the IR inside a pillowcase.
   c. Provide fluids to the patient by mouth or intravenously.
   d. Have emergency room personnel assist with the procedure.

10. Why should the left lateral decubitus position be used for demonstrating free air within the abdominal cavity?

    a. Free air will collect under the left hemidiaphragm.
    b. Fluid levels will collect under the right hemidiaphragm.
    c. The density of the liver provides good contrast for free air.
    d. The density of the stomach provides good contrast for free air.

11. How should a radiographer determine if an AP projection of the abdomen, left lateral decubitus position, is being requested for demonstrating free air or fluid levels?

    a. Ask the patient.
    b. Ask the attending physician.
    c. Examine for penetrating wounds.
    d. Examine for distended or firm abdomen.

12. When performing the AP projection of the abdomen, left lateral decubitus position, which of the following procedures should be performed when fluid levels are of primary interest?

    a. Ensure the entire left side is demonstrated.
    b. Ensure the entire right side is demonstrated.
    c. Center the IR 4 inches above the iliac crests to include the diaphragm.
    d. Have the patient drink one full glass of water before making the radiograph.

13. Which projection of the abdomen should be performed to demonstrate air or fluid levels when a trauma patient is unable to be positioned either upright or in the lateral recumbent position?

    a. AP
    b. Left AP oblique
    c. Right AP oblique
    d. Lateral, dorsal decubitus position

14. When performing the AP projection for the pelvis with a trauma patient, which of the following procedures should not be performed?

    a. Use a grid IR directly under the patient.
    b. Rotate the femurs 15 degrees medially.
    c. Transfer the patient to a radiographic table.
    d. Center the IR to a level of 2 inches inferior to the anterior superior iliac spine (ASIS).

15. Which action should a radiographer perform if a semiconscious head trauma patient begins vomiting during radiographic procedures?

    a. Obtain vital signs.
    b. Give the patient a plastic bag.
    c. Move the patient to a sitting position.
    d. Logroll the patient to the lateral recumbent position.

16. Which of the following procedures should a radiographer perform if a trauma patient with a head injury displays unequal pupils?

    a. Give the patient a drink of water.
    b. Remove restrictive immobilization devices.
    c. Immediately inform the attending physician.
    d. Logroll the patient into a lateral recumbent position.

17. Which of the following projections of the cranium would best demonstrate a suspected fracture of the posterior cranium?

    a. AP
    b. PA
    c. AP axial, Towne method
    d. Lateral, dorsal decubitus position

18. Which positioning line of the head should be nearly perpendicular to the IR when performing the acanthioparietal projection, reverse Waters method, for facial bones on a supine trauma patient?

    a. Mentomeatal
    b. Orbitomeatal
    c. Glabellomeatal
    d. Infraorbitomeatal

19. How should the central ray be directed when performing the acanthioparietal projection, reverse Waters method, for facial bones on a supine trauma patient?

    a. 37 degrees cephalad
    b. Perpendicular to the IR
    c. Parallel with the mentomeatal line
    d. Parallel with the IOML

20. Which of the following general rules should be followed when radiographing upper and lower limbs on trauma patients?

    a. Always obtain two radiographs, 90 degrees apart.
    b. Always position for true AP and lateral projections.
    c. When demonstrating long bones, always remove immobilization devices.
    d. When demonstrating long bones, always transfer the patient to the radiographic table.

14 Mouth and Salivary Glands

This exercise provides an anatomic review of the mouth and salivary glands and a cursory review of sialography. Identify structures, fill in missing words, provide a short answer, match columns, select the best choice, or choose true or false (explaining any statement you believe to be false) for each item.

1. Identify each lettered structure shown in Fig. 14-1.

   A. Posterior arch

   B. Anterior arch

   C. tonsil

   D. hard palate

   E. Uvula

   F. soft palate

   G. tongue

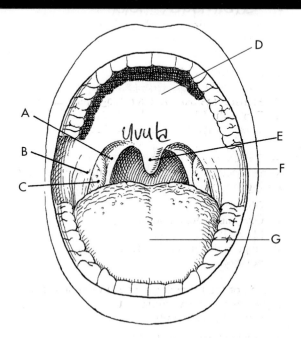

Fig. 14-1 Anterior aspect of the oral cavity.

2. Identify each lettered structure shown in Fig. 14-2.

A. orafice of the sub-mandibular duct
B. tongue
C. frenulum of the tongue
D. sublingual fold

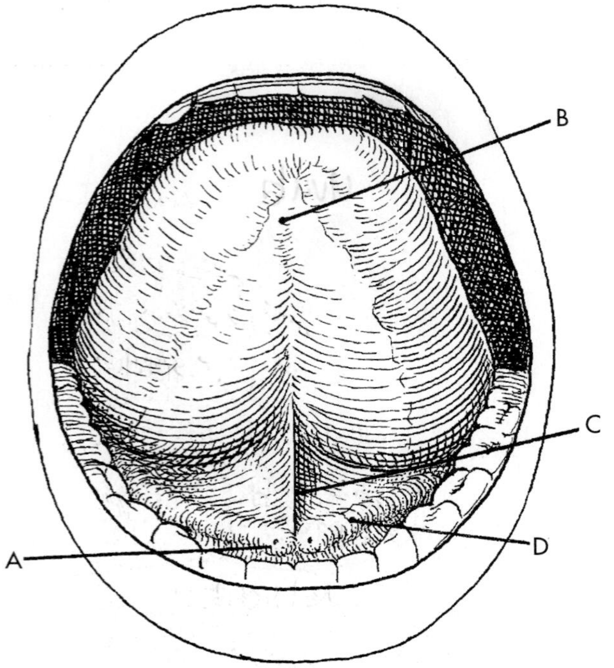

Fig. 14-2 Anterior view of the undersurface of tongue and floor of mouth.

3. Identify each lettered structure shown in Fig. 14-3.

A. parotid duct
B. sublingual (lingual) ducts
C. submandibular ducts
D. sublingual glands
E. parotid gland
F. submandibular gland

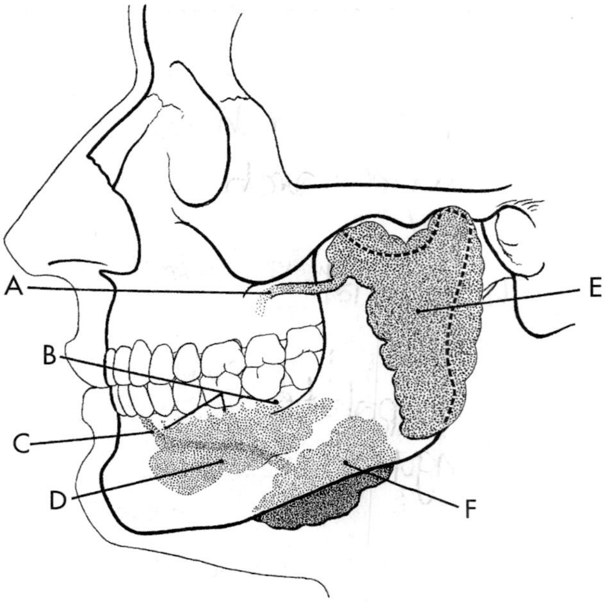

Fig. 14-3 The salivary glands from the left lateral aspect.

4. Identify each lettered structure shown in Fig. 14-4.

A. muscle tissue

B. ramus of the

C. parotid gland

D. tongue

E. dens

F. atlas (c1)

G. spinal cord

5. Identify each lettered structure shown in Fig. 14-5.

A. mandible

B. orthopharanyx

C. cervical vertebral body

D. sublingual gland

E. submandibular gland

F. tip of the parotid

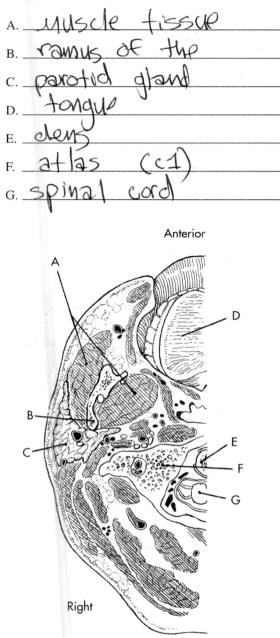

Fig. 14-4 Horizontal section of the face showing the relation of the parotid gland to the mandibular ramus.

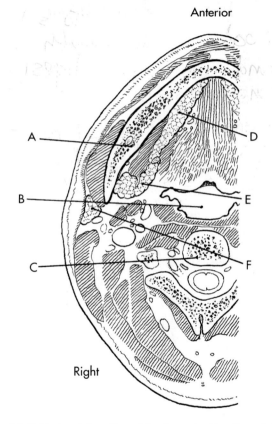

Fig. 14-5 Horizontal section of the face showing the relation of the submandibular and sublingual glands to surrounding structures.

6. What is the first division of the digestive system?

mouth

7. Define *mastication*. *The process of chewing and grinding food into small pieces.*

8. Which structures function in mastication?

teeth

9. What is the purpose of saliva? *To soften food, keep the mouth moist and contribute digestive enzymes*

10. Name the three pairs of salivary glands.

parotid, sublingual, submandibular

11. Define *sialography*. *radiographic exam of the salivary glands and ducts with the use of a contrast medium*

12. What type of contrast medium is used for sialography?

water soluble ionated medium.

13. Why can only one salivary gland at a time be examined by the sialographic method?

salivary gland pairs are in close proximity

14. List two reasons why preliminary radiographs are made before the introduction of the contrast medium. *To demonstrate any condition not demonstrable w/o the use of a contrast medium. & to establish optimal exposure factors*

15. Name the two projections that demonstrate the salivary glands and ducts.

tangential and lateral projections

16. Which salivary glands are demonstrated with the lateral projection?
    a. Parotid and sublingual
    b. Parotid and submandibular
    c. Sublingual and submandibular

17. How is the central ray directed for the tangential projection of a sialographic procedure?

⊥ to the IR at the lateral surface of the mandibular rami

18. True or False. The patient may be positioned prone or supine for the tangential projection.

True

19. True or False. The mandibular ramus should be parallel with the plane of the image receptor (IR) for the tangential projection.

True

20. True or False. Parotid glands on both sides of the face should be demonstrated with the same tangential exposure. Only 1 parotid gland on each tangential image projeting

21. Examine Fig. 14-6 and answer the questions that follow.

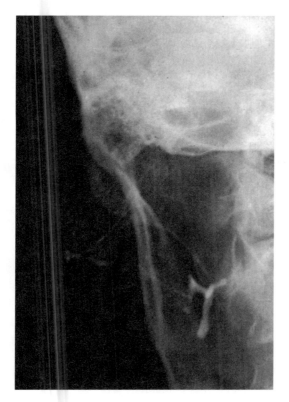

Fig. 14-6 Sialogram showing opacification of a gland.

a. Which projection does this image represent?

tangential projection

b. Which salivary gland is demonstrated?

parotid

c. What is the special breathing technique that can be performed by the patient to improve the radiographic demonstration of the gland with this type of projection?

the pt can fill the mouth with air, then puff out the cheeks AMAP

22. Examine Fig. 14-7 and answer the questions that follow.

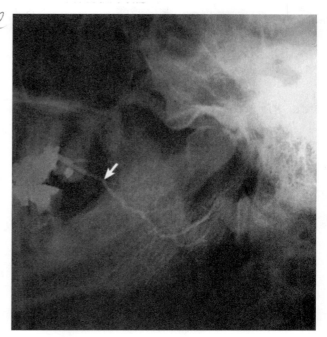

Fig. 14-7 Sialogram showing opacification of a gland.

a. Which projection does this image represent?

later projection

b. Which salivary gland is demonstrated?

parotid = lateral

c. To which duct does the arrow point?

parotid.

23. Examine Fig. 14-8 and answer the questions that follow.

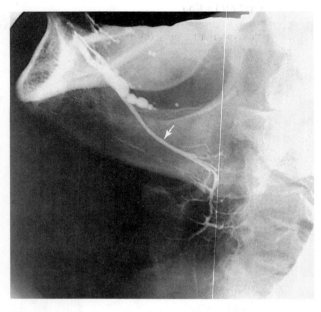

Fig. 14-8 Sialogram showing opacification of a gland.

a. Which projection does this image represent?

lateral projection

b. Which salivary gland is demonstrated?

submandibular

c. To which duct does the arrow point?

submandibular

SELF-TEST: MOUTH AND SALIVARY GLANDS

Answer the following questions by selecting the best choice.

1. What is the first division of the digestive system?
   a. Mouth
   b. Stomach
   c. Small intestine
   d. Salivary glands

2. Which salivary gland is the largest?
   a. Parotid
   b. Sublingual
   c. Submandibular

3. Which salivary glands are the smallest?
   a. Parotid
   b. Sublingual
   c. Submandibular

4. Which salivary glands are located along the lateral aspect of the mandibular ramus?
   a. Parotid
   b. Sublingual
   c. Submandibular

5. Which salivary duct opens into the oral vestibule opposite the second upper molar?
   a. Parotid
   b. Sublingual
   c. Submandibular

6. Which two imaging modalities have greatly reduced the frequency of sialography?
   a. Computed tomography and ultrasonography
   b. Computed tomography and magnetic resonance imaging
   c. Conventional tomography and ultrasonography
   d. Conventional tomography and magnetic resonance imaging

7. For sialography, into which structure is the contrast medium injected?
   a. Vein
   b. Artery
   c. Muscle
   d. Salivary duct

8. Which sialographic projection directs the central ray along the mandibular ramus?
   a. Lateral projection
   b. Tangential projection
   c. Verticosubmental projection
   d. Submentovertical projection

9. Which sialographic projection demonstrates a parotid gland superimposed over a mandibular ramus?
   a. Lateral projection
   b. Tangential projection
   c. Verticosubmental projection
   d. AP axial projection

10. Which two sialographic projections best demonstrate the parotid gland?
    a. Axial and lateral projections
    b. Axial and verticosubmental projections
    c. Tangential and lateral projections
    d. Tangential and verticosubmental projections

11. Which gland is demonstrated with tangential projections?
    a. Parotid
    b. Sublingual
    c. Submandibular

12. Which sialographic projection demonstrates parotid and submandibular glands?
    a. Lateral projection
    b. Tangential projection
    c. AP axial projection

13. Which salivary gland can be demonstrated with a lateral projection when the patient's head is adjusted so that the midsagittal plane is rotated approximately 15 degrees toward the IR from true lateral and the central ray is directed to a point 1 inch (2.5 cm) above the mandibular ramus?
    a. Parotid
    b. Sublingual
    c. Submandibular

14. Which salivary gland can be demonstrated with a lateral projection when the patient's head is positioned true lateral and a perpendicular central ray is directed to the inferior margin of the mandibular angle?
    a. Parotid
    b. Sublingual
    c. Submandibular

15. For the lateral projection demonstrating the submandibular gland, what is the purpose of pressing the tongue to the floor of the mouth?
    a. To hold the intraoral film in place
    b. To displace the submandibular gland below the mandible
    c. To prevent the tongue from superimposing the submandibular gland

13

Workbook for Merrill's Atlas of Radiographic Positioning and Procedures • Volume 2   Chapter **14** **Mouth and Salivary Glands**

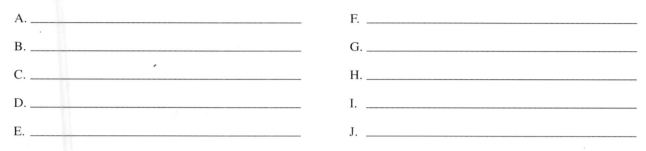

15 Anterior Part of the Neck

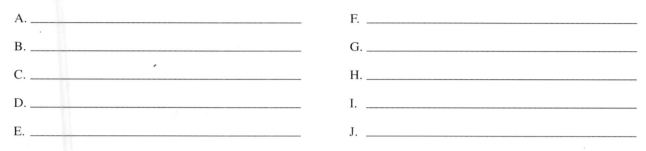

REVIEW

This exercise is a review of the anatomy and radiography of the anterior part of the neck. Identify structures, fill in missing words, or provide a short answer for each item.

1. Identify each lettered structure shown in Fig. 15-1.

A. _____   F. _____

B. _____   G. _____

C. _____   H. _____

D. _____   I. _____

E. _____   J. _____

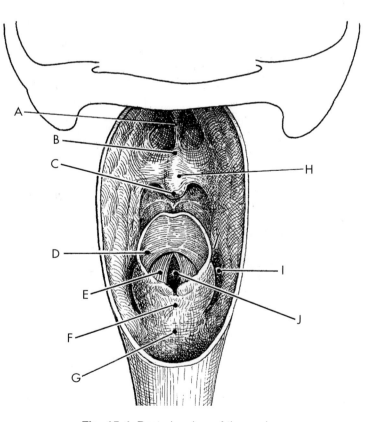

Fig. 15-1 Posterior view of the neck.

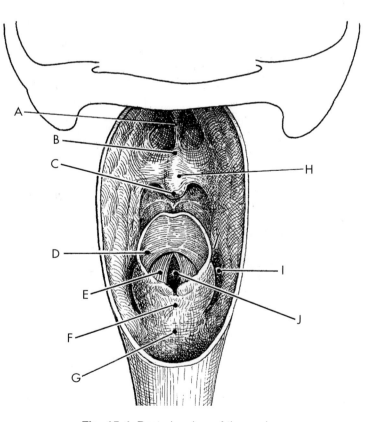15

2. Identify each lettered structure shown in Fig. 15-2.

A. _____

B. _____

C. _____

D. _____

E. _____

F. _____

G. _____

H. _____

I. _____

J. _____

K. _____

L. _____

M. _____

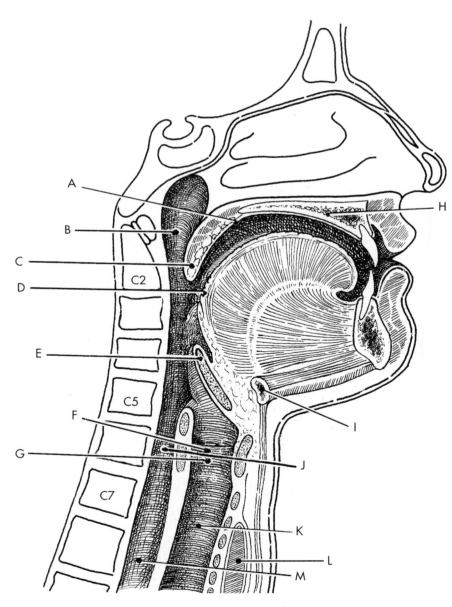

Fig. 15-2 Sagittal section of the face and neck.

3. Identify each lettered structure shown in Fig. 15-3.

A. _____

B. _____

C. _____

D. _____

E. _____

F. _____

G. _____

4. Identify each lettered structure shown in Fig. 15-4.

A. _____

B. _____

C. _____

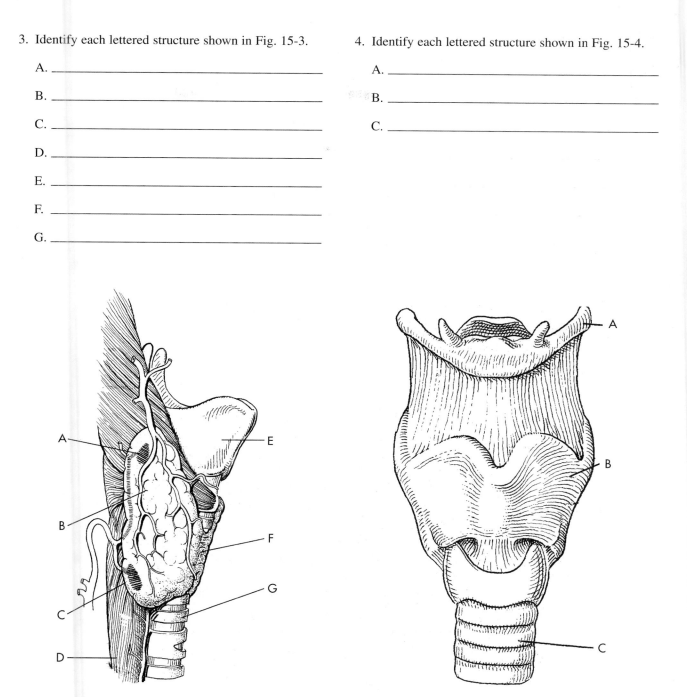

Fig. 15-3 Lateral aspect of the laryngeal area.

Fig. 15-4 Anterior aspect of the larynx.

5. Identify each lettered structure shown in Fig. 15-5.

A. _____

B. _____

C. _____

D. _____

E. _____

F. _____

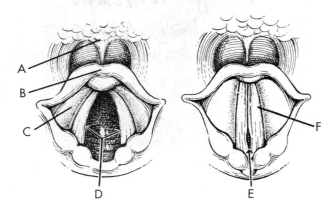

Fig. 15-5 Superior aspect of the larynx (open and closed true vocal folds).

6. For radiographic purposes, the neck is divided into

_____ and _____
portions.

7. The upper part of the respiratory system located in the

anterior part of the neck is the _____.

8. The upper part of the digestive system located in the

anterior part of the neck is the _____.

9. The two major glands located in the anterior part of the

neck are the _____ gland and the

_____ gland.

10. The structure of the upper neck that serves as a passage
for both food and air and is common to the respiratory

and digestive systems is the _____.

11. The portion of the pharynx located above the soft

palate is the _____.

12. The portion of the pharynx located from the soft

palate to the hyoid bone is the _____.

13. The organ of voice is the _____.

14. The structure that comprises the vocal apparatus of

the larynx is the _____.

15. The projections that demonstrate the pharynx and

larynx are _____ and _____.

16. During what four bodily functions are radiographs of
the pharynx and larynx made?

17. Identify the body position in which the patient
should be placed for each of the following examinations of the pharynx and larynx:

a. Tomographic studies:

_____

b. AP and lateral projections:

_____

18. For the AP projection, the central ray should be

directed perpendicular to the _____

_____.

19. Identify the x-ray tube and image receptor centering
points for the lateral projection of the following
structures:

a. Nasopharynx:_____

b. Oropharynx:_____

c. Larynx:_____

20. Identify each lettered structure shown in Fig. 15-6.

A. _____

B. _____

C. _____

D. _____

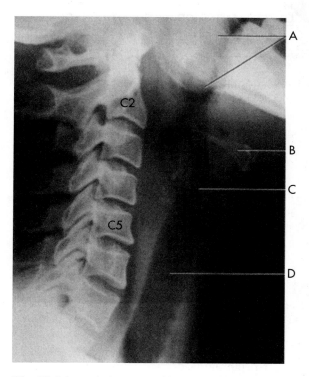

Fig. 15-6 Lateral pharynx and larynx (Valsalva maneuver).

SELF-TEST: ANTERIOR PART OF THE NECK

Answer the following questions by selecting the best choice.

1. What is the musculomembranous tubular structure located in front of the vertebrae and behind the nose, the mouth, and the larynx?

   a. Glottis
   b. Trachea
   c. Pharynx
   d. Esophagus

2. Which structure of the neck is approximately 1½ inches (4 cm) in length and is situated below the root of the tongue and in front of the laryngeal pharynx?

   a. Larynx
   b. Trachea
   c. Esophagus
   d. Oropharynx

3. Which structure forms the laryngeal prominence?

   a. Epiglottis
   b. True vocal cord
   c. Cricoid cartilage
   d. Thyroid cartilage

4. Which structure prevents leakage into the larynx during swallowing?

   a. Pharynx
   b. Epiglottis
   c. Cricoid cartilage
   d. Thyroid cartilage

5. What is the most superiorly located structure of the neck?

   a. Larynx
   b. Glottis
   c. Pharynx
   d. Epiglottis

6. For the AP projection that demonstrates the pharynx and larynx, to which level of the patient should the central ray be directed?

   a. C1
   b. C7
   c. Mandibular angles
   d. Laryngeal prominence

7. For preliminary AP and lateral projections that demonstrate the pharynx and larynx, when should the exposures be made to ensure filling the throat passages with air?

   a. During expiration
   b. During inspiration
   c. After suspended expiration
   d. After suspended inspiration

8. Which body position should be used for tomographic examinations of the pharynx and larynx?

   a. Prone
   b. Supine
   c. Upright lateral
   d. Recumbent lateral

9. For the lateral projection that demonstrates the oropharynx, to which level of the patient should the central ray be directed?

   a. C7
   b. Mandibular angles
   c. Laryngeal prominence
   d. External acoustic meatuses

10. Which procedure should the patient perform for tomographic studies of pharyngolaryngeal structures?

    a. Quiet inspiration through the nose
    b. Phonation of a high-pitched *"e-e-e"*
    c. Suspended respiration after expiration
    d. Suspended respiration after inspiration

16 Digestive System: Abdomen and Biliary Tract

SECTION 1

ANATOMY OF THE DIGESTIVE SYSTEM: ABDOMEN AND BILIARY TRACT

Exercise 1

This exercise pertains to the abdominal contents. Identify structures for each question.

1. Identify each lettered structure shown in Fig. 16-1.

A. left lobe of the liver

B. falciform ligament

C. right lobe of the liver

D. gall bladder

E. ascending colon

F. illeum

G. appendix

H. diaphraghm

I. esophogus

J. stomach

K. spleen

L. pancreas

M. descending colon

N. transverse colon

O. small intestine

P. urinary bladder

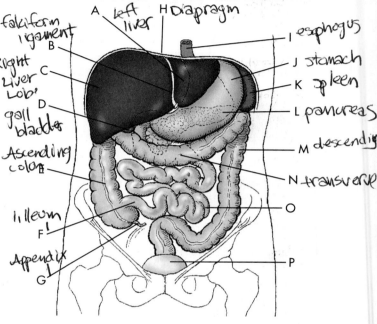

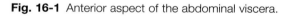

Fig. 16-1 Anterior aspect of the abdominal viscera.

2. Identify each lettered structure shown in Fig. 16-2.

A. toungue
B. sublingual gland
C. submandibular gland
D. gall bladder
E. bilary ducts
F. visceral surface of the liver
G. vermaform appendix
H. parotid gland

I. pharanyx
J. esophagus
K. stomach
L. spleen
M. pancreas
N. large intestine
O. small intestine

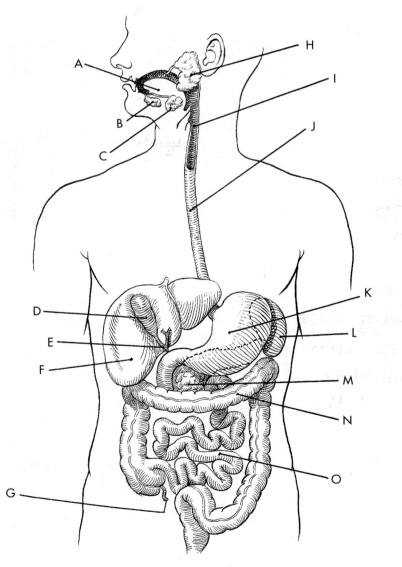

Fig. 16-2 Alimentary tract and its accessory organs.

3. Identify each lettered structure shown in Fig. 16-3.

A. Hepopancreatic ampulla

B. cystic duct

C. right lobe of the liver

D. gall bladder

E. liver

F. falciform ligament

G. quadrate lobe of the liver

H. left lobe of the liver

I. Left hepatic duct

J. caudate lobe of the liver

K. left lobe of the liver   common hepatic duct

L. left hepatic duct   common bile duct

M. pancreatic duct

N. pancreas

O. duodenum

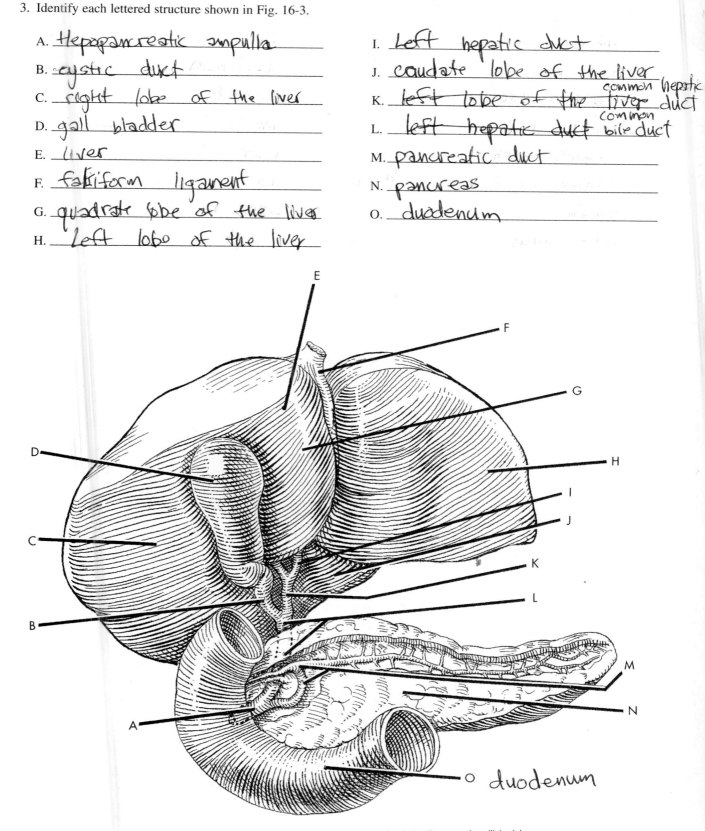

Fig. 16-3 Visceral surface (inferoposterior aspect) of the liver and gallbladder.

4. Identify each lettered structure shown in Fig. 16-4.

A. cut surface of the liver

B. gall bladder

C. cystic duct

D. right kidney

E. common hepatic duct

F. common bile duct

G. spleen

H. left kidney

I. pancreas

J. duodenum

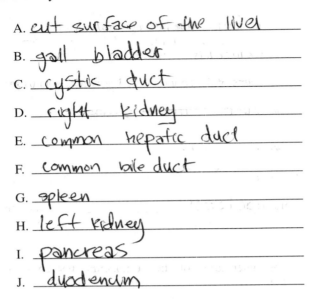

Fig. 16-4 Visceral (inferoposterior) surface of gallbladder and bile ducts.

5. Identify each lettered structure shown in Fig. 16-5.

A. liver

B. duodenum

C. stomach

D. inferior vena cava

E. right kidney

F. aorta

G. pancreas

H. left kidney

I. spleen

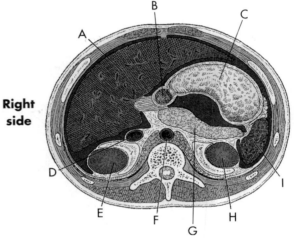

Fig. 16-5 Sectional image of the upper abdomen showing the relationship of digestive system components.

Exercise 2

Match the pathology terms in Column A with the appropriate definition in Column B. Not all choices from Column B should be selected.

Column A

<u>b</u> 1. Ileus

<u>e</u> 2. Pancreatic pseudocyst

<u>i</u> 3. Cholecystitis

<u>a</u> 4. Cholelithiasis

<u>c</u> 5. Biliary stenosis

<u>k</u> 6. Pancreatitis

<u>d</u> 7. Bowel obstruction

<u>f</u> 8. Choledo-cholithiasis

<u>g</u> 9. Pneumoperi-toneum

<u>h</u> 10. Abdominal aortic aneurysm

Column B

a. The presence of gallstones

b. Failure of bowel peristalsis

c. Narrowing of the bile ducts

d. Blockage of the bowel lumen

e. Complication of acute pancreatitis that results in a collection of debris, fluid, pancreatic enzymes, and blood

f. Calculus in the common bile duct

g. Presence of air in the peritoneal cavity

h. Localized dilatation of the abdominal aorta

i. Acute or chronic inflammation of the gallbladder

j. Transfer of a cancerous lesion from one area to another

k. Acute or chronic inflammation of the pancreas

Exercise 3

This exercise pertains to the liver, biliary system, pancreas, and spleen. Fill in missing words, provide a short answer, or choose true or false (explaining any statement you believe to be false) for each item.

1. The name of the double-walled seromembranous sac that lines the abdominal cavity is the

   peritoneum.

2. The names of the two layers of the peritoneum are

   the parietal layer and the

   visceral layer.

3. The outer layer of the peritoneum that contacts the underside of the diaphragm is called the

   parietal layer.

4. The inner layer of the peritoneum that contacts various organs is called the visceral layer.

5. The organ that occupies most of the right hypochondrium and the epigastrium regions of the abdomen is

   the liver.

6. The largest organ in the abdominal cavity is the

   liver.

7. The radiographically significant physiologic function

   of the liver is the production of bile.

8. The right and left hepatic ducts join to form the

   common hepatic duct.

9. The cystic duct enables bile from the liver to be stored

   in the gall bladder.

10. The gallbladder is usually located on the inferior side

    of the right lobe of the liver.

11. The common hepatic duct unites with the cystic duct to form the _common bile duct_ _____.

12. In 20% of subjects, before entering the duodenum, the common bile duct joins with the _pancreatic duct_.

13. The muscular contraction of the gallbladder is activated by a hormone called _cholecystokinin_.

14. Another name for the ampulla of Vater is the _hepatopancreatic ampulla_.

15. The gland that produces insulin is the _pancreas_ _____.

16. True or False. In a hypersthenic patient, the gallbladder is situated high and well away from the midsagittal plane. _true_

17. True or False. The gallbladder is located posterior to the liver in the retroperitoneal space. _False - GB on inferior surface on Right lobe of liver_

18. True or False. The pancreas cannot be demonstrated using plain radiography. _True_

19. True or False. The spleen is an organ of the lymphatic system. _True_

20. True or False. The pancreas and the liver secrete specialized digestive juices into the small intestine. _True_

POSITIONING OF THE ABDOMEN AND BILIARY TRACT

Exercise 1: Positioning for the Abdomen

A variety of radiographic procedures are used to demonstrate the abdomen and its contents. A patient is usually first examined with plain radiography before specialized studies using contrast media are performed. This exercise reviews the positions and projections commonly used to produce radiographs of the abdomen without the introduction of a contrast medium. Fill in missing words, provide a short answer, select answers from a list, or choose true or false (explaining any statement you believe to be false) for each item.

Items 1 through 5 pertain to general procedures for abdominal radiography.

1. What three projections usually comprise the three-way or acute abdomen series?

   Supine KUB
   AP upright Adm.
   PA chest

2. Why is a chest radiograph included as part of the acute abdomen series?

   To dem. free air that may accumulate underneath the diapraghm.

3. In the acute abdomen series, what radiograph should be substituted for the upright abdomen radiograph when the patient is unable to stand?

   Left lateral decublitus

4. List the three considerations for the use of gonadal shielding in abdominal radiography.

   · exam not comprimised
   · if part is 2½ inches of exam
   · youth

5. Visualizing the sharply defined outline of what muscle group is an excellent criterion for judging the quality of an abdomen radiograph?

   Psoas

27

Workbook for Merrill's Atlas of Radiographic Positioning and Procedures • Volume 2   Chapter 16   Digestive System: Abdomen and Biliary Tract

Items 6 through 15 pertain to *anteroposterior* (AP) and *posteroanterior* (PA) projections. Examine Fig. 16-6 as you answer the following questions.

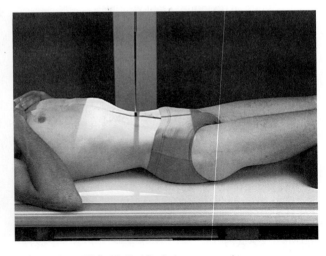

Fig. 16-6 AP abdomen, supine.

6. What is the commonly used acronym that refers to the AP projection of the abdomen with the patient supine?

    KUB

7. Which plane of the body should be centered to the midline of the image receptor (IR)?

    midsaggital

8. For the AP projection with the patient supine, to what level of the patient should the IR be centered?

    illiac crests

9. List the two levels of the patient to which the IR should be centered when the patient is positioned upright, and give the reason for the difference in IR placement.

    2" superior to illiac crest
    diapraghm to bladder

10. What structure of the upper abdomen should be seen on the abdomen radiograph when the patient is upright? Explain why.

    diapraghm - to demonstrate free air

11. What breathing instructions should be given the patient?

    Suspend respiration upon expiration

12. What is the advantage of exposing abdominal radiographs at the suspension of the recommended phase of respiration as compared with the other respiration phase?

    So that the organs of the abd. do not appear compressed

13. What two identification markers should be seen on the radiograph when the patient is upright?

    upright tag
    R or L marker

28

Chapter **16** **Digestive System: Abdomen and Biliary Tract**   Workbook for Merrill's Atlas of Radiographic Positioning and Procedures • Volume 2

14. With reference to radiation protection, what is the advantage of the PA projection over the AP projection?

A reduction of the rad. exposure to the gonads

15. From the following list, circle the three evaluation criteria that indicate the patient was properly positioned without rotation for a KUB radiograph.

a. Intervertebral foramina should be open.
b. Alae or wings of the ilia should be symmetric.
c. Lumbar vertebrae pedicles should be superimposed.
d. If seen, ischial spines of the pelvis should be symmetric.
e. Spinous processes should be in the center of the lumbar vertebrae.

Items 16 through 26 pertain to the *AP projection, left lateral decubitus position.* Examine Fig. 16-7 as you answer the following questions.

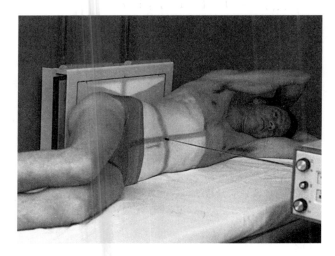

Fig. 16-7 AP abdomen, left lateral decubitus position.

16. What is the advantage of the left lateral decubitus position compared with the supine position AP abdomen?

demonstration of free- air levels

17. Why is the left lateral decubitus position preferred over the right lateral decubitus position when the patient is unable to stand?

free air will be visualized the stomach will not obscure view

18. Describe the position of the patient for left lateral decubitus position.

recumbent lateral w/ left side down

19. Why is it advisable to let the patient remain in the lateral recumbent position for several minutes before making the exposure?

To allow air to rise to its highest level

20. With reference to the patient, describe the placement and centering of the IR.

vertical IR on pt's posterior side at the level of the illiac crests

21. What breathing instructions should be given to the patient?

suspend after full expiration

22. Describe how and to where the central ray should be directed.

↓ to mid IP
CR entering at level of illiac crests

23. Which side of the abdomen—the "up" side or the "down" side—should be demonstrated if only one side can be imaged and the patient is suspected of having fluid levels within the abdominal cavity?

The dependent side "down"

24. Which side of the abdomen—the "up" side or the "down" side—should be demonstrated if only one side can be imaged and the patient may have free air in the abdomen?

The dependent side "up"

25. What structure of the upper abdomen should be demonstrated on the radiograph?

diaphragm

26. What identification markers should be seen on the radiograph?

Marker indicate the side of pt that is up.

Items 27 through 33 pertain to the *lateral projection*. Examine Fig. 16-8 as you answer the following questions.

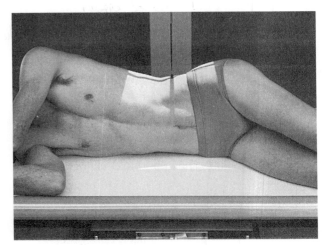

Fig. 16-8 Right lateral abdomen.

27. True or False. A lateral projection of the abdomen can be performed with the patient placed in either the right lateral recumbent position or the left lateral recumbent position.

True

28. True or False. The midsagittal plane should be perpendicular and centered to the IR.

False - midcoronal plane ⊥ to IP

29. True or False. The exposure should be made after the patient has suspended respiration after full inspiration.

False - expiration

30. To what level of the patient should the IR be centered?

@ illiac crest or
2" superior to illiac crest
to include the diaphragm

31. If a compression band is needed to immobilize the patient, where should it be placed?

Across the pelvis

32. Where exactly should the central ray enter the patient?

To mid coronal plane @ the illiac crests

33. What two areas of the image can be closely examined to determine if the patient was rotated?

pelvis & lumbar vertebrae

Items 34 through 40 pertain to the *lateral projection, dorsal decubitus position.* Examine Fig. 16-9 as you answer the following questions.

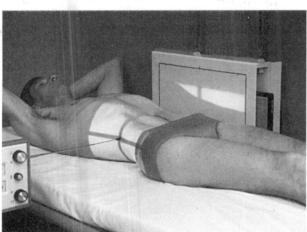

Fig. 16-9 Lateral abdomen, left dorsal decubitus position.

34. What is the name of the radiographic position that produces a lateral image of the abdomen with the patient in the supine position?

Dorsal decub.

35. What purpose is served by having the patient slightly flex his or her knees?

To releive the strain on the pt's back

36. To what level of the patient should the long axis of the IR be centered?

Mid coronal

37. How far above the level of the iliac crests should the central ray enter the patient?

2"

38. True or False. The exposure should be made after the patient has suspended respiration at the end of inspiration.
local anethesia

39. True or False. The central ray should be directed horizontally and perpendicular relative to the center of the film.
True

40. From the following list, circle the three evaluation criteria that indicate the patient was correctly positioned for a lateral projection while placed in the dorsal decubitus position.

   a. The wings of the ilia should be symmetric.
   b. The entire abdomen should be demonstrated.
   c. The diaphragm should be included without motion.
   d. The abdominal contents should be seen with soft-tissue gray tones.
   e. The spinous processes should be seen in the center of the lumbar vertebrae.
   f. The ribs and pelvis should be equidistant to the edge of the IR on both sides.

Exercise 2: Contrast Studies for the Biliary Tract

This exercise pertains to radiographic demonstration of the biliary tract using a contrast medium. Fill in missing words, provide a short answer, or choose true or false (explaining any statement you believe to be false) for each item.

1. Radiographic visualization of the gallbladder after the introduction of a contrast medium is termed

   ~~tongue~~ cholestography

2. Cholangiography is defined as the radiographic study of the ~~sublingual gland~~ Bilary Ducts

3. Sonography is the imaging modality of choice for demonstration of the gallbladder and biliary tract.

4. Name two other imaging modalities that have reduced the need for radiographic procedures of the biliary tract: CT, MRI

5. The abbreviation *PTC* stands for Percutaneus transhepatic cholangiography

6. PTC is used for the treatment of obstructive jaundice.

7. In what position is the patient placed to begin a PTC procedure?
   a. Supine ⟵
   b. Prone
   c. 45 degree LPO
   d. 45 degree RPO

8. True or False. PTC is performed using surgical aseptic technique.

9. True or False. PTC is performed with the patient under conscious sedation.

   A local anesthetic is used

10. True or False. If stones are identified on PTC, surgery is the only removal option.

    retrieval baskets can be used once drainage catheter is in pbc

11. List three reasons postoperative (T-tube) cholangiography is performed.
    1. Demonstrat patency & colibur of bilary ducts
    2. Dem. the status of the sphincter of the hepopancreatic ampulla
    3. Dem. the presence of residual or previously undetected stons in the bilary ducts.

12. In which of the following biliary ducts is the T-tube placed for drainage?
    a. Right and left hepatic ducts
    b. Right hepatic duct and common hepatic duct
    c. Common hepatic duct and common bile duct ⟵
    d. Cystic duct and common bile duct.

13. What is the purpose of clamping the T-tube the day before the cholangiogram procedure?

    To allow the tube to fill w/bile to minimize the possibility of air bubbles entering the ducts. Air bubbles can mimic cholesterol (radiolucent stones)

14. What type of contrast media is used for postoperative cholangiography?

    water soluable, ionated

15. After the preliminary scout radiograph of the abdomen has been obtained, the patient is positioned in the RPO position with the RUQ centered to the midline of the grid.

16. What procedure is referred to by the abbreviation *ERCP?*

    Endoscopic retrograde cholangiopancreatography.

17. List two specifications in which ERCP is a useful diagnostic method.

When the bilary ducts are not dilated and when ampulla is not obstructed.

18. _Sonagraphy_ is often used before ERCP to rule out the presence of _pancreatic psedocysts._.

19. Where is the endoscope positioned during ERCP?

The duodenum.

20. What are the proper postprocedure instructions for the patient?

No food or drink (NPO) 1 hr post exam to allow for the local anesthetic to wear off.

33

Workbook for Merrill's Atlas of Radiographic Positioning and Procedures • Volume 2   Chapter **16   Digestive System: Abdomen and Biliary Tract**

SELF-TEST: ABDOMEN AND BILIARY TRACT

Answer the following questions by selecting the best choice.

1. Which organ produces bile?
   a. Liver
   b. Spleen
   c. Pancreas
   d. Gallbladder

2. Which body function does the pancreas perform?
   a. Filtration of blood
   b. Production of bile
   c. Production of lymphocytes
   d. Production of digestive juices

3. Which organ stores and concentrates bile?
   a. Liver
   b. Spleen
   c. Pancreas
   d. Gallbladder

4. Which substance activates the muscular contraction of the gallbladder?
   a. Bile
   b. Cholecystokinin
   c. Pancreatic juices
   d. Cholecystolithiasis

5. The spleen is part of which body system?
   a. Urinary
   b. Digestive
   c. Endocrine
   d. Lymphatic

6. In which organ are clusters of islet cells found?
   a. Liver
   b. Spleen
   c. Pancreas
   d. Gallbladder

7. How many major lobes does the liver have?
   a. One
   b. Two
   c. Three
   d. Four

8. Which structure forms the mesentery and omenta folds?
   a. Liver
   b. Pancreas
   c. Gallbladder
   d. Peritoneum

9. Which organ's blood is supplied by the portal vein?
   a. Liver
   b. Spleen
   c. Pancreas
   d. Gallbladder

10. Which duct is formed by the merging of the right and left hepatic ducts?
    a. Cystic
    b. Pancreatic
    c. Common bile
    d. Common hepatic

11. Which duct is formed by the union of the cystic duct with the common hepatic duct?
    a. Pancreatic
    b. Left hepatic
    c. Right hepatic
    d. Common bile

12. Where do the pancreatic and common bile ducts terminate?
    a. Ileum
    b. Duodenum
    c. Gallbladder
    d. Large intestine

13. Which duct connects the gallbladder to the common hepatic duct?
    a. Cystic
    b. Pancreatic
    c. Right hepatic
    d. Common bile

14. Which three projections usually comprise the acute abdomen series for ambulatory patients?
    a. Supine KUB, AP upright abdomen, and PA chest
    b. Supine KUB, right lateral decubitus abdomen, and PA chest
    c. Left lateral decubitus abdomen, dorsal decubitus abdomen, and PA chest
    d. Right lateral decubitus abdomen, left lateral decubitus abdomen, and dorsal decubitus abdomen

15. To which level of the patient should the IR be centered for the KUB?
    a. T10 vertebral body
    b. L3 vertebral body
    c. 2 inches (5 cm) above the iliac crests
    d. Iliac crests

16. For the AP upright abdomen radiograph of an adult of average size, why should the IR be slightly raised above the centering level used for the supine KUB radiograph?

    a. To include the bladder
    b. To include the diaphragm
    c. To visualize gallstones
    d. To visualize kidney stones

17. For the KUB radiograph, when should respiration be suspended, and what effect will that have on the patient?

    a. On full expiration; elevate the diaphragm
    b. On full expiration; depress the diaphragm
    c. On full inspiration; elevate the diaphragm
    d. On full inspiration; depress the diaphragm

18. Why is it desirable to include the diaphragm in the upright abdomen radiograph?

    a. To demonstrate free air in the abdomen
    b. To demonstrate fluid levels in the thorax
    c. To demonstrate fluid levels in the abdomen
    d. To demonstrate calculi in the gallbladder and kidneys

19. Which of the following guidelines is not necessary to follow when deciding whether to use gonadal shielding for the KUB radiograph?

    a. The patient has reasonable reproductive potential.
    b. The gonads lie within 2 inches (5 cm) of the primary beam.
    c. The purpose for performing the examination is not compromised.
    d. The permission to use gonadal shielding is granted by the patient.

20. Which projection should be used to demonstrate free air within the abdominal cavity when the patient is unable to stand for an upright abdomen radiograph?

    a. AP projection with the patient supine
    b. Lateral projection, dorsal decubitus position
    c. AP projection, left lateral decubitus position
    d. AP projection, right lateral decubitus position

21. Which projection does not demonstrate free air levels within the abdomen?

    a. AP projection with the patient supine
    b. AP projection with the patient upright
    c. Lateral projection, dorsal decubitus position
    d. AP projection, left lateral decubitus position

22. What is the major advantage of the PA projection of the abdomen over the AP projection of the abdomen?

    a. The PA projection reduces the exposure dose to the gonads.
    b. The PA projection magnifies gallstones for better visualization.
    c. The PA projection demonstrates the pubic rami below the urinary bladder.
    d. The PA projection reduces the object–to–image-receptor distance of the kidneys.

23. Which radiographic position of the abdomen requires that the patient be placed in the lateral recumbent position on his or her left side and that the central ray be directed along the midsagittal plane, entering the anterior surface of the patient's abdomen at the level of the iliac crests?

    a. Dorsal decubitus
    b. Ventral decubitus
    c. Left lateral decubitus
    d. Right lateral decubitus

24. Which radiographic position of the abdomen requires that the patient be supine and that the central ray be directed to a lateral side of the patient, entering slightly anterior to the midcoronal plane?

    a. Dorsal decubitus
    b. Ventral decubitus
    c. Left lateral decubitus
    d. Right lateral decubitus

25. Which radiographic position of the abdomen requires that the patient be placed in the lateral recumbent position on his or her left side, that the IR be placed under the patient and centered to the abdomen at the level of the iliac crests, and that the central ray be directed to enter the right side of the patient slightly anterior to the midcoronal plane?

    a. Left lateral
    b. Right lateral
    c. Left lateral decubitus
    d. Right lateral decubitus

26. The lateral projection with the patient placed in the dorsal decubitus position, the left lateral projection, and the left lateral decubitus position of the abdomen all require which of the following?

    a. The central ray should enter the left side of the patient.
    b. The patient should suspend respiration after expiration.
    c. The patient should suspend respiration after inspiration.
    d. The central ray should enter the anterior side of the abdomen.

27. For the lateral projection with the patient placed in the dorsal decubitus position, where should the central ray enter the patient?

    a. 2 inches (5 cm) anterior to the midcoronal plane at the level of the iliac crests
    b. 2 inches (5 cm) anterior to the midcoronal plane and 2 inches above the level of the iliac crests
    c. 2 inches (5 cm) posterior to the midcoronal plane at the level of the iliac crests
    d. 2 inches (5 cm) posterior to the midcoronal plane and 2 inches above the level of the iliac crests

28. For the lateral projection with the patient placed in the dorsal decubitus position, which procedure should be performed to ensure that the entire abdomen is included on the radiograph?

    a. Use support cushions to elevate the patient.
    b. Center the IR to the level of the xiphoid process.
    c. Center the IR to the anterior surface of the abdomen.
    d. Direct the central ray to a point 2 inches (5 cm) below the iliac crests.

29. Which structures should be examined to see whether the patient was rotated for a lateral projection of the abdomen?

    a. Pelvis and lumbar vertebrae
    b. Pelvis and thoracic vertebrae
    c. Diaphragm and lumbar vertebrae
    d. Diaphragm and thoracic vertebrae

30. The radiographic study of the biliary ducts is known as:

    a. Cholegraphy
    b. Cystography
    c. Cholecystography
    d. Cholangiography

31. Which of the following is indicated for patients with jaundice and dilated biliary ducts?

    a. ERCP
    b. T-tube cholangiography
    c. Acute abdominal series
    d. PTC

32. Which of the following is used to detect residual stones in the biliary ducts?

    a. Acute abdominal series
    b. PTC
    c. ERCP
    d. T-tube cholangiography

33. Air bubbles present in the T-tube during cholangiography can mimic:

    a. Inflammation
    b. Cholesterol stones
    c. Malignancy
    d. Obstruction

34. The patient is placed in the _____ position for postoperative cholangiographic images.

    a. LPO
    b. RPO
    c. Supine
    d. Prone

35. Which of the following is indicated when the biliary ducts are not dilated and the ampulla is not obstructed?

    a. ERCP
    b. Postoperative cholangiography
    c. PTC
    d. Acute abdominal series

17 Digestive System: Alimentary Canal

SECTION 1

ANATOMY OF THE ALIMENTARY CANAL

Exercise 1

This exercise pertains to the digestive system. Identify structures for each question.

1. Identify each lettered structure shown in Fig. 17-1.

A. tongue

B. sublingual gland

C. submandibular gland

D. gall bladder

E. bilary ducts

F. vermaform appendix

G. rectum

H. parotid gland

I. pharanyx

J. esophogus

K. stomach

L. spleen

M. pancreas

N. large intestine

O. small intestine

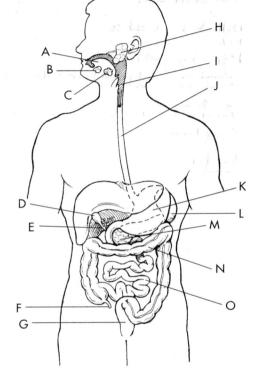

Fig. 17-1 The alimentary canal and its accessory organs.

2. Identify each lettered structure shown in Fig. 17-2.

A. cardiac antrum

B. cardia

C. lesser curvature

D. angular notch

E. pyloric sphincter

F. duodenum

G. pyloric canal

H. pyloric antrum

I. greater curvature

J. cardiac notch

K. fundus

L. body

3. Identify each lettered structure shown in Fig. 17-3.

A. cardiac sphincter

B. pyloric sphincter

C. duodenum

D. pyloric canal

E. rugae

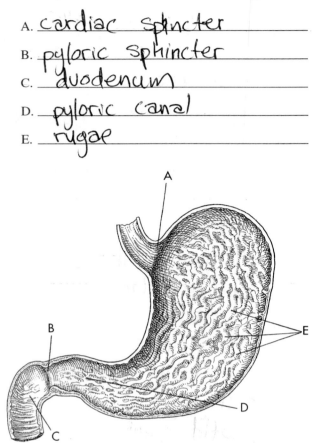

Fig. 17-3 Section of the stomach showing rugae.

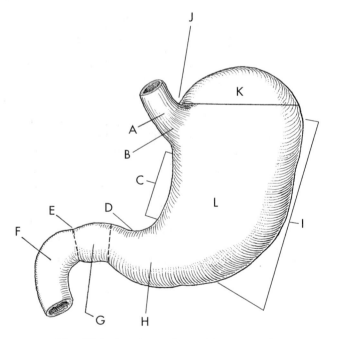

Fig. 17-2 Anterior surface of the stomach.

4. Identify each lettered structure shown in Fig. 17-4. *(or face of biliary & pancreatic ducts)*

A. major duodenal papilla

B. hepatopancreatic ampulla

C. gall bladder

D. cystic duct

E. common hepatic duct

F. common bile duct

G. pylorus

H. stomach

I. pancreatic duct

J. pancreas

K. duodenum

5. Identify each lettered structure shown in Fig. 17-5.

A. illeum

B. veneform appendix

C. cecum

D. ascending colon

E. right coloc flexure

F. transverse colon

G. left colic fixture

H. descending colon

I. sigmoid colon

J. rectum

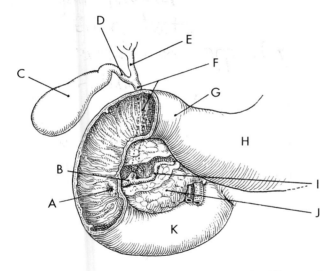

Fig. 17-4 The duodenal loop in relation to the biliary and pancreatic ducts.

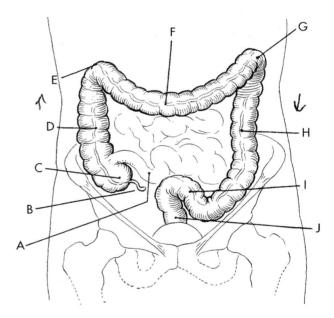

Fig. 17-5 Anterior aspect of the large bowel.

6. Identify each lettered structure shown in Fig. 17-6.

A. sacrum

B. anal canal

C. rectum

D. rectal ampulla

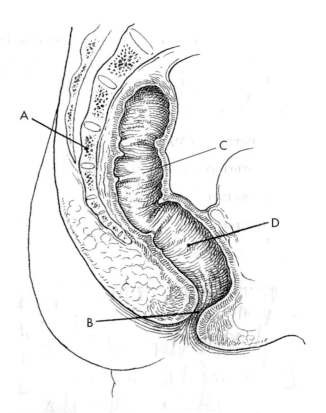

Fig. 17-6 Sagittal section showing the anal canal and rectum.

Exercise 2

Use the following clues to complete the crossword puzzle. All answers refer to the alimentary canal.

Across

1. Stores bile   *gall bladder*
5. Gastric folds
8. Attached to cecum
10. Terminates alimentary canal
11. Widest part of alimentary canal
15. Contraction waves
18. Proximal part of small bowel
19. Left colic flexure
22. Between cecum and right colic flexure
23. Average body build
24. Precedes anal canal

Down

2. Digestive juice   *bile*
3. Musculomembranous tube
4. Upper part of stomach
6. Lower than sthenic
7. Proximal part of large intestine   *cecum*
9. Precedes esophagus
12. Large body build
13. Middle part of small bowel
14. Very slender body build
16. Intestinal bend
17. Between left colic flexure and sigmoid
20. Produces bile   *liver*
21. Distal part of small bowel

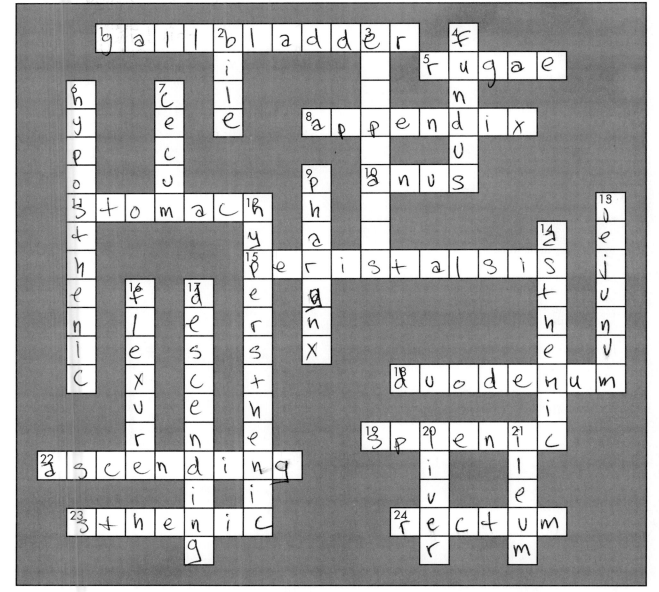

41

Exercise 3

Match the structures or portions of organs found in the alimentary canal from the list in Column A with the major organs to which they most closely relate as listed in Column B.

Column A   **Column B**

_b_ 1. Bulb   a. Stomach

_a_ 2. Body   b. Small intestine

_a_ 3. Rugae   c. Large intestine

_b_ 4. Ileum

_c_ 5. Cecum

_c_ 6. Rectum

_a_ 7. Fundus

_a_ 8. Pylorus

_c_ 9. Sigmoid

_b_ 10. Jejunum

_b_ 11. Duodenum

_c_ 12. Transverse

_c_ 13. Ascending

_c_ 14. Descending

_a_ 15. Lesser curvature

_a_ 16. Greater curvature

_b_ 17. Hepatopancreatic ampulla

_a_ 18. Cardiac sphincter

_c_ 19. Left colic flexure

_c_ 20. Right colic flexure

Exercise 4

Match the pathology terms in Column A with the appropriate definition in Column B. Not all choices from Column B should be selected.

Column A   **Column B**

_f_ 1. Ulcer   a. Inflammation of the colon

_e_ 2. Polyp   b. Twisting of a bowel loop on itself

_g_ 3. Gastrointestinal reflux   c. Protrusion of the bowel into the groin

_ga_ 4. Colitis   d. Inflammation of the lining of the stomach

_d_ 5. Gastritis   e. Growth or mass protruding from a mucous membrane

_b_ 6. Volvulus   f. Depressed lesion of the surface of the alimentary canal

_k_ 7. Diverticulum   g. Backward flow of the stomach contents into the esophagus

_h_ 8. Diverticulosis   h. Diverticula in the colon without inflammation or symptoms

_i_ 9. Intussusception   i. Prolapse of a portion of the bowel into the lumen of an adjacent part

_c_ 10. Inguinal hernia   j. Protrusion of the stomach through the esophageal hiatus of the diaphragm

                                      k. Pouch created by the herniation of the mucous membrane through the muscular coat

Exercise 5

This exercise pertains to the alimentary canal and its related organs. Fill in missing words or provide a short answer for each question.

1. The musculomembranous passage that extends from the pharynx to the stomach is the _esophogus_.

2. The expanded part of the distal end of the esophagus is the _cardiac antrum_.

3. The opening into the stomach through which food and liquids pass is the _cardia oraface_.

4. The organ in which gastric digestion begins is the _stomach_.

5. The gastric folds of the stomach are the _rugae_.

6. The border of the stomach with the lesser curvature is the _right (medial)_ border.

7. The lesser curvature extends from the esophagogastric junction to the _pylorus_.

8. The left and inferior borders of the stomach are the _greater curvature_.

9. Fig. 17-7 shows four diagrams, each representing a different body habitus. Indicate in the blanks provided which of the following body habitus type each diagram represents: sthenic, asthenic, hyposthenic, or hypersthenic.

   a. Diagram A: _hypersthenic_
   b. Diagram B: _sthenic_
   c. Diagram C: _hyposthenic_
   d. Diagram D: _asthenic_

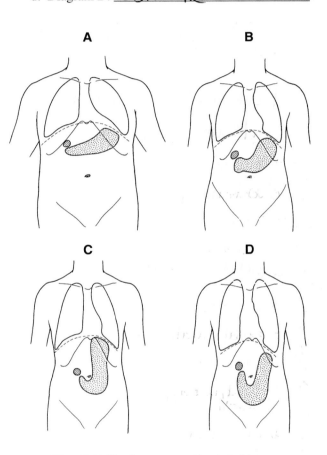

A   **B**

C   **D**

Fig. 17-7 The four types of body habitus.

10. Name the four parts of the stomach.

43

Workbook for Merrill's Atlas of Radiographic Positioning and Procedures • Volume 2   Chapter 17 Digestive System: Alimentary Canal

11. The part of the stomach immediately surrounding the esophageal opening is the _Cardia_.

12. The most superior part of the stomach is the _Fundus_.

13. The most inferior part of the stomach is the _pyloric_ portion.

14. The opening between the stomach and the small intestine is the _pyloric oraface_.

15. The three parts of the small intestine are the _duodenum_, _jejunum_, and _ileum_.

16. The proximal part of the small intestine is the _duodenum_.

17. The radiographically significant first segment of the proximal part of the small intestine is the _duodenal bulb_.

18. The small intestine terminates at the _illeo-cecal valve_.

19. The common bile and the pancreatic ducts empty into the _duodenum_.

20. The middle part of the small intestine is the _jejunum_.

21. The distal part of the small intestine is the _illeum_.

22. The shortest part of the small intestine is the _duodenum_; the longest part is the _ileum_.

23. The longer of the two intestines is the _small_ intestine.

24. The passage from the small intestine to the large intestine is the _illeocecal valve_.

25. The proximal part of the large intestine is the _cecum_.

26. The vermiform appendix attaches to the large intestine at the _cecum_.

27. Located between the ascending colon and the transverse colon is the _right colic_ flexure.

28. The part of the colon that extends from the cecum to the right colic flexure is the _ascending_ colon.

29. The part of the colon that extends between the two flexures is the _transverse_ colon.

30. Located between the transverse colon and the descending colon is the _left colic_ flexure.

31. The part of the colon that extends inferiorly from the left colic flexure is the _descending_ colon.

32. The sigmoid colon is located between the two parts of the large intestine known as the _descending colon_ and the _rectum_.

33. The sigmoid colon terminates in the _rectum_.

34. The part of the large intestine that extends between the rectum and the anus is the _anal canal_.

35. The external opening at the terminal end of the anal canal is the _anus_.

POSITIONING OF THE ALIMENTARY CANAL

Exercise 1: Positioning for the Esophagus

The esophagus can be radiographically examined after a contrast medium has been introduced. This exercise pertains to procedures used to obtain the required radiographs of the esophagus. Fill in missing words, provide a short answer, or choose true or false (explaining any statement you believe to be false) for each item.

1. List the projections that comprise the typical esophageal study.

   AP & PA proj.
   AP or PA oblique proj (RAO or LAO pos) and lateral proj.

2. What two types of contrast media are used for double-contrast esophageal studies?

   A high density barium study product and CO_2 crystals

3. Why is the PA oblique projection, left anterior oblique (LAO) position, not included in the typical esophageal study?

   The LAO position may superimpose vertebral shadows w/the distal esophagus.

4. When demonstrating the entire esophagus, to what level of the patient should the image receptor (IR) be centered?

   T5-T6 (the top of the IR should be level w/the mouth)

5. What two oblique positions can be used to demonstrate the entire esophagus effectively?

   RAO & LPO

6. Why is the recumbent right anterior oblique (RAO) position preferred over the upright position?

   It allows more complete contrast filling of the esophagus.

7. For anteroposterior (AP) or posteroanterior (PA) projections, how is it determined that the selection of exposure factors was acceptable?

   The esophagus should be adequately demonstrated through the S.I. thoracic vertebrae

8. In relation to the surrounding structures, where should the esophagus appear in images with the patient in the RAO position?

   To the left of the vertebral column, between the thoracic vertebrae & the heart.

9. In radiographs of a contrast-filled esophagus with the patient in the RAO position, how does the esophagus appear in relation to the surrounding structures when rotation of the patient was insufficient?

   partially obscured by the thoracic vertebrae.

45

Workbook for Merrill's Atlas of Radiographic Positioning and Procedures • Volume 2   Chapter **17** Digestive System: Alimentary Canal

10. In the lateral projection radiograph, what structures are used to determine whether the patient was rotated? How should these structures appear?

posterior ribs, they should be S.I.

11. For radiographs with the patient in the RAO position, the patient should be rotated approximately

35° to *40°* degrees.

12. The esophagus should be clearly seen from the lower neck to the *cardiac orafice* .

13. (True) or False. Single-contrast and double-contrast studies can be used to demonstrate the esophagus.

14. (True) or False. A barium sulfate mixture is the preferred contrast medium for esophagrams.

15. True or (False.) The most important requirement for the contrast medium is that the weight per volume should be rated greater than 50%.

A 30% to 50% weight per volume suspension is acceptable. The most important criterion for the barium is that the flow must be sufficient to coat the esophageal walls.

Exercise 2: The Gastrointestinal Series

One of the more commonly performed studies employing contrast media is the gastrointestinal (GI) series. This exercise pertains to gastrointestinal studies. Identify structures, fill in missing words, provide a short answer, select from a list, or choose true or false (explaining any statement you believe to be false) for each item.

Items 1 through 20 pertain to upper gastrointestinal (UGI) examination procedures.

1. What acronym refers to the upper gastrointestinal series?

UGI.

2. As part of patient preparation, why should the patient maintain a soft, low-residue diet for two days?

To reduce the production of intestinal gas and fecal matter

3. How can the UGI study be affected if the patient smokes cigarettes shortly before the examination?

The coating ability of the barium could be diminished because of the secretion of gastic juices may be stimulated

4. What type of radiopaque contrast medium usually is used in routine UGI studies?

A barium sulfate product of 30-50% weight per volumn concentration

5. List the two general GI examination procedures routinely used to examine the stomach.

single-contrast examinations

6. What is the range of weight per volume concentration for the barium sulfate suspension usually used for single-contrast examinations?

30 – 60% lesions

7. List two advantages of performing the double-contrast examination.

Small lesions are readily demonstrated, and the mucosal lining of the stomach can be more clearly demonstrated

8. What are the two types of contrast media used in double-contrast procedures?

High density barium sulfate suspension and gas producing substance

9. True or False. Both the single-contrast and double-contrast procedures should begin with the patient in the lateral recumbent position.

The exam should begin w/the pt. upright

10. True or False. After the patient consumes the barium sulfate suspension for a double-contrast examination, all radiographs should be performed with the patient in the upright position.

Most radiographs are obtains are obtained w/ the pt recumbent (coating of mucosal surface)

11. True or False. The barium sulfate suspension used for double-contrast examinations should have a higher weight per volume ratio than the barium sulfate suspension used for single-contrast examinations.

True

12. Why should patients undergoing double-contrast examinations turn from side to side or roll over a few times during the procedure?

To coat the mucosal lining of the stomach

13. During double-contrast examinations, what instructions should be given to the patient after the patient swallows the carbon dioxide crystals or tablets to ensure a double-contrast effect?

The pt should be instructed not to belch

14. What is the purpose of using glucagon during the double-contrast examination?

To relax the gastric tract enabling gastric structures to expand, thus enabling it to be better demonstrated

15. What is a biphasic GI examination?

A UGI examination is an exam done by first examining double contrast, after which a low weight per volume BaSO₄ is administered and the pt is administered w/a single contrast procedure

16. Which method of examination—the single-contrast or double-contrast—is performed first as part of a biphasic examination?

Double contrast

17. What are the two methods of performing hypotonic duodenography?

w/intubation & w/o intubation

18. True or False. Hypotonic duodenography originally required that the contrast medium be introduced directly through a tube placed into the duodenum.

19. True or False. The tubeless hypotonic duodenography examination is performed after a drug has temporarily paralyzed the duodenum.

20. True or False. Other imaging modalities such as sonography and computed tomography have largely replaced hypotonic duodenography.

Items 21 through 31 pertain to the *PA projection*. Examine Fig. 17-8 as you answer the following questions.

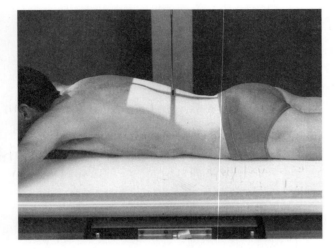

Fig. 17-8 PA stomach and duodenum.

21. True or False. Routine radiographs of the stomach and duodenum should be made with the patient in the upright position. *The pt should be recumbent*

22. True or False. The PA projection with the patient in the prone position demonstrates the contour of the barium-filled stomach and duodenal bulb.

23. True or False. The PA projection with the patient in the upright position shows the size, shape, and relative position of the barium-filled stomach.

24. True or False. A compression band may be placed across the patient's abdomen to immobilize the patient and reduce involuntary movement of the viscera.
A compression band should not be used to immobilize the pt. because it can cause filling defects and interefere with the filling and emptying of the duodenal bulb.

25. How should the prone position of the patient be adjusted to prevent the full weight of the abdomen from causing the stomach and duodenum to press against the vertebral column?
The pt's weight should be supported.

26. How should the patient's position be adjusted to center the stomach over the midline of the table?
Center over midline of grid w/ saggital plane passing halfway between the vertebral column and the left lateral border of the abdomen.

27. When performing the PA projection on a prone patient, to what level of the patient should the IR be centered? *centered about 1 or 2" above the lower rib margin at the level L1-L2.*

28. How should the centering of the IR be adjusted if the patient is repositioned from the prone position to the upright position?
Center the IR 3-6" lower.

29. With which body habitus does the greatest visceral movement occur between the prone position and the upright position?

asthenic

30. What breathing instructions should be given to the patient when making the exposure?

suspend respiration after expiration.

31. How and to where should the central ray be directed?

⊥ to center of IR

2" above the lower margin of the ribs.

Items 32 through 37 pertain to the *PA oblique projection, RAO position.* Examine Fig. 17-9 as you answer the following questions.

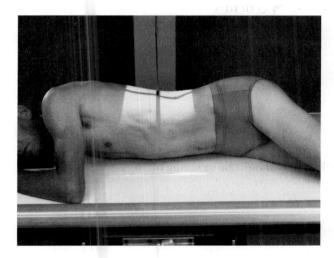

Fig. 17-9 PA oblique stomach and duodenum, RAO position.

32. Describe how the patient should be adjusted from the prone position to the RAO position.

pt turned toward left raised left side - supported w/forearm raised left knee.

33. How and to where should the central ray be directed?

⊥ to center of IR.

34. How many degrees should the patient be rotated from the prone position?
   a. 10 to 15
   b. 20 to 35
   c. 40 to 70

35. Which type of body habitus requires the most rotation?
   a. Sthenic
   b. Hyposthenic
   c. Hypersthenic

36. True or False. For the average patient, the PA oblique projection, RAO position produces the best image of the pyloric canal and the duodenal bulb filled with barium. *True*

37. True or False. The PA oblique projection, RAO position radiograph should be exposed when the patient has suspended respiration after full inspiration.

False

suspend respiration upon full expiration.

Items 38 through 45 pertain to the *AP oblique projection, left posterior oblique (LPO) position.* Examine Fig. 17-10 as you answer the following questions.

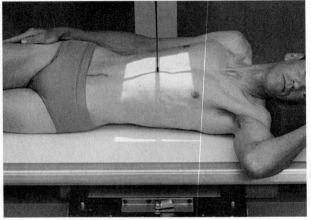

Fig. 17-10 AP oblique stomach and duodenum, LPO position.

38. The AP oblique projection, LPO position, is best performed if the patient is adjusted from the

    _supine_____ (supine or prone) position.

39. The side of the patient that should be elevated away

    from the table is the ___right_____ (right or left) side.

40. For the AP oblique projection, LPO position, most

    patients should be rotated ____45_____ degrees.

41. To what level of the patient should the IR be centered?

    midway between the xiphoid pro-
    cess and the lower lateral
    margin of the ribs.

42. Where exactly should the central ray enter the patient?

    To a point midway between the
    MSP and left lateral margin
    of the abdomen
    Also to the level midway between xiphoid
    & lower lateral margin of the ribs.

43. True or False. The AP oblique projection, LPO position, demonstrates the fundic portion of the stomach filled with barium.

    True

44. True or False. The AP oblique projection, LPO position, demonstrates the pyloric canal and duodenal bulb filled with barium. An Air contrast image
    LPO
    ↳ of pyloric valve canal and duodenal bulb

45. Identify each lettered structure shown in Fig. 17-11.

    A. distal esophogus
    B. fundus
    C. body
    D. pylorus
    E. duodenum

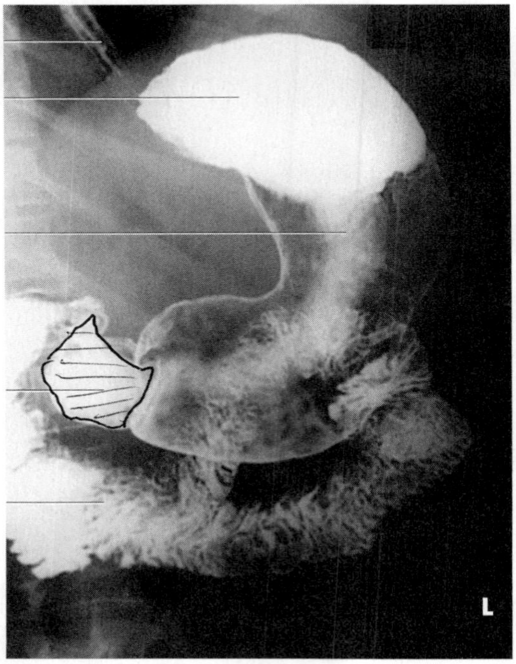

Fig. 17-11 AP oblique stomach and duodenum, LPO position.

Items 46 through 53 pertain to the *right lateral projection.*
Examine Fig. 17-12 as you answer the following questions.

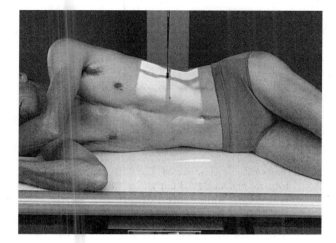

Fig. 17-12 Right lateral stomach and duodenum.

46. Which radiographic body position should be used to best demonstrate the duodenal loop and the duodenojejunal junction filled with contrast medium?

    a. Upright RAO position
    b. Recumbent LPO position
    c. Upright left lateral position
    d. Recumbent right lateral position

47. At which vertebral level should the central ray enter the patient if the patient is in the recumbent position?

    a. T10-T11
    b. L1-L2
    c. L5-S1

48. Approximately how many inches above the lower rib margin should the IR be centered to the recumbent patient?

    a. 1 to 2
    b. 3 to 4
    c. 5 to 6

49. At which vertebral level should the central ray enter the patient if the patient is moved from the recumbent position to the upright lateral position?

    a. T12
    b. L1
    c. L3
    d. L5

50. When examining right lateral projection radiographs, which osteologic structures should be examined to determine whether the patient was rotated?

    a. Ribs
    b. Vertebrae
    c. Pelvic bones

51. Describe how and to where the central ray should be directed to the IR and the patient.

    ⊥ to the center of the IR and midway between the MCP and ~~lateral margin~~ anterior surface of the abdomen

52. Examine Fig. 17-13 and indicate whether the following gastric structures are mostly barium-filled or mostly gas-filled:

a. Stomach fundus: _gas filled_

b. Duodenal bulb: _barium filled_

c. Duodenum: _barium filled_

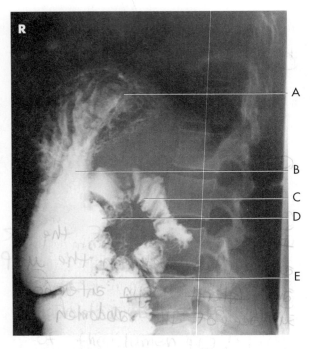

Fig. 17-13 Right lateral stomach.

53. Identify each lettered structure shown in Fig. 17-13.

A. _fundus_

B. _body_

C. _duodenum_

D. _duodenal bulb._

E. _pyloric portion_

Items 54 through 60 pertain to the *AP projection*. Examine Fig. 17-14 as you answer the following questions.

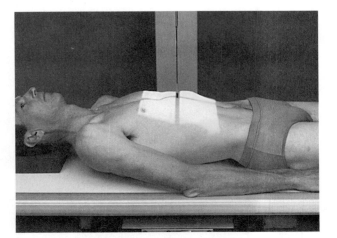

Fig. 17-14 AP stomach and duodenum.

54. Which body position should be used?

a. Prone
b. Supine
c. Upright

55. Which procedure should be performed to help demonstrate a diaphragmatic herniation (hiatal hernia)?

a. Tilt the table to Fowler's angulation.
b. Place the patient in the upright position.
c. Tilt the table to the Trendelenburg angulation.
d. Place the patient in the right lateral recumbent position.

56. Describe how the patient should be centered to the grid when using a 35- × 43-cm IR.

center the MSP to the center of the grid.

57. Describe how the patient should be centered to the grid when using a 30- × 35-cm IR.

center @ saggital plane passing midway between the MSP and the lateral margin. of the left ribs. to the midline of the ribs

58. When using the 30- × 35-cm IR, to what level of the patient should it be centered?

midway between the tip of the xiphoid process and the lower margin of the ribs.

59. How should each of the following structures be demonstrated—barium-filled or gas-filled (double-contrast)?

a. Body: gas-filled (double contrast)

b. Fundus: barium-filled

c. Pylorus: gas-filled (double contrast

d. Duodenal bulb: gas-filled (double contrast)

60. Identify each lettered structure shown in Fig. 17-15.

A. fundus

B. body

C. _____

D. _____

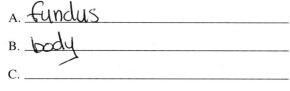

Fig. 17-15 AP stomach and duodenum.

Exercise 3: Small Intestine Examination

The small intestine can be radiographically examined by more than one method, often after the stomach is examined. This exercise pertains to the small intestine examination, often referred to as the small bowel series. Provide a short answer or select the answer from a list for each item.

1. List the three methods by which a barium sulfate mixture can be administered for a small bowel series.

   orally, reflux, filling and intubation (direct injection)

2. Which small bowel series method is most commonly used?

   a. Oral
   b. Enteroclysis
   c. Complete reflux

3. Select the four instructions from the following list that are usually given to patients preparing for the oral method of performing a small bowel series.

   a. Have a cleansing enema.
   b. Do not eat breakfast on the morning of the examination.
   c. Do not eat an evening meal the night before the examination.
   d. Swallow laxatives the morning of the examination.
   e. Drink 3 to 4 glasses of water the morning of the examination.
   f. Consume nothing by mouth after the evening meal the night before the examination.
   g. Eat a restricted diet (soft, low-residue foods) for up to 2 days before the examination.

4. Why is a time marker displayed on each radiograph made during the oral method small bowel series?

   a. To show the time of the day the exposure was made
   b. To indicate the interval between the exposure of the radiograph and the previous one
   c. To indicate the interval between the exposure of the radiograph and the ingestion of the barium

5. How should the patient be placed for timed radiographs when compression of the abdominal contents is desired?

   a. Prone
   b. Supine
   c. Lateral recumbent

6. Approximately how long after the patient swallows the barium sulfate mixture should the first radiograph be made?

   a. 5 minutes
   b. 15 minutes
   c. 30 minutes

7. Approximately how long after the exposure of the first radiograph should subsequent radiographs be exposed?

   a. 5 to 10 minutes
   b. 15 to 30 minutes
   c. 35 to 45 minutes

8. How might the oral method of small bowel examination be affected by giving the patient a cup of cold water after the administration of the contrast medium?

   a. Peristalsis is accelerated.
   b. Peristalsis is slowed down.
   c. The stomach becomes distended.

9. Which small bowel series method often requires the administration of glucagon or diazepam (Valium) to relax the intestine and reduce patient discomfort during the initial filling of the small intestine?

   a. Oral
   b. Enteroclysis
   c. Complete reflux

10. How should the patient be positioned when the small intestine is to be filled by the complete reflux method?

    a. Prone
    b. Supine
    c. Lateral recumbent

11. Which small bowel series method injects contrast medium through an intestinal tube?

    a. Oral
    b. Enteroclysis
    c. Complete reflux

12. Where in the small intestine should the tube be inserted for the enteroclysis method of performing a small bowel series?

    a. Ileum
    b. Jejunum
    c. Duodenum

13. Which method of performing a small bowel series does not use a cleansing enema as part of patient preparation?

    a. Oral
    b. Enteroclysis
    c. Complete reflux

Items 14 through 20 pertain to the *AP or PA projection.* Examine Fig. 17-16 as you answer the following questions.

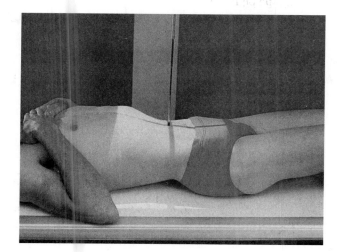

Fig. 17-16 AP small intestine.

14. For the AP projection demonstrating the small intestine, which plane of the body should be centered to the grid?

    a. Horizontal
    b. Midsagittal
    c. Midcoronal

15. For the AP projection demonstrating the small intestine of a sthenic patient within 30 minutes after the administration of contrast, to which level of the patient should the IR be centered?

    a. T12
    b. L2
    c. L5

16. For delayed AP projections demonstrating the small intestine of a sthenic patient, to which level of the patient should the IR be centered?

    a. T12
    b. L2
    c. Iliac crests

17. For the AP projection, when should the exposure be made?

    a. At the end of expiration
    b. At the end of inspiration

18. How should the central ray be directed?

    a. Perpendicularly
    b. Angled caudally
    c. Angled cephalically

19. When visualized on a small bowel series radiograph, which structure usually indicates adequate demonstration of the entire small intestine?

    a. Cecum
    b. Jejunum
    c. Duodenum

20. From the following list, circle the seven evaluation criteria that indicate small bowel series radiographs were properly performed.

    a. The patient should not be rotated.
    b. A time marker should be included.
    c. No ribs should be seen below the diaphragm.
    d. The exposure factors should demonstrate the anatomy.
    e. The stomach should be included on the initial radiographs.
    f. The vertebral column should be in the middle of the radiograph.
    g. The entire small intestine should be included on each radiograph.
    h. The entire alimentary canal should be included on each radiograph.
    i. The examination is usually completed when barium is visualized in the cecum.
    j. The examination is usually completed when barium is visualized in the jejunum.
    k. The postevacuation film is accomplished after the administration of a cleansing enema.

Exercise 4: Large Intestine Examination

The large intestine is frequently examined radiographically after the introduction of a suitable contrast medium. This type of examination is called the barium enema (BE). This exercise pertains to the procedures and radiographs used for the two methods of BEs. Identify structures, fill in missing words, provide a short answer, match columns, select from a list, or choose true or false (explaining any statement you believe to be false) for each item.

1. What are the two basic methods of performing a BE?
   a. Oral and double-contrast
   b. Oral and enteroclysis (intubation)
   c. Single-contrast and double-contrast
   d. Single-contrast and enteroclysis (intubation)

2. What is the most common type of contrast medium used for a BE?

   Barium Sulfate

3. Why should a high-density barium product be used as the contrast medium for double-contrast studies?

   To obtain better coating of the lumen

4. What two radiolucent contrast media can be used during the double-contrast study?

   Air and CO₂ (carbon dioxide)

5. When might an orally administered, water-soluble, iodinated contrast medium be used in place of a barium sulfate mixture?

   When the pt. can not tolerate retrograde filling of the colon

6. What should be included in the instructions generally given to a patient in preparation for a BE?

   restrictive diet
   cleansing enemas
   laxatives

7. What is considered the most important aspect of patient preparation for the BE?

   The entire colon should be as clean as possible
   no fecal material present

8. What should the temperature of the barium be when the administration of a warm barium solution is desirable?

   approximately 85-90° F.

9. How could the patient be affected if the barium solution is too warm?

   Too warm - could be debilitating to the pt.
   may injure internal structures
   may release Ba SO₄
   (facilitate

10. What should the temperature of the barium be when administering cold barium solution?

41° F

11. What are the advantages of filling the large intestine with a cold barium solution?

- less irritation
- relaxes colon
- stimulates tonal contraction of anal sphincter
- improves BaSO₄ retention

12. List three instructions that can be given to the patient to help the patient retain the barium during the examination.

- maintain tight contraction of the anal sphincter
- ↑ pt comfort
- relax ab muscles
- concentrate on deep oral breathing

13. What is the maximum height above the level of the anus that a BE bag may be placed on an IV stand?

24 "

14. Approximately how far into the rectum should an enema tip be inserted?

3½ - 4½ "

3½ - 4 inches

15. What wording refers to the last radiograph usually performed as part of a BE examination?

postevac. image

Items 16 through 19 pertain to the *PA projection*. Examine Fig. 17-17 as you answer the following questions.

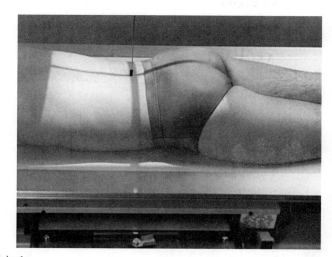

Fig. 17-17 PA large intestine.

16. How should the patient be placed for the PA projection?
    a. Prone
    b. Supine
    c. Upright
    d. Lateral recumbent

17. To which level of the patient should the IR be centered?
    a. T12
    b. L2
    c. Iliac crests
    d. Symphysis pubis

18. How should the central ray be directed for the PA projection?
    a. Perpendicularly
    b. Angled caudally
    c. Angled cephalically

19. Identify each lettered structure shown in Fig. 17-18.

A. _Left colic Flexure_ _____ (flexure)

B. _right colic flexure_ _____ (flexure)

C. _transverse colon_ _____

D. _descending colon_ _____

E. _ascending colon_ _____

F. _cecum_ _____

G. _Sigmoid_ _____

H. _rectum_ _____

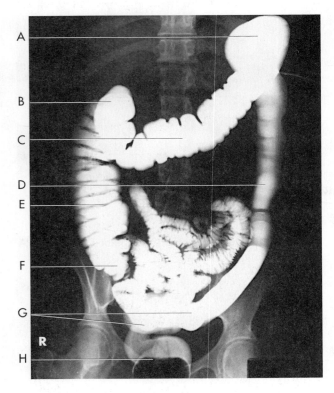

Fig. 17-18 PA large intestine.

Items 20 through 25 pertain to the *PA axial projection.* Examine Fig. 17-19 as you answer the following questions.

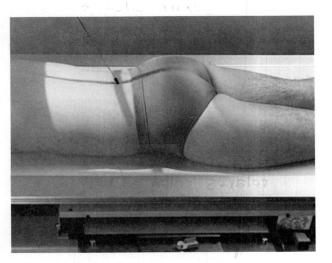

Fig. 17-19 PA axial large intestine.

20. For the PA axial projection, which plane of the body should be centered to the midline of the table?

   a. Transverse
   b. Midsagittal
   c. Midcoronal

21. To which level of the patient should the central ray be directed for the PA axial projection?

   a. L2
   b. Symphysis pubis
   c. Anterior superior iliac spines

22. How should the central ray be directed for the PA axial projection?

   a. Perpendicularly
   b. Angled caudally
   c. Angled cephalically

23. Which area of the large intestine is best demonstrated with the PA axial projection?

   a. Ileocecal
   b. Superior
   c. Rectosigmoid

24. True or False. Both colic flexures should be seen with the PA axial projection.

superior colic flexion

both flexures
trans verse need not
be dem

25. Identify each lettered structure shown in Fig. 17-20.

A. _left colic Flexure_ (flexure)

B. _transverse colon_

C. _sigmoid_

D. _rectum_

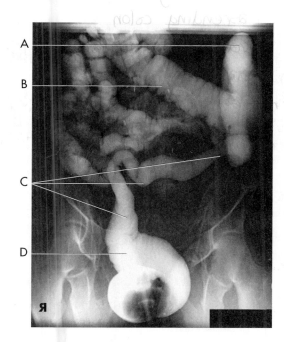

Fig. 17-20 PA axial large intestine.

Items 26 through 30 pertain to the *PA oblique projection, RAO position*. Examine Fig. 17-21 as you answer the following questions.

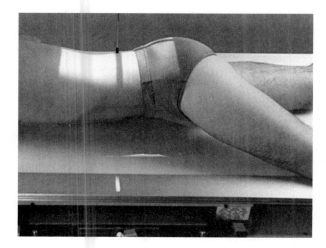

Fig. 17-21 PA oblique large intestine, RAO position.

26. True or False. For the PA oblique projection, RAO position, the patient should be rotated 35 to 45 degrees from the prone position.

27. True or False. For the PA oblique projection, RAO position, the central ray should be directed 35 to 45 degrees caudally. _⊥ to center IR_

28. True or False. Both colic flexures should be seen in the RAO position radiograph.

29. True or False. The PA oblique projection, RAO position is performed primarily to demonstrate the right colic flexure.

30. Identify each lettered structure shown in Fig. 17-22.

A. _Left colic flexure_ (flexure)

B. _right colic flexure_ (flexure)

C. _descending colon_

D. _ascending colon_

E. _sigmoid_

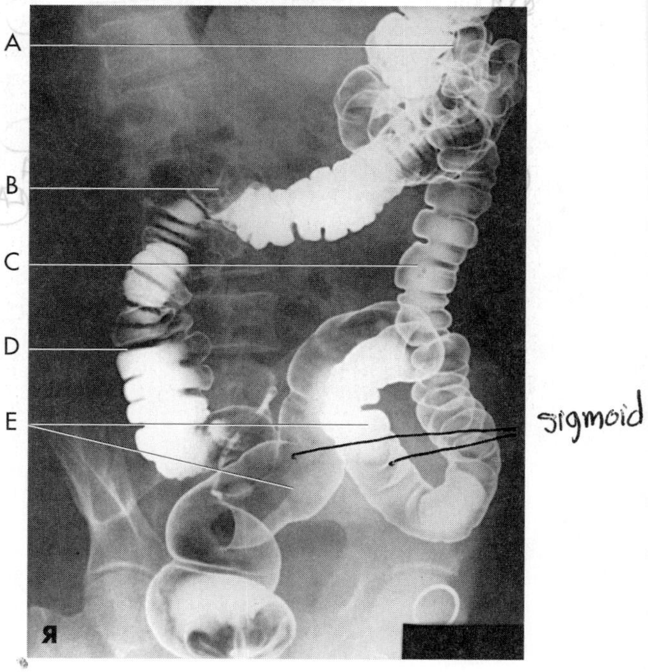

Fig. 17-22 PA oblique large intestine, RAO position.

Items 31 through 33 pertain to the *PA oblique projection, LAO position*. Examine Fig. 17-23 as you answer the following questions.

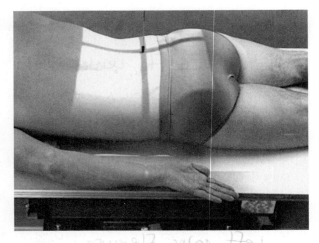

Fig. 17-23 PA oblique large intestine, LAO position.

31. To which level of the patient should the IR be centered for the PA oblique projection, LAO position?

    a. T12
    b. L2
    c. Iliac crests
    d. Symphysis pubis

32. Which two structures of the large intestine are demonstrated primarily with the PA oblique projection, LAO position?

    a. Left colic flexure and ascending colon
    b. Left colic flexure and descending colon   PA
    c. Right colic flexure and ascending colon   LAO
    d. Right colic flexure and descending colon

33. Identify each lettered structure shown in Fig. 17-24.

    A. left colic flexure _____ (flexure)
    B. right colic flexure _____ (flexure)
    C. transverse colon _____
    D. descending colon _____
    E. ascending colon _____
    F. vermaform appendix _____
    G. sigmoid _____

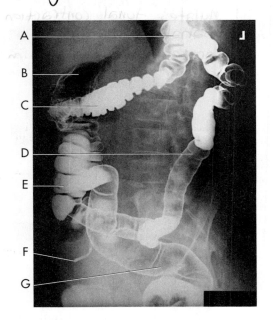

Fig. 17-24 PA oblique large intestine, LAO position.

Items 34 through 38 pertain to the *lateral projection*. Examine Fig. 17-25 as you answer the following questions.

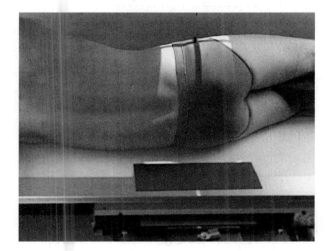

Fig. 17-25 Left lateral rectum.

34. For the lateral projection, to what level of the patient should an IR that is 24 × 30 cm be centered?

To the level of ASIS

35. In the image of the left lateral projection, how is it determined that the patient was not rotated?

hips & femurs should be Super Imposed.

36. Which portions of the large intestine are of prime interest with the lateral projection?
   a. Sigmoid and rectum
   b. Cecum and ascending colon
   c. Left colic flexure and descending colon
   d. Right colic flexure and ascending colon

37. For the lateral projection, which plane of the body should be centered to the midline of the table?
   a. Transverse
   b. Midsagittal
   c. Midcoronal

38. Identify each lettered structure shown in Fig. 17-26.

   A. Sigmoid
   B. sacrum
   C. rectum
   D. pubic symphysis

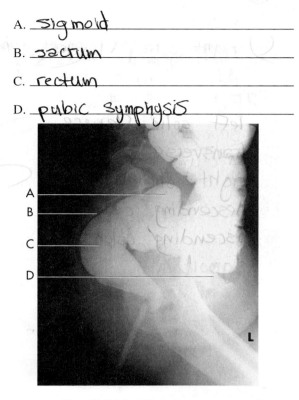

Fig. 17-26 Left lateral rectum.

Items 39 through 43 pertain to the *AP projection*. Examine Fig. 17-27 as you answer the following questions.

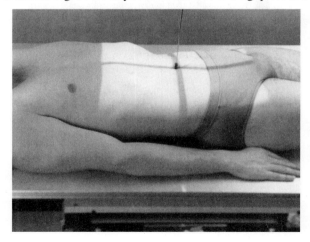
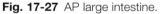

Fig. 17-27 AP large intestine.

39. Which plane of the body should be centered to the grid for the AP projection?

Midsagittal

40. To what level of the patient should the IR be centered?

Illiac crests

41. ~~True~~ or False. The patient should suspend respiration for the exposure.

42. ~~True~~ or False. The entire colon should be demonstrated for the AP projection.

43. Identify each lettered structure shown in Fig. 17-28.

A. _left colic flexure_ (flexure)

B. _transverse colon_

C. _right colic flexure_ (flexure)

D. _descending colon_

E. _ascending colon_

F. _sigmoid_

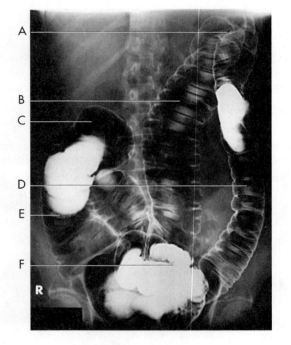

Fig. 17-28 AP large intestine.

Items 44 through 48 pertain to the *AP axial projection*. Examine Fig. 17-29 as you answer the following questions.

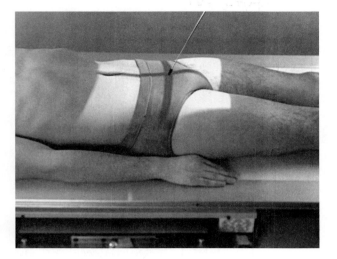

Fig. 17-29 AP axial large intestine.

44. Which projection produces an image similar to the AP axial projection?

   a. AP projection
   b. PA axial projection
   c. PA oblique projection, LAO position
   d. PA oblique projection, RAO position

45. In which direction and how many degrees should the central ray be directed?

   a. Caudally 10 to 20 degrees
   b. Caudally 30 to 40 degrees
   c. Cephalically 10 to 20 degrees
   d. Cephalically 30 to 40 degrees

46. For the AP axial projection, where on the patient's anterior surface should the central ray enter when a 35- × 43-cm IR is used?

2" below the level of the ASIS's.

47. To produce a coned-down image of the AP axial projection on an IR that is 24 × 30 cm, where on the patient should the central ray enter?

The inferior margin of the the pubic symphysis

48. Identify each lettered structure shown in Fig. 17-30.

A. descending colon

B. sigmoid

C. rectum

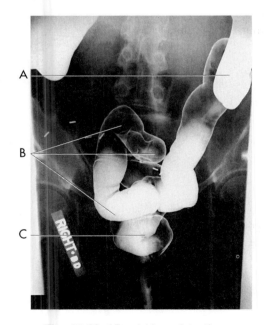

Fig. 17-30 AP axial large intestine.

Items 49 through 53 pertain to the *AP oblique projection, LPO position*. Examine Fig. 17-31 as you answer the following questions.

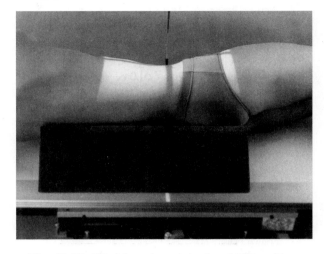

Fig. 17-31 AP oblique large intestine, LPO position.

49. The AP oblique projection, LPO position, produces an image similar to the PA oblique projection (RAO position).

50. For the AP oblique projection, LPO position, the patient should be rotated 35 to 45 degrees.

51. For the AP oblique projection, LPO position, which side of the patient—right or left—should be elevated away from the x-ray table?

right

52. Which flexure—right colic or left colic—should be well demonstrated with the AP oblique projection, LPO position?

right colic flexure

53. Identify each lettered structure shown in Fig. 17-32.

A. _left colic flexure_ (flexure)

B. _right colic flexure_ (flexure)

C. _descending colon_

D. _ascending colon_

E. _sigmoid_

F. _rectum_

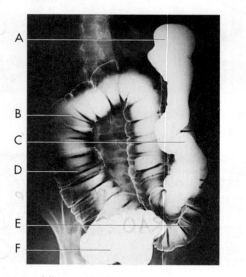

Fig. 17-32 AP oblique large intestine, LPO position.

Items 54 through 57 pertain to the *AP oblique projection, right posterior oblique (RPO) position.* Examine Fig. 17-33 as you answer the following questions.

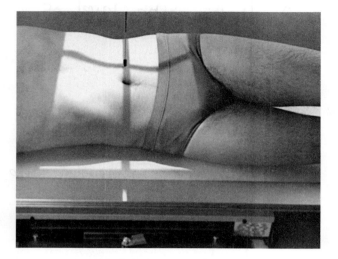

Fig. 17-33 AP oblique large intestine, RPO position.

54. What other oblique position produces an image similar to the AP oblique projection, RPO position?

LAO

55. Which flexure—right colic or left colic—should be well demonstrated with the AP oblique projection, RPO position?

Left colic

56. How many degrees should the patient be rotated from the supine position for the AP oblique projection, RPO position?

$35^\circ - 45^\circ$

57. Identify each lettered structure shown in Fig. 17-34.

A. left colic _____ (flexure)

B. transverse colon

C. right colic _____ (flexure)

D. descending colon

E. ascending colon

F. sigmoid

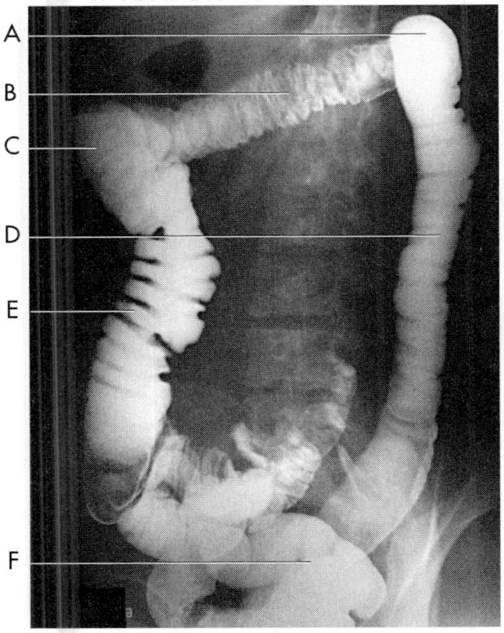

Fig. 17-34 AP oblique large intestine, RPO position.

Items 58 through 64 pertain to *AP or PA projections, right and left lateral decubitus positions.* Examine Figs. 17-35 and 17-36 as you answer the following questions.

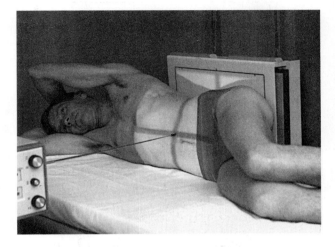

Fig. 17-35 AP large intestine, right lateral decubitus position.

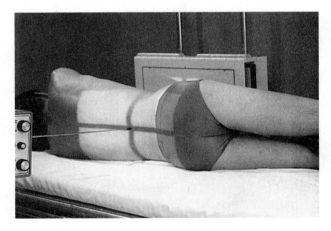

Fig. 17-36 PA large intestine, left lateral decubitus position.

58. Which BE projection requires that the patient be placed in the right lateral recumbent position and that a horizontal central ray be directed to the midline of the patient at the level of the iliac crests?

a. Right lateral
b. AP oblique, RPO position
c. PA oblique, RAO position
d. AP, right lateral decubitus position

59. For lateral decubitus positions, what should be accomplished to ensure that the dependent side of the patient is demonstrated?

support the pt on a radio-lucent pad.

60. How much of the colon should be demonstrated in the image of a lateral decubitus position?

area from the flextures to the colon. rectum

61. Name the lateral decubitus position that best demonstrates each of the following intestinal structures.

a. Left colic flexure: *right lat. decub-*

b. Right colic flexure: *left lat. decub*

62. Figs. 17-37 and 17-38 are lateral decubitus radiographs. Examine the images and answer the questions that follow.

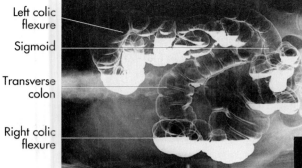

Left colic flexure
Sigmoid
Transverse colon
Right colic flexure

Fig. 17-37 Radiograph of the large intestine, lateral decubitus position.

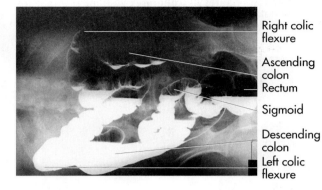

Right colic flexure
Ascending colon
Rectum
Sigmoid
Descending colon
Left colic flexure

Fig. 17-38 Radiograph of the large intestine, lateral decubitus position.

a. Which image shows the left lateral decubitus position?

_____ 38 _____

b. Which image shows the right lateral decubitus position?

_____ 37 _____

c. Which image best demonstrates the left colic flexure?

_____ 37 _____

d. Which image best demonstrates the right colic flexure?

_____ 38 _____

e. Which image requires that the patient be placed in the left lateral recumbent position?

_____ 38 _____

f. Which image requires that the patient be placed in the right lateral recumbent position?

_____ 37 _____

Questions 63 and 64 pertain to BE radiographs performed with the patient in the upright position.

63. For upright frontal, oblique, and lateral projections, how is the centering of the IR adjusted from that used for the recumbent positions? Why is this compensation necessary?

its lower (2"-3")

64. Examine Fig. 17-39 and answer the questions that follow.

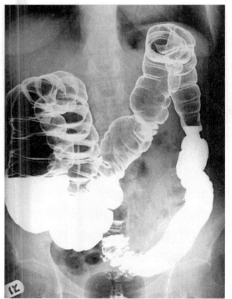

Fig. 17-39 AP large intestine.

a. What body position was used to make this radiograph?

upright

b. What image characteristics led you to that conclusion?

liquid BaSO4 can be seen settling in lower levels of colon.

65. Figs. 17-40 through 17-47 represent different projections used to obtain BE radiographs. Examine the images, then match the figures in Column A with the positions/projections in Column B.

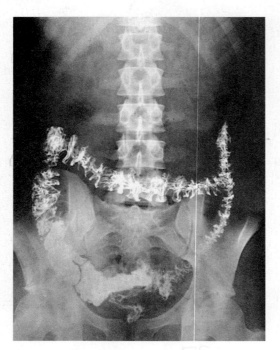

Fig. 17-40 BE radiograph.

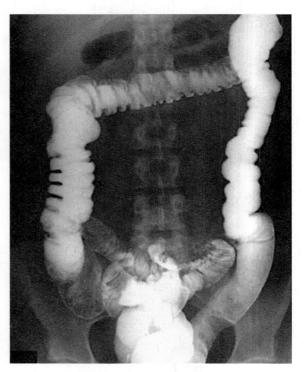

Fig. 17-42 BE radiograph.

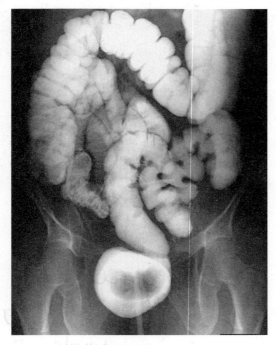

Fig. 17-41 BE radiograph.

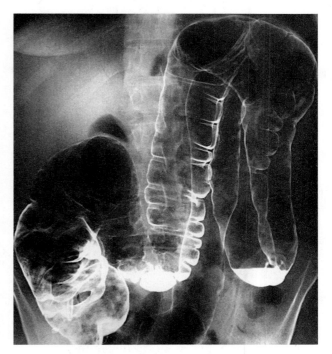

Fig. 17-43 BE radiograph.

68

Chapter 17 Digestive System: Alimentary Canal   Workbook for Merrill's Atlas of Radiographic Positioning and Procedures • Volume 2

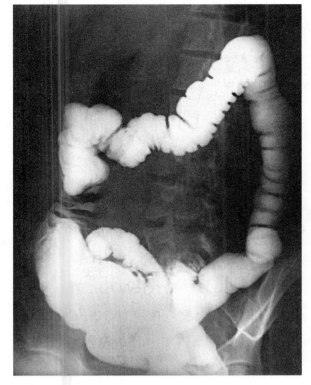

Fig. 17-44 BE radiograph.

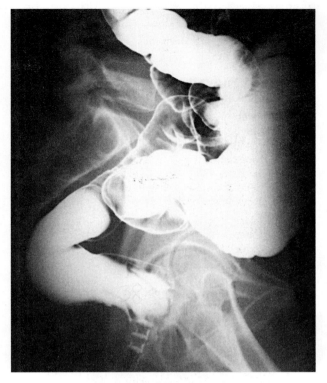

Fig. 17-46 BE radiograph.

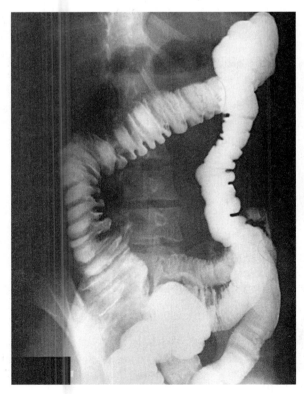

Fig. 17-45 BE radiograph.

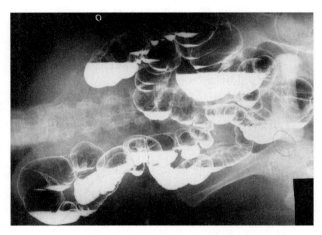

Fig. 17-47 BE radiograph.

Column A	Column B
_____ 1. Fig. 17-40	a. LAO position
_____ 2. Fig. 17-41	b. LPO position
_____ 3. Fig. 17-42	c. AP axial projection
_____ 4. Fig. 17-43	d. PA, upright position
_____ 5. Fig. 17-44	e. AP, recumbent position
_____ 6. Fig. 17-45	f. Left lateral position
_____ 7. Fig. 17-46	g. Postevacuation
_____ 8. Fig. 17-47	h. Lateral decubitus position

SELF-TEST: ANATOMY AND POSITIONING OF THE ALIMENTARY CANAL

Answer the following questions by selecting the best choice.

1. In which body habitus type is the stomach almost horizontal and high in the abdomen?
   a. Sthenic
   b. Asthenic
   c. Hyposthenic
   d. Hypersthenic

2. Which curvature is located on the right (medial) border of the stomach?
   a. Lesser
   b. Greater
   c. Inferior
   d. Superior

3. Which area is the most superior part of the stomach?
   a. Head
   b. Body
   c. Fundus
   d. Pylorus

4. Which area is the most inferior part of the stomach?
   a. Body
   b. Cardia
   c. Fundus
   d. Pylorus

5. The distal esophagus empties its contents into which of the following?
   a. Duodenum
   b. Pyloric canal
   c. Duodenal bulb
   d. Cardiac antrum

6. Which opening is located between the stomach and small intestine?
   a. Cardiac orifice
   b. Pyloric orifice
   c. Ileocecal orifice
   d. Hepatopancreatic ampulla

7. Which opening is at the distal end of the small intestine?
   a. Anus
   b. Cardiac orifice
   c. Pyloric orifice
   d. Ileocecal orifice

8. Which structure is the proximal part of the small intestine?
   a. Ileum
   b. Pylorus
   c. Jejunum
   d. Duodenum

9. Which structure is the distal part of the small intestine?
   a. Ileum
   b. Cecum
   c. Jejunum
   d. Duodenum

10. In which abdominal region does the large intestine originate?
    a. Left iliac
    b. Right iliac
    c. Left lumbar
    d. Right lumbar

11. Which structure is the proximal part of the large intestine?
    a. Ileum
    b. Cecum
    c. Rectum
    d. Sigmoid

12. Which part of the large intestine is located between the ascending and descending parts of the colon?
    a. Cecum
    b. Rectum
    c. Sigmoid
    d. Transverse colon

13. Which structure is located between the ascending colon and the transverse colon?
    a. Sigmoid
    b. Left colic flexure
    c. Right colic flexure
    d. Descending colon

14. Where in the large intestine is the left colic flexure located?
    a. Between the cecum and the ascending colon
    b. Between the ascending colon and the transverse colon
    c. Between the transverse colon and the descending colon
    d. Between the descending colon and the sigmoid

15. Which structure is the pouchlike part of the large intestine situated below the junction of the ileum and the colon?
    a. Cecum
    b. Rectum
    c. Sigmoid
    d. Vermiform appendix

70

Chapter **17** **Digestive System: Alimentary Canal**   Workbook for Merrill's Atlas of Radiographic Positioning and Procedures • Volume 2

16. Where in the large intestine is the sigmoid located?

    a. Between the cecum and the transverse colon
    b. Between the ascending colon and the transverse colon
    c. Between the descending colon and the rectum
    d. Between the transverse colon and the descending colon

17. Approximately how long does it usually take a barium meal to reach the ileocecal valve?

    a. 30 minutes to 1 hour
    b. 2 to 3 hours
    c. 4 to 5 hours
    d. 24 hours

18. Approximately how long does it usually take a barium meal to reach the rectum?

    a. 2 to 3 hours
    b. 4 to 5 hours
    c. 6 to 8 hours
    d. 24 hours

19. Which two imaging modalities are most commonly used to examine the alimentary canal after the introduction of a barium product?

    a. Fluoroscopy and sonography
    b. Fluoroscopy and radiography
    c. Computed tomography and sonography
    d. Computed tomography and radiography

20. Which type of contrast medium is most commonly used for examining the upper GI tract?

    a. An oily, viscous compound
    b. A barium sulfate suspension
    c. A nonionic injectable compound
    d. A water-soluble, iodinated solution

21. To best demonstrate the swallowing function, in which position should the patient be placed to begin the fluoroscopic phase of single-contrast examinations of the esophagus?

    a. Upright
    b. Left lateral decubitus
    c. Recumbent LAO
    d. Recumbent RPO

22. Which two recumbent oblique positions can be used to best demonstrate an unobstructed image of a barium-filled esophagus between the vertebrae and the heart?

    a. LAO and LPO
    b. LAO and RPO
    c. RAO and LPO
    d. RAO and RPO

23. Which of the following is a major advantage of the double-contrast UGI examination over the single-contrast UGI examination?

    a. The patient can better tolerate the procedure.
    b. Radiation exposure to the patient is reduced.
    c. Small lesions on the mucosal lining are better demonstrated.
    d. The examination can be performed with the patient upright instead of recumbent

24. Which description refers to the biphasic GI examination?

    a. A single-contrast study of the entire alimentary canal
    b. A single-contrast study of the upper GI tract
    c. A double-contrast study of the upper GI tract
    d. A combination single-contrast and double-contrast study of the upper GI tract

25. Which body habitus produces the greatest visceral movement when a patient is moved from the prone position to the upright position?

    a. Sthenic
    b. Asthenic
    c. Hyposthenic
    d. Hypersthenic

26. For the PA projection as part of the UGI examination, why should the lower lung fields be included on a 35- × 43-cm IR?

    a. To demonstrate pneumothorax
    b. To demonstrate a possible hiatal hernia
    c. To demonstrate fluid levels in the thorax
    d. To demonstrate the gas bubble in the fundus of the stomach

27. For the double-contrast UGI examination, which projection produces the best image of a gas-filled duodenal bulb and pyloric canal?

    a. AP oblique projection, upright LPO position
    b. AP oblique projection, recumbent LPO position
    c. PA oblique projection, upright RAO position
    d. PA oblique projection, recumbent RAO position

28. For the single-contrast UGI examination with the patient recumbent, which projection produces the best image of a barium-filled pyloric canal and duodenal bulb in patients whose habitus approximates the sthenic type?

    a. AP projection
    b. Left lateral projection
    c. AP oblique projection, LPO position
    d. PA oblique projection, RAO position

29. For the UGI examination with the patient recumbent, which projection best stimulates gastric peristalsis to better demonstrate the pyloric canal and duodenal bulb?

    a. AP projection
    b. Left lateral projection
    c. AP oblique projection, LPO position
    d. PA oblique projection, RAO position

30. Which breathing procedure should the patient perform when UGI radiographs are exposed?

    a. Slow, deep breathing
    b. Quick, panting breaths
    c. Suspended expiration
    d. Suspended inspiration

31. For the double-contrast UGI examination with the patient recumbent, which projection produces the best image of a gas-filled fundus?

    a. Left lateral projection
    b. AP projection, left lateral decubitus position
    c. AP oblique projection, LPO position
    d. PA oblique projection, RAO position

32. For the UGI examination with the patient recumbent, which projection best demonstrates the right retrogastric space?

    a. Right lateral projection
    b. AP projection, right lateral decubitus position
    c. AP oblique projection, LPO position
    d. PA oblique projection, RAO position

33. For the AP projection with the patient supine (as part of the UGI examination), which procedure should be performed to best demonstrate a diaphragmatic herniation (hiatal hernia)?

    a. Angle the central ray 30 to 35 degrees caudally.
    b. Tilt the table and patient into a full Trendelenburg position.
    c. Instruct the patient to suspend respiration after full inspiration.
    d. Place radiolucent cushions under the thorax to elevate the shoulders.

34. To which level of the patient should the central ray be directed for the PA oblique projection, RAO position, as part of the UGI examination?

    a. T9-T10
    b. T11-T12
    c. L1-L2
    d. L3-L4

35. Which examination of the alimentary canal requires that a series of radiographs be taken at specific time intervals after the ingestion of the contrast medium?

    a. UGI series
    b. BE
    c. Esophagography
    d. Small bowel series

36. For a small bowel series of a patient with hypomotility of the small intestine, which procedure should be performed to accelerate peristalsis?

    a. Roll the patient 360 degrees.
    b. Instruct the patient to drink a glass of ice water.
    c. Instruct the patient to perform the Valsalva maneuver.
    d. Tilt the table and patient into a full Trendelenburg position.

37. Which structure, when visualized on a radiograph as part of a small bowel series, usually indicates the completion of the exam?

    a. Ileum
    b. Cecum
    c. Jejunum
    d. Duodenum

38. What is the proper sequence for filling the large intestine with barium when performing a BE?

    a. Rectum, sigmoid, ascending colon, transverse colon, and descending colon
    b. Rectum, sigmoid, descending colon, transverse colon, and ascending colon
    c. Sigmoid, rectum, ascending colon, transverse colon, and descending colon
    d. Sigmoid, rectum, descending colon, transverse colon, and ascending colon

39. Which procedure should be used during a BE to relax the large intestine and enable the patient to better retain the barium sulfate suspension?

    a. Instruct the patient to perform the Valsalva maneuver.
    b. Raise the barium bag to 24 inches above the rectum.
    c. Administer cold (41° F) barium sulfate suspension.
    d. Administer warm (95° F) barium sulfate suspension.

40. Before the enema tip is inserted during a BE, why should a small amount of barium sulfate mixture be allowed to run into a waste basin?

    a. To lubricate the enema tip
    b. To remove air from the tube
    c. To determine if the mixture is too warm or too cold
    d. To ensure that the consistency of the mixture is adequate

41. Which procedure should be accomplished when inserting the enema tip for a BE?

   a. Lubricate the tip with petroleum jelly.
   b. Place the patient in the Trendelenburg position.
   c. Inflate the air-filled retention tip before insertion.
   d. Ensure that the tip is inserted no more than 3½ to 4 inches (8.9 to 10 cm).

42. For the PA projection during a BE, what is the advantage of placing the x-ray table and patient in a slight Trendelenburg position?

   a. To demonstrate the ileocecal valve
   b. To enable more air to be injected into the colon
   c. To help separate overlapping loops of distal bowel
   d. To move the transverse colon higher in the abdomen

43. Which structures of the large intestine are of primary interest with AP axial or PA axial projections during a BE?

   a. Sigmoid and rectum
   b. Cecum and ileocecal valve
   c. Left and right colic flexures
   d. Ascending and descending colons

44. How many degrees and in which direction should the central ray be directed for the PA axial projection during a BE?

   a. 20 to 25 degrees caudal
   b. 20 to 25 degrees cephalic
   c. 30 to 40 degrees caudal
   d. 30 to 40 degrees cephalic

45. Which structure of the large intestine is of primary interest for the PA oblique projection, RAO position, during BE examinations?

   a. Anal canal
   b. Left colic flexure
   c. Right colic flexure
   d. Descending colon

46. Which two oblique projections can be performed to best demonstrate the left colic flexure during a BE?

   a. PA oblique projection, LAO position; and AP oblique projection, LPO position
   b. PA oblique projection, LAO position; and AP oblique projection, RPO position
   c. PA oblique projection, RAO position; and AP oblique projection, LPO position
   d. PA oblique projection, RAO position; and AP oblique projection, RPO position

47. Which structure of the large intestine is best demonstrated if the patient is rotated 45 degrees from a supine position to move the right side of the abdomen away from the x-ray table during a BE?

   a. Ileum
   b. Cecum
   c. Left colic flexure
   d. Right colic flexure

48. For the right lateral decubitus position as part of a BE, which procedure should be done to ensure that the ascending colon is demonstrated in the image?

   a. Center the IR to the iliac crests.
   b. Elevate the patient on a radiolucent support.
   c. Tilt the table and patient into a full Trendelenburg position.
   d. Make the exposure after the patient suspends respiration.

49. Which BE projection requires that a 24- × 30-cm IR be placed lengthwise and centered to the level of the anterior superior iliac spine (ASIS)?

   a. AP projection
   b. Lateral projection
   c. AP projection, left lateral decubitus position
   d. AP oblique projection, LPO position

50. Which BE projection does not require colic flexures to be included in the image?

   a. AP projection
   b. Lateral projection
   c. AP projection, lateral decubitus position
   d. PA oblique projection, RAO position

18 Urinary System

SECTION 1

ANATOMY OF THE URINARY SYSTEM

Exercise 1

This exercise pertains to urinary structures. Identify structures for each question.

1. Identify each lettered structure shown in Fig. 18-1.

A. right kidney

B. inferior vena cava

C. aorta

D. left kidney

E. left ureter

F. urinary bladder

2. Identify each lettered structure shown in Fig. 18-2.

A. right kidney

B. right ureter

C. urinary bladder

D. rectum

E. prostate

F. anal canal

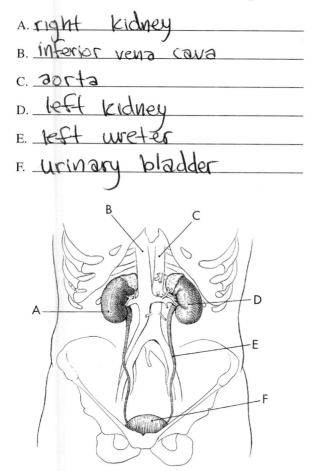

Fig. 18-1 Anterior aspect of the urinary system in relation to the surrounding structures.

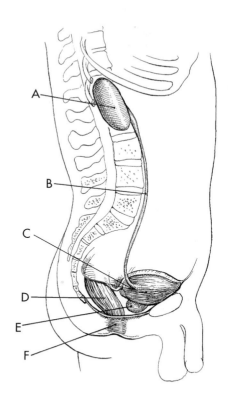

Fig. 18-2 Lateral aspect of the male urinary system in relation to the surrounding structures.

3. Identify each lettered part of the kidney shown in Fig. 18-3.

A. <u>Hilum</u>

B. <u>renal papilla</u>

C. <u>renal pelvis</u>

D. <u>renal cortex</u>

E. <u>renal sinus</u>

F. <u>renal medulla</u>

G. <u>renal pyramid</u>

H. <u>minor calyx</u>

I. <u>major calyx</u>

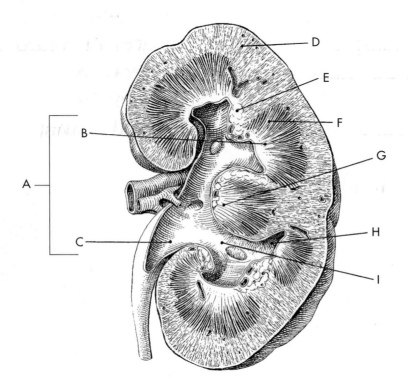

Fig. 18-3 Midcoronal section of a kidney.

4. Identify each lettered structure shown in Fig. 18-4.

A. cortex

B. medulla

C. afferent arteriole

D. efferent arteriole

E. glomerulus

F. distal convoluted tubule

G. glomular capsule

H. proximal convoluted capsule

I. descending limb of Henle's loop

J. ascending limb of Henle's loop

K. collecting duct

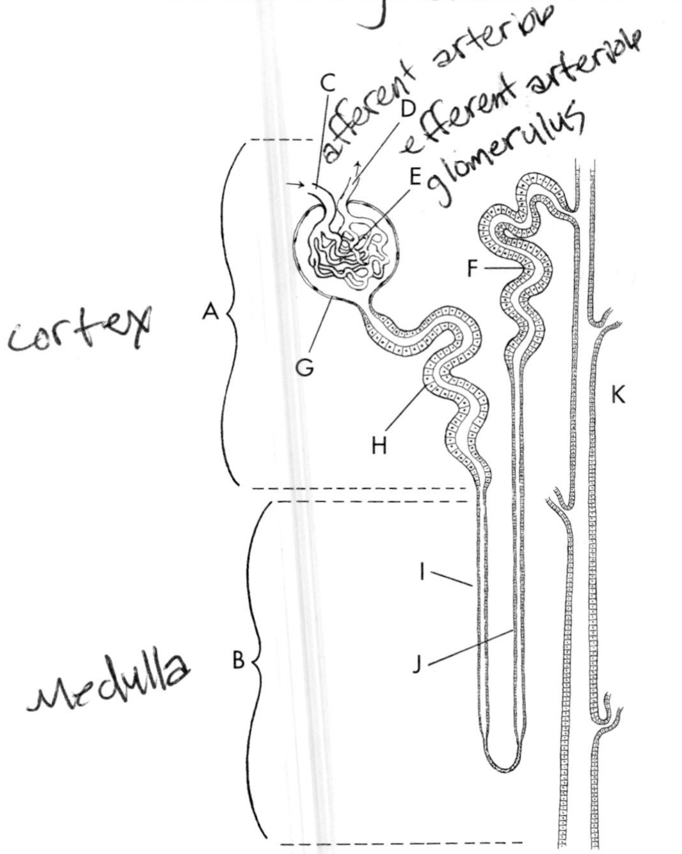

5. Identify each lettered structure shown in Fig. 18-5.

A. ovary

B. uterine tube

C. uterus

D. bladder

E. pubic symphysis

F. urethra

G. vagina

H. rectum

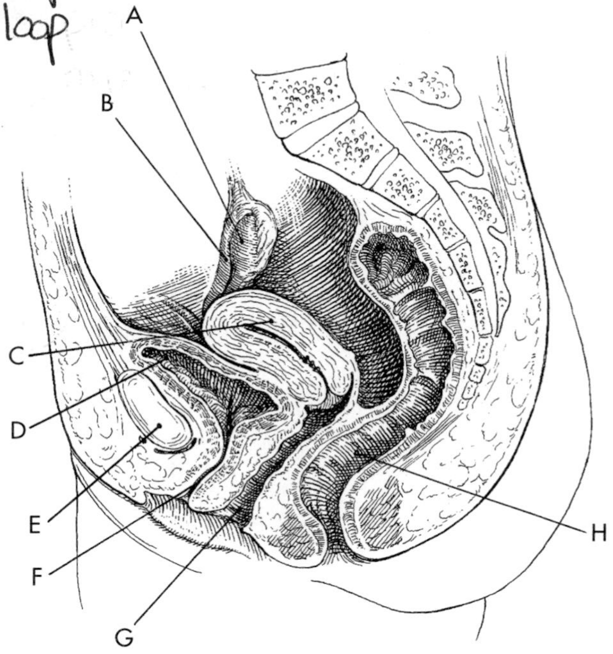

Fig. 18-4 Diagram of a nephron and collecting duct.

Fig. 18-5 Midsagittal section through the female pelvis.

6. Identify each lettered structure shown in Fig. 18-6.

A. bladder

B. pubic symphysis

C. urethra

D. sacrum

E. rectum

F. prostate

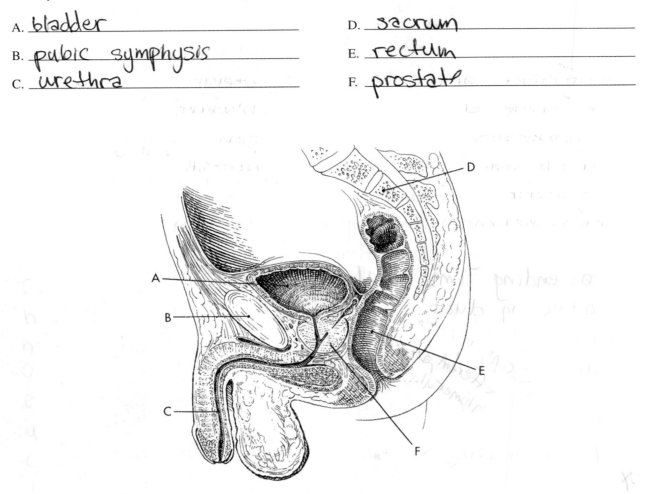

Fig. 18-6 Midsagittal section through the male pelvis.

Exercise 2

Use the following clues to complete the crossword puzzle. All answers refer to the urinary system.

Across

3. Outer renal tissue
4. This arteriole leaves the capsule
6. Filtrate derivative
7. Another term for suprarenal
8. Urine vessel from glomerular capsule
10. Cup-shaped urine receivers
12. Cone-shaped renal segments
15. Cluster of blood vessels
16. Urinary reservoir
17. Functional renal unit
18. Musculomembranous excretory duct
19. Medial opening of a kidney

Down

1. This arteriole enters the capsule
2. Inner renal tissue
3. Membranous cup; Bowman's _____
5. Central renal cavity
6. External excretory tube
9. Male gland
11. Gland that is found on a kidney
13. Glomerular fluid
14. Primary organ of urinary system

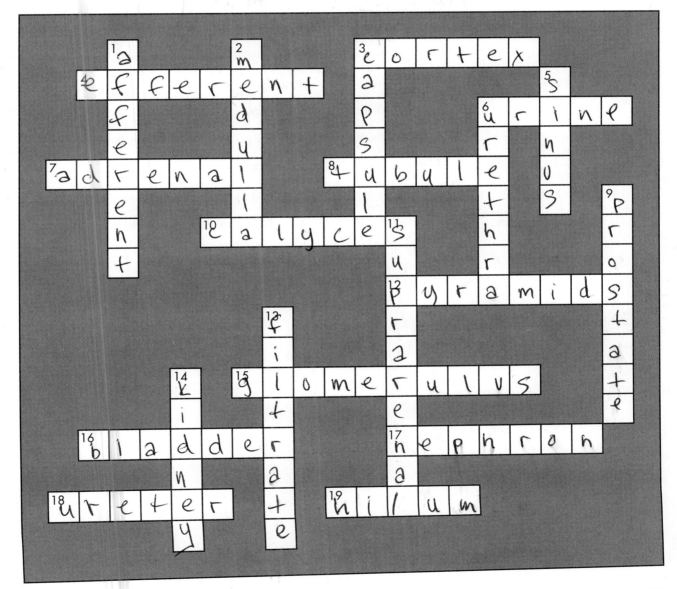

Exercise 3

Match the pathology terms in Column A with the appropriate definition in Column B. Not all choices from Column B should be selected.

Column A

_l_ 1. Tumor

_p_ 2. Fistula

_a_ 3. Cystitis

_d_ 4. Stenosis

_k_ 5. Calculus

_g_ 6. Carcinoma

_j_ 7. Ureterocele

_f_ 8. Pyelonephritis

_h_ 9. Hydronephrosis

_n_ 10. Polycystic kidney

_o_ 11. Renal obstruction

_e_ 12. Renal hypertension

_m_ 13. Glomerulonephritis

_c_ 14. Congenital anomaly

_i_ 15. Vesicoureteral reflux

Column B

a. Inflammation of the bladder

b. Enlargement of the prostate

c. Abnormality present since birth

d. Narrowing or contraction of a passage

e. Increased blood pressure to the kidneys

f. Inflammation of the kidney and renal pelvis

g. Malignant new growth composed of epithelial cells

h. Distension of the renal pelvis and calyces with urine

i. Backward flow of urine from the bladder into the ureters

j. Ballooning of the lower end of the ureter into the bladder

k. Abnormal concretion of mineral salts, often called a stone

l. New tissue growth where cell proliferation is uncontrolled

m. Inflammation of the capillary loops in the glomeruli of the kidneys

n. Massive enlargement of the kidney with the formation of many cysts

o. Condition preventing the normal flow of urine through the urinary system

p. Abnormal connection between two internal organs or between an organ and the body surface

Exercise 4

This exercise pertains to the anatomy of the urinary system. Fill in missing words for each question.

1. The kidneys and ureters are part of the ___urinary___ system.

2. The organ that removes waste products from the blood is the ___kidney___.

3. The gland that sits on the superior pole of each kidney is the ___suprarenal___ gland.

4. Blood vessels, nerves, and the ureter enter a kidney through an opening known as the ___hilum___.

5. The hilum is located on the ___medial___ border of the kidney.

6. In the average (sthenic) person, the superior pole of the kidney is located at the ___T12___ vertebral level.

7. The microscopic functional unit of the kidney is the ___nephron___.

8. Nephron units are found in the layer of renal tissue known as the ___cortex___.

9. The proximal portion of a nephron consisting of a double-walled membranous cup is the ___glomerular___ capsule.

10. A cluster of blood capillaries surrounded by a Bowman's capsule is a ___glomerulus___.

11. A glomerulus branches off the ___renal___ artery.

12. The blood vessel entering a glomerular capsule is the ___afferent___ arteriole; the blood vessel leaving a glomerular capsule is the ___efferent___ arteriole.

13. The fluid that passes from the glomerulus to the glomerular capsule is ___glomerular filtrate___.

14. Urine from collecting ducts drains into minor ___calyces___.

15. Minor calyces drain urine into major ___calyces___.

16. Major calyces unite to form the expanded, funnel-shaped renal ___pelvis___.

17. The long tubes that transport urine from the kidneys are the ~~pelves~~ ___ureters___.

18. Ureters transport urine from kidneys to the ___urinary bladder___.

19. The musculomembranous tube that conveys urine from the urinary bladder to outside the body is the ___urethra___.

20. The gland that surrounds the proximal part of the male urethra is the ___prostate___.

Exercise 5: Abbreviations

This exercise provides practice in the use of the common abbreviations related to urinary system radiography and the imaging profession. Write out the expanded form beside each abbreviation.

1. VCUG: voiding cystourethrogram

2. BUN: blood urine nitrogen

3. IV: intravenus

4. ACR: american college of radiology

5. BPH: benign prostate hyperplasia

Exercise 6: Venipuncture and IV Contrast Media Administration

This exercise pertains to venipuncture and intravenous (IV) contrast media administration. Items require you to write a short answer or select from a list.

1. Which condition should be prevented if strict aseptic techniques are used when administering medications intravenously?

   a. The patient lapsing into shock
   b. Introducing infection into the patient
   c. Injecting an excessive amount of medication

2. How does the use of an IV filter affect a bolus injection?

   a. The rate of injection will be reduced.
   b. The introduction of foreign matter will increase.
   c. The time required to inject the medication will be reduced.

3. What are the three parts of a syringe?

   a. Tip, barrel, and bevel
   b. Tip, barrel, and plunger
   c. Hub, cannula, and bevel
   d. Hub, cannula, and plunger

4. What are the three parts of a hypodermic needle?

   a. Tip, barrel, and bevel
   b. Tip, barrel, and plunger
   c. Hub, cannula, and bevel
   d. Hub, cannula, and plunger

5. To what does the term *needle gauge* refer?

   a. The angle of the bevel
   b. The length of the needle
   c. The diameter of the needle

6. What injection apparatus is preferred for most IV administrations?

   a. Butterfly set
   b. Over-the-needle cannula
   c. Seldinger-technique needle

7. Which procedure should be performed to maintain a closed system with a multiple-dose vial of medication?

   a. Discard the vial after the second use.
   b. Inject into the bottle an amount of air equal to the amount of fluid to be withdrawn.
   c. Inject into the bottle an amount of sterile saline solution equal to the amount of fluid to be withdrawn.

8. When assessing vessels for venipuncture, why should a vessel not be used if a pulse is detected?

   a. A pulse indicates the vessel is an artery.
   b. A pulse indicates the patient is hypertensive.
   c. A pulse indicates the patient has low blood pressure.
   d. A pulse indicates the patient has a fistula in that vessel.

9. From the following list, circle the four sites that are most often used for establishing IV access.

   a. Anterior hand
   b. Posterior hand
   c. Femoral artery
   d. Anterior forearm
   e. Posterior forearm
   f. Ulnar aspect of the wrist
   g. Radial aspect of the wrist
   h. Anterior aspect of the elbow

10. Describe how the skin should be prepared before inserting a needle into a vein.

    using tincture of iodine 1% to 2% or iso-propyl alcohol 70%, wipe skin w/ circular motion (2" diameter) w/o lifting the swab until the process is completed.

11. How far above the site of a venipuncture should the tourniquet be placed?

    6-8 inches

12. How should the IV needle be inserted—bevel up or bevel down?

    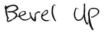
    Bevel Up

13. When inserting an IV needle into the patient, what angle should exist between the needle and the patient's skin surface?

45°

14. What is the significance of a backflow of blood into the syringe during a venipuncture procedure?

The vein has successfully been penetrated by the needle

15. What procedure should a radiographer perform if the needle has punctured both walls of the vein?

remove the needle & apply direct pressure to the puncture site

16. What is infiltration?
    a. The procedure for using an IV filter in tubing
    b. The introduction of a hypodermic needle into a vein
    c. The process of injecting fluid into tissues instead of a vein

17. Which other term refers to infiltration?
    a. Extraction
    b. Extirpation
    c. Extravasation

18. Which procedure should a radiographer perform after a needle has been removed from a vein?
    a. Apply a tourniquet 3 to 4 inches above the puncture site.
    b. Using a 2- × 2-inch pad of gauze, apply pressure directly to the injection site.
    c. Clean the area using a circular motion covering an area that is approximately 2 inches in diameter.

19. From the following list, circle the four symptoms that may indicate the occurrence of infiltration.
    a. Pain
    b. Burning
    c. Redness
    d. Swelling
    e. Dyspnea
    f. Sneezing
    g. Rapid pulse
    h. Hypotension

20. From the following list, circle the five golden rules of medication administration.
    a. The right time
    b. The right route
    c. The right patient
    d. The right syringe
    e. The right amount
    f. The right medication
    g. The right technologist
    h. The right body position

POSITIONING OF THE URINARY SYSTEM

Exercise 1: Excretory Urography

Radiography of the urinary system comprises numerous specialized procedures. The most common radiographic examination of the urinary system is the excretory urogram. This exercise pertains to excretory urography. Identify structures, fill in missing words, select from a list, provide a short answer, or choose true or false (explain any item you believe to be false) for each question.

Questions 1 through 22 pertain to general information concerning excretory urography.

1. The radiographic investigation of the renal drainage system is accomplished by various procedures classified under the general term __Urography__.

2. Which two terms refer to the excretory urogram examination?
   a. Cystourethrography and retrograde urography
   b. Cystourethrography and intravenous pyelography
   c. Intravenous urography and retrograde urography
   d. (circled) Intravenous urography and intravenous pyelography

3. From the following list, circle four terms that identify the typical contrast media currently used in excretory urography.
   a. (circled) Ionic
   b. (circled) Nonionic
   c. (circled) Iodinated
   d. Noniodinated
   e. (circled) Injectable
   f. Noninjectable

4. From the following list, circle the mild adverse reactions to iodinated contrast medium administration.
   a. (circled) Hives
   b. Death
   c. (circled) Nausea
   d. Dyspnea
   e. (circled) Vomiting
   f. (circled) Warm feeling
   g. Cardiac arrest
   h. Renal shutdown
   i. Respiratory arrest
   j. (circled) Flushed appearance
   k. (circled) Edema of the respiratory mucous membranes

5. How soon after the injection of a contrast medium are symptoms of a reaction most likely to occur?
   a. (circled) Within 5 minutes
   b. Between 5 to 10 minutes
   c. More than 10 minutes

6. From the following list, circle the four typical procedures that a patient might ideally experience when preparing for the intravenous urography (IVU) examination.
   a. (circled) Laxative
   b. Cleansing enema
   c. (circled) Light evening meal
   d. Liquid diet for 3 to 4 days
   e. (circled) Low-residue diet for 1 or 2 days
   f. Drinking 32 ounces of water to fill the bladder
   g. (circled) Nothing by mouth (NPO) after midnight on the day of the examination

7. What is the purpose of giving a child 12 ounces of carbonated beverage just before the start of IVU?
   To distend the stomach w/gas providing a negative density that better dem.

8. Why should an immobilization band not be applied across the patient's upper abdomen in an effort to control motion during IVU? renal structures
   Inappropriate Abd. pressure might retard the excretion of fluid from the kidneys & might cause distortion of ureteral structures

9. What is the purpose of applying compression over the distal ends of the ureters?
   To retard the flow of opacified urine into the bladder allowing renal structures to be visualized

10. Where on the abdomen should compression pads be located to compress the ureters?
    Anterior surface of Abd. About 2" ↑ Pubic Symphsis

11. When ureteral compression is used, why should the pressure be slowly released when the compression device is no longer needed?
    rapid release will rupture the viscera

12. Why is ureteral compression currently not often used in excretory urography?
    ↑ c.m. better dem. the ureters

13. Why might an upright anteroposterior (AP) projection of the abdomen be made before the injection of the contrast medium?
    Dem. the mobility of Kidneys

14. What identification data should be included on every postinjection radiograph?
    Pt Data, Marker, timy & pos. label

15. Why is it desirable to have the patient remove his or her underwear?
    unwanted data & skin folds

16. Why should the patient be instructed to empty his or her bladder just before IVU is to begin?

    a. To locate the ureteral openings
    b. To measure the capacity of the bladder
    c. To prevent dilution of the opacified urine

17. From the following list, circle the five reasons that AP projections with the patient recumbent are performed as the scout radiograph.

    a. To demonstrate the bladder
    b. To identify the location of the kidneys
    c. To demonstrate the presence of calculi
    d. To demonstrate the contour of the kidneys
    e. To check the radiographic exposure factors
    f. To demonstrate the mobility of the kidneys
    g. To examine for radiopaque artifacts on the positioning table
    h. To determine how well the patient's gastrointestinal (GI) tract was cleaned

18. What can be done to enhance the filling of renal structures with contrast medium when the patient is supine?

    a. Place supports under the patient's knees.
    b. Place a support under the patient's lumbar region.
    c. Direct the central ray 20 to 25 degrees caudally.
    d. Tilt the x-ray table and patient to the Trendelenburg position.

19. Approximately how long after a bolus injection of the contrast medium should the exposure be made to best demonstrate a nephrogram?

    a. 30 seconds
    b. 3 minutes
    c. 5 minutes

20. How long after the completion of the contrast medium injection does the contrast agent usually begin to appear in the renal pelvis?

    a. 30 seconds to 1 minute
    b. 2 to 8 minutes
    c. 10 to 14 minutes
    d. 15 to 20 minutes

21. How long after the injection of the contrast medium does the greatest concentration usually appear within the kidneys?

    a. 30 seconds to 1 minute
    b. 2 to 8 minutes
    c. 15 to 20 minutes
    d. 30 to 45 minutes

22. A postvoiding radiograph is usually the last radiograph taken to demonstrate which structure(s)?

    a. Ureters
    b. Bladder
    c. Kidneys

Items 23 through 32 pertain to the *AP projection*. Examine Fig. 18-7 as you answer the following questions.

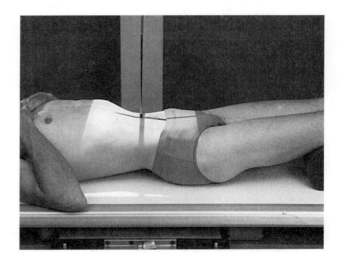

Fig. 18-7 Supine urogram, AP projection.

23. True or False. The AP projection may be obtained with the patient either supine or upright.

24. True or False. Preliminary (scout) radiographs are most often obtained with the patient supine.

25. True or False. Postinjection radiographs are most often obtained with the patient upright.

    False - post injection = supine

26. What is the most likely purpose for obtaining an AP projection radiograph with the patient standing?

    a. To elongate the ureters
    b. To demonstrate ureteral reflux
    c. To demonstrate air–fluid levels
    d. To demonstrate the mobility of the kidneys

27. What adjustment in the supine patient's position can be made to help demonstrate the distal ends of the ureters?

    a. Place supports under the patient's knees.
    b. Place a support under the patient's lumbar region.
    c. Tilt the table and patient 15 to 20 degrees toward the Trendelenburg position.
    d. Position a compression band around the patient's abdomen.

28. What should be done to reduce the lordotic curvature when performing the AP projection with the patient recumbent?

a. Place supports under the patient's knees.
b. Tilt the table and patient 10 to 15 degrees toward the Trendelenburg position.
c. Position a compression band around the patient's abdomen.

29. Which procedure should be performed if the bladder is not seen in the AP projection to demonstrate the entire urinary system?

a. Center the image receptor (IR) to the level of L3.
b. Direct the central ray 10 to 15 degrees cephalically.
c. Make a separate AP projection radiograph of the bladder.
d. Tilt the table and patient 10 to 15 degrees toward the Trendelenburg position.

30. Why is it desirable to include the area below the pubic symphysis for older male patients?

a. To demonstrate distal ureters
b. To demonstrate ureteral reflux
c. To demonstrate the prostate region
d. To demonstrate urinary bladder calculi

31. If a device is used for ureteral compression, to which level of the patient should it be centered?

a. L1-L3
b. At the level of the ASIS
c. 2 inches (5 cm) above the iliac crests
d. 1 inch (2.5 cm) above the superior border of the pubic symphysis

32. Identify each lettered structure shown in Fig. 18-8.

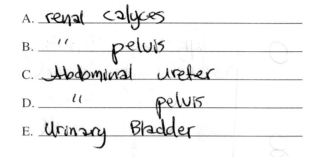

A. renal calyces
B. " pelvis
C. Abdominal ureter
D. " pelvis
E. Urinary Bladder

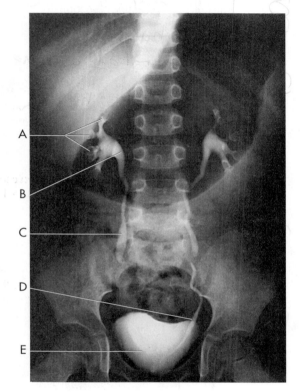

Fig. 18-8 AP projection of the urinary system.

Questions 33 through 38 pertain to *AP oblique projections*. Examine Fig. 18-9 as you answer the following questions.

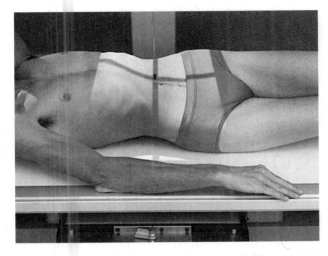

Fig. 18-9 Urogram, AP oblique projection (RPO position).

33. Into which position should the patient be placed when beginning to position for either type of AP oblique projection?

   a. Prone
   b. Supine
   c. Lateral recumbent

34. When performing the AP oblique projection, right posterior oblique (RPO) position, which kidney will be parallel with the plane of the IR?

   a. Left
   b. Right

35. Approximately how many degrees should the patient be rotated from the supine position to an oblique position to demonstrate renal and urinary structures?

   a. 10 degrees
   b. 20 degrees
   c. 30 degrees
   d. 40 degrees

36. Which structure should be centered to the grid for the AP oblique projection, left posterior oblique (LPO) position?

   a. Left kidney
   b. Right kidney
   c. Vertebral column

37. To which level of the patient should the IR be centered?

   a. L3
   b. Iliac crests
   c. Anterior superior iliac crests
   d. Pubic symphysis

38. Where should the central ray enter the patient?

   a. 2 inches lateral to the midline on the elevated side
   b. 2 inches lateral to the midline on the dependent side
   c. Centered to the midline 2 inches below the iliac crests

Items 39 through 43 pertain to the *lateral projection (lateral recumbent position)*. Examine Fig. 18-10 as you answer the following questions.

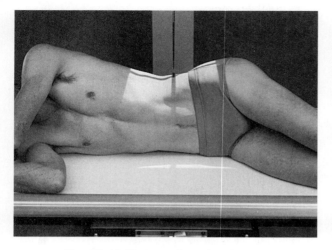

Fig. 18-10 Urogram, lateral projection.

39. Which plane of the body should be centered to the grid?

     MCP

40. Describe how the patient's arms and hands should be placed.

     Arms extended
     Elbows flexed
     Hands under head

41. Which areas of the patient should be examined to ensure that the patient is not rotated?

     Pelvis & Lumbar vertebrae

42. The exposure should be made at the end of

     expiraton (inspiration or expiration).

43. Exposure factors should produce a _____ (long or short) scale of contrast.

Items 44 through 50 pertain to the *lateral projection (dorsal decubitus position)*. Examine Fig. 18-11 as you answer the following questions.

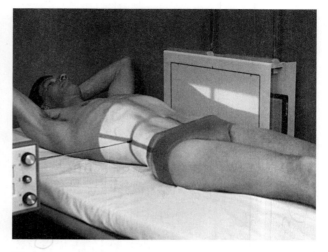

Fig. 18-11 Urogram, lateral projection (dorsal decubitus position).

44. The dorsal decubitus position requires that the patient be _____ (prone or (supine)).

45. The long axis of the IR should be centered to the _____*MCP*_____ plane.

46. Which area of the patient should be closest to the grid?
    a. Side
    b. Anterior
    c. Posterior

47. To which level of the patient should the IR be centered?
    a. L3
    b. Iliac crests
    c. Anterior superior iliac spines
    d. Pubic symphysis

48. (True) or False. Only male patients should have gonadal shielding for this type of projection.

49. True or False. The exposure should be made at the end of inspiration. On Expiration

50. True or False. The central ray should be directed horizontal and perpendicular to the center of the IR.

Exercise 2: Retrograde Urography

Retrograde urography is a radiographic procedure that demonstrates certain urinary structures. This exercise pertains to retrograde urography. Provide a short answer, select from a list, or choose true or false (explaining any statement you believe to be false) for each item.

Examine Fig. 18-12 as you answer the following questions about retrograde urography.

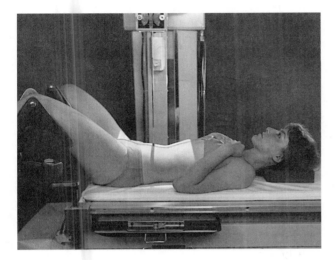

Fig. 18-12 Patient positioned on the table for retrograde urography.

1. True or False. Retrograde urography differs from excretory urography in that the contrast medium is injected directly into the kidney by means of a percutaneous injection through the skin.
   catheters thru, urethra, bladder ureters then kidneys

2. True or False. Retrograde urography is performed on a regular x-ray table. special tables used for R.U. exams

3. At the beginning of the retrograde urographic examination, the patient should be placed in the modified _____ position.

   a. Prone
   b. Upright
   c. Lithotomy
   d. Lateral recumbent

4. Which IR size should be used for urograms of the typical adult?

   a. 18 × 24 cm
   b. 24 × 30 cm
   c. 35 × 43 cm

5. Who should inject the contrast medium?

   a. Urologist
   b. Radiologist
   c. Radiographer

6. Describe how a kidney function test can be performed during retrograde urography.

   Urologist injects a color dye

7. List the three AP projection radiographs that usually comprise a retrograde urographic examination.

   1 scout
   2 pyelogram
   3. urogram

8. Why might the head of the x-ray table be lowered 10 to 15 degrees during the retrograde pyelography procedure?

   Renal Pelvis will be enhanced

9. Which retrograde urographic radiograph sometimes requires that the head of the table be elevated 35 to 40 degrees?

   a. Pyelogram
   b. Ureterogram
   c. Preliminary radiograph showing catheter insertion

10. After necessary AP projections are made, which oblique positions are often used for oblique projections?

   a. RPO and LPO
   b. RPO and LAO
   c. RAO and LPO
   d. RAO and LAO

Exercise 3: Retrograde Cystography

Projections obtained during retrograde cystography often include an AP projection, both AP oblique projections (RPO and LPO positions), and a lateral projection. This exercise pertains to those projections. Fill in missing words or provide a short answer for each item.

1. Describe how the contrast medium is introduced into the patient for retrograde cystography.

   catheter thru urethra Into kidneys

Questions 2 through 11 pertain to *AP axial or posteroanterior (PA) axial projections*. Examine Fig. 18-13 as you answer the following questions.

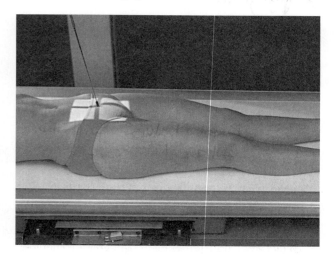

Fig. 18-13 AP axial bladder.

2. For the typical adult, which size IR should be used to demonstrate the bladder, and how should it be placed in the IR holder?

   a. 18 × 24 cm; crosswise
   b. 18 × 24 cm; lengthwise
   c. 24 × 30 cm; crosswise
   d. 24 × 30 cm; lengthwise

3. Which structures are sometimes better demonstrated with the head of the table lowered 15 to 20 degrees?

   a. Prostate gland and urethra
   b. Lower (distal) ends of the ureters
   c. Upper (proximal) ends of the ureters

4. Why should patients in the supine position extend the lower limbs?

   a. To demonstrate ureteral reflux
   b. To retard the excretion of opacified urine from the bladder
   c. To enable the lumbar lordotic curve to arch the pelvis enough to tilt the pubic bones inferiorly

5. Which breathing instructions should be given to the patient?

   a. Breathe slowly.
   b. Suspend breathing after expiration.
   c. Suspend breathing after inspiration.

6. To demonstrate the bladder during cystography, how many degrees and in which direction should the central ray be directed for the AP axial projection?

   a. 5 degrees caudal
   b. 5 degrees cephalic
   c. 10 to 15 degrees caudal
   d. 10 to 15 degrees cephalic

7. To which level of the patient should the central ray enter for the AP axial projection?

   a. The iliac crests
   b. 2 inches (5 cm) above the upper border of the pubic symphysis
   c. 2 inches (5 cm) below the upper border of the pubic symphysis

8. How should the patient be positioned to best demonstrate the prostate?

   a. Prone
   b. Supine
   c. Upright
   d. Lateral recumbent

9. How should the central ray be directed to best demonstrate the prostate?

   a. Caudally
   b. Cephalically
   c. Perpendicularly

10. If minor reflux is present at the bladder, what other structures most likely will be demonstrated?

    a. Both kidneys
    b. Distal ureters
    c. Prostate gland

11. How should the pubic bones be demonstrated in the image of the AP axial projection?

   a. They should superimpose both the bladder neck and the proximal urethra.

   b. They should be projected above both the bladder neck and the proximal urethra.

   c. They should be projected below both the bladder neck and the proximal urethra.

Items 12 through 16 pertain to *AP oblique projections.* Examine Fig. 18-14 as you answer the following questions.

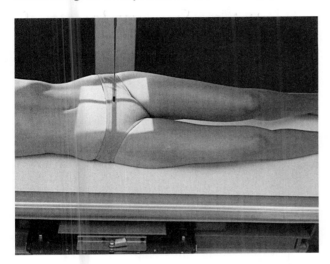

Fig. 18-14 Retrograde cystogram, AP oblique projection (RPO position).

12. In which position should the patient be placed?

   a. Semiprone

   b. Semisupine

   c. Lateral recumbent

13. How should the patient's uppermost thigh be positioned to prevent it from superimposing the bladder in AP oblique projections?

   a. Crossed over the other thigh

   b. Flexed and placed at right angles to the abdomen

   c. Extended and abducted enough to prevent its superimposition on the bladder area

14. How many degrees should the patient be rotated for AP oblique projections?

   a. 10 to 15

   b. 20 to 30

   c. 40 to 60

15. From the following list, circle the two ways that the central ray can be directed for AP oblique projections.

   a. Perpendicularly

   b. 10 degrees caudally

   c. 10 degrees cephalically

   d. 20 degrees caudally

   e. 20 degrees cephalically

16. With reference to the pubic bones, where should the bladder neck be seen in the AP oblique projection radiograph, RPO position?

   a. Above

   b. Below

   c. To the left side

   d. To the right side

Questions 17 through 20 pertain to the *lateral projection.* Examine Fig. 18-15 as you answer the following questions.

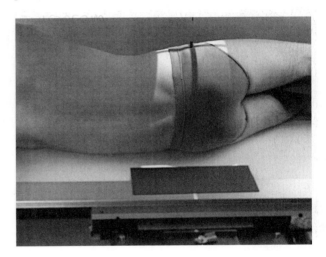

Fig. 18-15 Cystogram, lateral projection.

17. Which body position should be used for the lateral projection for cystography?

   a. Upright lateral

   b. Lateral recumbent

   c. Ventral decubitus (prone)

   d. Dorsal decubitus (supine)

18. Where should the IR be centered for the lateral projection?

   a. At the level of the iliac crests

   b. At the level of the pubic symphysis

   c. 2 inches (5 cm) above the iliac crests

   d. 2 inches (5 cm) above the pubic symphysis

19. How should the central ray be directed?

    a. Horizontally
    (b.) Perpendicularly
    c. Angled caudally
    d. Angled cephalically

20. Which imaged structures can determine whether the patient was rotated from the lateral position?

    a. Lumbar vertebrae
    b. Crests of the ilia
    (c.) Hips and femora

Exercise 4: Male Cystourethrography

This exercise pertains to male cystourethrography. Provide a short answer, select from a list, or choose true or false (explaining any statement you believe to be false) for each item. Examine Fig. 18-16 *as you answer the following questions.*

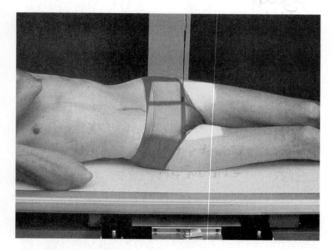

Fig. 18-16 Cystourethrogram, AP oblique projection (RPO position).

1. Define *cystourethrography.*

    exam. of bladder post contrast injextion

2. Describe how the contrast medium is introduced into the urinary structures of interest.

    catheter from uretal canal thru to ~~kidneys~~ bladder,

3. After the contrast medium is introduced into the patient, in which two positions can the patient be placed to demonstrate urinary structures?

    a. RAO and LAO
    b. RAO and LPO
    c. RPO and LAO
    (d.) PO and LPO

4. How many degrees should the patient be rotated for the desired oblique projection?

    a. 15 to 20 degrees
    b. 25 to 30 degrees
    (c.) 35 to 40 degrees

5. To which level of the patient should the IR be centered?

    a. Crests of the ilia
    b. Anterior superior iliac spines
    c. 2 inches (5 cm) above the superior border of the pubic symphysis
    (d.) Superior border of the pubic symphysis

6. True or False. To ensure adequate coverage, the IR should be placed lengthwise.

7. True or False. To ensure that the entire urethra is filled, the exposure should be made while the physician is injecting the contrast medium.

8. True or False. After the bladder is filled with contrast medium, the voiding film can be exposed with the patient in either a posterior oblique or an upright position.

9. True or False. The radiation field should be large enough to include the entire urinary system on all radiographs. *bladder & urethra in full view.*

10. Identify each lettered structure shown in Fig. 18-17.

A. *bladder*

B. *prostatic urethra*

C. *membranous urethra*

D. *spongy (cavernous) urethra*

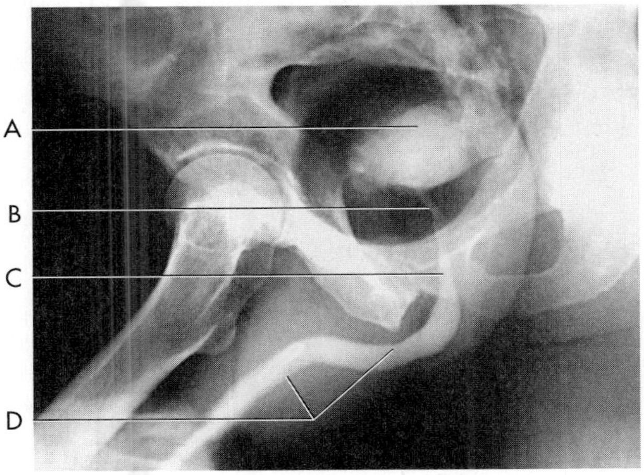

Fig. 18-17 Cystourethrogram, AP oblique projection (RPO position).

Exercise 5: Identifying Urinary System Radiographs

Identify each of the following radiographs by selecting the best choice from the list provided for each image.

1. Fig. 18-18:
   a. Excretory urogram, AP projection
   b. Retrograde urogram, AP projection
   c. Excretory cystogram, AP projection
   d. Preliminary (scout) radiograph, AP projection

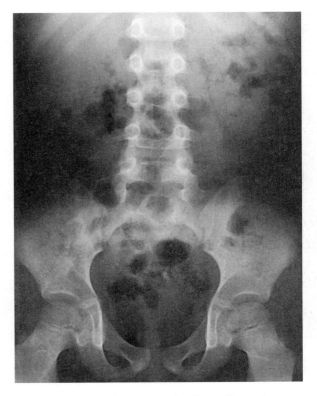

Fig. 18-18 Urinary examination radiograph.

2. Fig. 18-19:

    (a.) Excretory urogram, AP projection
    b. Retrograde urogram, AP projection
    c. Excretory cystogram, AP projection
    d. Preliminary (scout) radiograph, AP projection

3. Fig. 18-20:

    a. Excretory urogram, AP projection
    (b.) Retrograde urogram, AP projection
    c. Excretory cystogram, AP projection
    d. Preliminary (scout) radiograph, AP projection

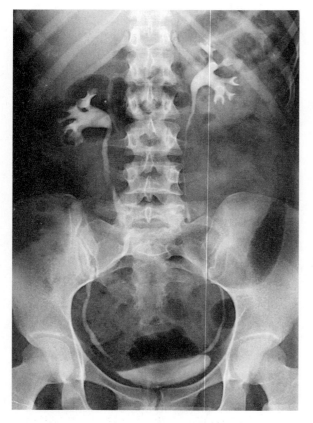

Fig. 18-19 Urinary examination radiograph.

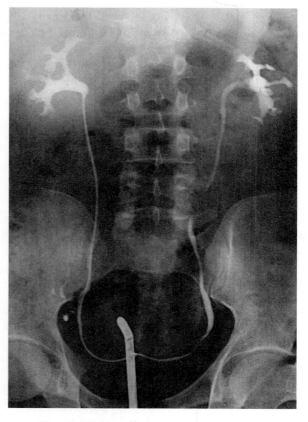

Fig. 18-20 Urinary examination radiograph.

4. Fig. 18-21:

    a. Excretory urogram, AP oblique projection, LPO position

    b. Excretory urogram, AP oblique projection, RPO position

    c. Retrograde cystogram, AP oblique projection, LPO position

    d. Retrograde cystogram, AP oblique projection, RPO position

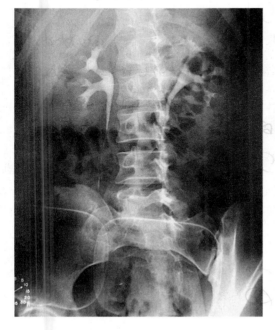

Fig. 18-21 Urinary examination radiograph.

5. Fig. 18-22:

    a. Urogram, lateral projection

    b. Urogram, left lateral decubitus

    c. Excretory urogram, AP oblique projection, RPO position

    d. Excretory urogram, AP oblique projection, LPO position

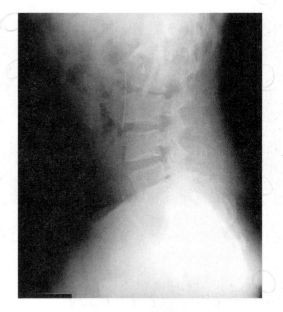

Fig. 18-22 Urinary examination radiograph.

6. Fig. 18-23:

    a. Prevoiding filled bladder, AP projection

    b. Postvoiding emptied bladder, AP projection

    c. Retrograde cystogram, AP oblique projection, RPO position

    d. Injection cystourethrogram, AP oblique projection, RPO position

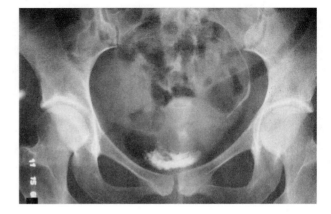

Fig. 18-23 Urinary examination radiograph.

7. Fig. 18-24:
   a. Prevoiding filled bladder, AP projection
   b. Postvoiding emptied bladder, AP projection
   c. Retrograde cystogram, AP oblique projection, RPO position
   d. Injection cystourethrogram, AP oblique projection, RPO position

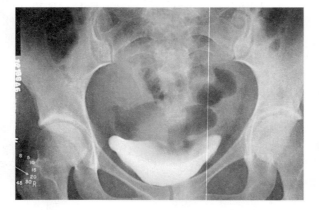

Fig. 18-24 Urinary examination radiograph.

8. Fig. 18-25:
   a. Excretory cystogram, AP projection
   b. Retrograde cystogram, AP projection
   c. Postvoiding emptied bladder, AP projection
   d. Retrograde cystogram, AP oblique projection, RPO position

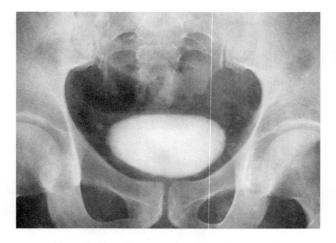

Fig. 18-25 Urinary examination radiograph.

9. Fig. 18-26:
   a. Excretory cystogram, AP projection
   b. Retrograde cystogram, AP projection
   c. Postvoiding emptied bladder, AP projection
   d. Retrograde cystogram, AP oblique projection, RPO position

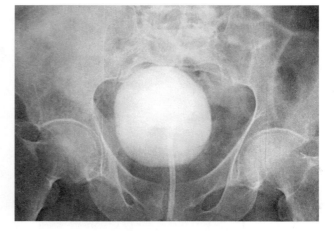

Fig. 18-26 Urinary examination radiograph.

10. Fig. 18-27:
    a. Excretory cystogram, AP projection
    b. Retrograde cystogram, AP projection
    c. Postvoiding emptied bladder, AP projection
    d. Retrograde cystogram, AP oblique projection, RPO position

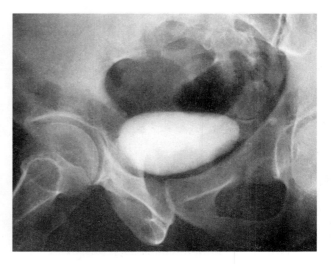

Fig. 18-27 Urinary examination radiograph.

SELF-TEST: ANATOMY AND POSITIONING OF THE URINARY SYSTEM

Answer the following questions by selecting the best choice.

1. Which renal structure filters the blood?
   a. Glomerulus
   b. Major calyx
   c. Efferent arteriole
   d. Afferent arteriole

2. Which urinary excretory duct conveys urine from the bladder to outside the body?
   a. Ureter
   b. Urethra
   c. Efferent arteriole
   d. Afferent arteriole

3. Which body organ filters blood and produces urine as a by-product of waste material?
   a. Liver
   b. Spleen
   c. Kidney
   d. Pancreas

4. At which vertebral level is the superior border of the kidneys usually found?
   a. T10
   b. T12
   c. L2
   d. L4

5. What is the name of the opening on the medial border of a kidney?
   a. Pole
   b. Base
   c. Apex
   d. Hilum

6. Which of the following is an excretory examination used to demonstrate the upper urinary tract?
   a. Cystourethrography
   b. Retrograde urography
   c. Intravenous urography
   d. Retrograde cystography

7. Which examination has the ability to produce a radiographic image demonstrating renal cortical tissue well saturated with contrast medium?
   a. Cystourethrography
   b. Retrograde urography
   c. Intravenous urography
   d. Retrograde cystography

8. Which projection best demonstrates the mobility of the kidneys?
   a. AP projection with the patient supine
   b. AP projection with the patient upright
   c. Lateral projection with the patient lateral recumbent
   d. Lateral projection with the patient in dorsal decubitus position

9. In intravenous urography, what is the purpose of applying compression pads over the distal ends of both ureters?
   a. To demonstrate ureteral reflux
   b. To demonstrate the mobility of the kidneys
   c. To retard the flow of opacified urine into the bladder
   d. To retard the flow of opacified urine from the bladder

10. Which of the following is not a reason for obtaining a scout radiograph with the patient recumbent for excretory urography?
   a. To evaluate exposure factors
   b. To demonstrate urinary calculi
   c. To determine the location of the kidneys
   d. To demonstrate the mobility of the kidneys

11. For excretory urography, what should an adult patient do just before getting on the examination table?
   a. Empty the bladder.
   b. Remove all jewelry.
   c. Drink 12 ounces of cold water.
   d. Drink 12 ounces of carbonated beverage.

12. What is the purpose of obtaining an AP projection radiograph of the kidneys 30 seconds after the bolus injection of a contrast medium in excretory urography?
   a. To demonstrate ureteral reflux
   b. To demonstrate opacified renal cortex
   c. To demonstrate opacified renal arteries
   d. To demonstrate the mobility of the kidneys

13. What is the purpose of tilting the patient and table 15 to 20 degrees toward the Trendelenburg position for the AP projection during excretory urography?
   a. To demonstrate distal ureters
   b. To demonstrate opacified renal cortex
   c. To demonstrate the base of the bladder
   d. To demonstrate the mobility of the kidneys

14. How many degrees should the patient be rotated for AP oblique projections, posterior oblique positions, during excretory urography?
   a. 15
   b. 30
   c. 45
   d. 60

15. For intravenous urography of a child, what should the patient be given when the scout radiograph shows an excessive amount of intestinal gas overlying the kidneys?

    a. A laxative
    b. A cleansing enema
    c. 12 ounces of iced water
    d. 12 ounces of carbonated beverage

16. Which examination requires that the patient be placed on a special urographic–radiographic examination table?

    a. Cystourethrography
    b. Retrograde urography
    c. Intravenous urography
    d. Retrograde cystography

17. Which renal structures are not demonstrated during retrograde urographic examinations?

    a. Ureters
    b. Nephrons
    c. Minor calyces
    d. Major calyces

18. In addition to the AP projection, which projection would most likely be included in the radiographs for retrograde urography?

    a. PA projection
    b. PA oblique projection
    c. AP oblique projection
    d. AP projection, lateral decubitus position

19. What is the purpose of tilting the table 10 to 15 degrees toward the Trendelenburg position for retrograde urography?

    a. To demonstrate the ureters
    b. To demonstrate the mobility of the kidneys
    c. To produce a nephrogram effect in the kidneys
    d. To prevent contrast medium from escaping the kidneys

20. What is the purpose of raising the head of the table 35 to 40 degrees for retrograde urography?

    a. To demonstrate the ureters
    b. To position the patient for catheterization
    c. To produce a nephrogram effect in the kidneys
    d. To prevent contrast medium from escaping the kidneys

21. Which condition would most likely be demonstrated during voiding cystography?

    a. Renal cyst
    b. Renal calculi
    c. Ureteral reflux
    d. Hydronephrosis

22. For the AP axial projection of the bladder, how many degrees and in which direction should the central ray be directed?

    a. 15 degrees caudal
    b. 15 degrees cephalic
    c. 25 degrees caudal
    d. 25 degrees cephalic

23. For retrograde cystography, which projection should be performed to demonstrate the anterior and posterior walls of the bladder?

    a. Upright AP projection
    b. Recumbent AP projection
    c. Direct lateral projection
    d. AP projection, lateral decubitus position

24. For cystourethrography with an adult male patient, to which level of the patient should the IR be centered?

    a. T12 vertebra
    b. L3 vertebra
    c. L5 vertebra
    d. Pubic symphysis

25. For cystourethrography with an adult male patient, which of the following should be used to obtain a radiograph while the patient is urinating?

    a. Recumbent PA projection
    b. Dorsal decubitus position
    c. Lateral decubitus position
    d. Recumbent AP oblique projection

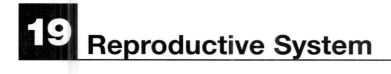

Reproductive System

SECTION 1

ANATOMY OF THE REPRODUCTIVE SYSTEM

Exercise 1

This exercise pertains to the anatomy of the female reproductive system. Identify structures, fill in missing words, provide a short answer, or match columns for each item.

1. Identify each lettered structure shown in Fig. 19-1.

A. _fundus_

B. _round ligament_

C. _ovarian ligament_

D. _uterine tube_

E. _ovary_

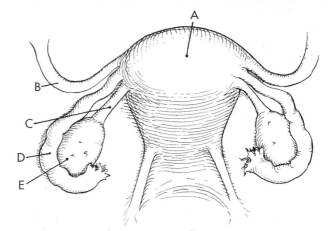

Fig. 19-1 Superoposterior view of the uterus, ovaries, and uterine tubes.

2. Identify each lettered structure shown in Fig. 19-2.

A. _____   G. _____

B. _____   H. _____

C. _____   I. _____

D. _____   J. _____

E. _____   K. _____

F. _____   L. _____

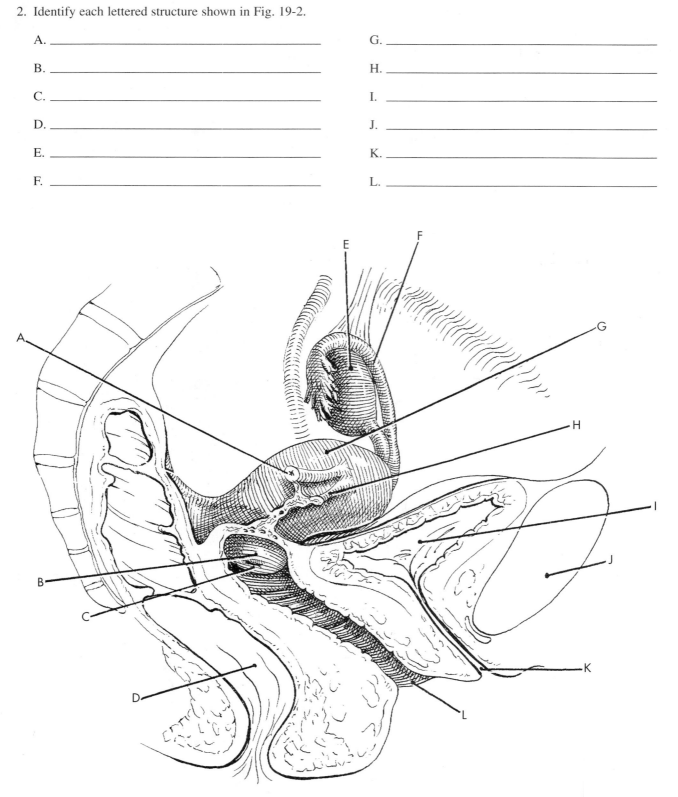

Fig. 19-2 Sagittal section showing the relation of the internal genitalia to the surrounding structures.

3. The female gonads are called the _____.

4. Female reproductive cells are called _____.

5. The structure that conveys an ovum from a gonad to the uterus is the _____ tube.

6. The number of uterine tubes in the typical adult female is _____.

7. The pear-shaped muscular organ of the female reproductive system is the _____.

8. Name the four main parts of the uterus.

9. What part of the uterus is referred to as the neck?

10. Match the uterine structures in Column A with the definitions in Column B.

Column A

____ 1. Body

____ 2. Fundus

____ 3. Cervix

____ 4. Isthmus

____ 5. Endometrium

Column B

a. Superiormost portion

b. Cylindrical vaginal end

c. Mucosal lining of the uterine cavity

d. Constricted area adjacent to the vaginal end

e. Where ligaments attach the uterus within the pelvis

Exercise 2

This exercise pertains to the anatomy of the male reproductive system. Identify structures or fill in missing words for each item.

1. Identify each lettered structure shown in Fig. 19-3.

A. _____

B. _____

C. _____

D. _____

E. _____

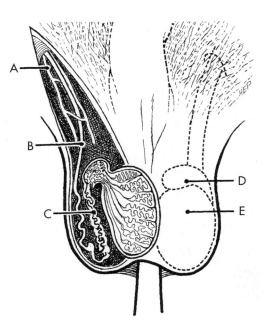

Fig. 19-3 Frontal section of the testes and ductus deferens.

2. Identify each lettered structure in Fig. 19-4.

A. _____

B. _____

C. _____

D. _____

E. _____

F. _____

G. _____

3. Identify each lettered structure shown in Fig. 19-5.

A. _____

B. _____

C. _____

D. _____

E. _____

F. _____

G. _____

H. _____

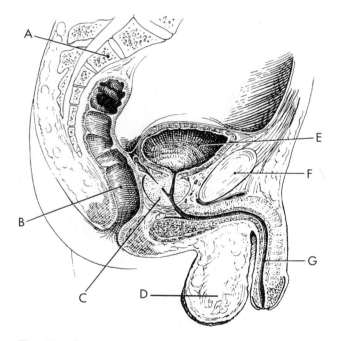

Fig. 19-4 Sagittal section showing the male genital system.

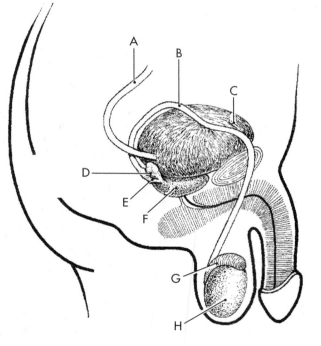

Fig. 19-5 Sagittal section through the male pelvis.

4. The male gonads are called the _____.

5. Male reproductive cells are called _____.

6. The oblong structure attached to each testicle is the

   _____.

7. The excretory channel that allows male germ cells to pass from a gonad to the urethra is the

   _____.

8. The union of the ductus deferens and the seminal

   vesicle duct forms the _____ duct.

9. The accessory genital organ that is composed of muscular and glandular tissues is the

   _____.

10. The ducts from the prostate open into the proximal

    portion of the _____.

RADIOGRAPHY OF THE REPRODUCTIVE SYSTEM

Exercise 1: Radiography of the Female Reproductive System

Although other imaging modalities have reduced the demand for radiographic examinations of the female reproductive system, some facilities still radiographically demonstrate female reproductive structures. This exercise pertains to radiographic visualization of the female reproductive system. Match columns of relevant information or select the correct answer from a list for each item.

1. Match each radiographic examination from Column A with the type of patient from Column B who is most likely to undergo that type of examination.

Column A	Column B
____ 1. Fetography	a. Pregnant patient
____ 2. Pelvimetry	b. Nongravid patient
____ 3. Vaginography	
____ 4. Placentography	
____ 5. Pelvic pneumography	
____ 6. Hysterosalpingography	

2. Match the descriptions in Column A with the corresponding type of examination in Column B. Some descriptions may have more than one examination associated with them. Examinations will be used more than once.

Column A

_____ 1. Determines pelvic diameters

_____ 2. Uses a Colcher-Sussman ruler

_____ 3. Helps determine placenta previa

_____ 4. Requires a gaseous contrast agent

_____ 5. Requires the use of a contrast agent

_____ 6. Requires a radiopaque contrast agent

_____ 7. Investigates the patency of uterine tubes

_____ 8. Largely replaced by diagnostic ultrasound

_____ 9. Performed to demonstrate a fetus in utero

_____ 10. Introduces a contrast agent into the vaginal canal

_____ 11. Introduces a contrast agent through a uterine cannula

_____ 12. Introduces a contrast agent directly into the peritoneal cavity

_____ 13. Should be performed about 10 days after the onset of menstruation

_____ 14. Performed to determine the size, shape, and position of the uterus and uterine tubes

_____ 15. Performed to demonstrate congenital abnormalities of the muscular structure that extends from the cervix to the external genitalia

Column B

a. Fetography

b. Pelvimetry

c. Vaginography

d. Placentography

e. Pelvic pneumography

f. Hysterosalpingography

3. Figs. 19-6 through 19-10 are representative examinations of the female reproductive system. Examine the images, then select the best answer from the list provided for each image.

i. Fig. 19-6:
   a. Pelvimetry
   b. Vaginography
   c. Pelvic pneumography
   d. Hysterosalpingography

Uterine tube

Normal contrast "spill" into peritoneal cavity

Body of uterus

Speculum

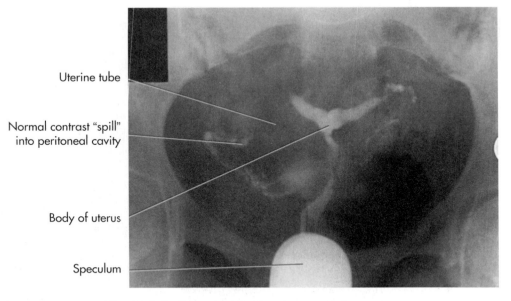
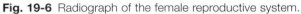

Fig. 19-6 Radiograph of the female reproductive system.

ii. Fig. 19-7:
   a. Fetography
   b. Vaginography
   c. Pelvic pneumography
   d. Hysterosalpingography

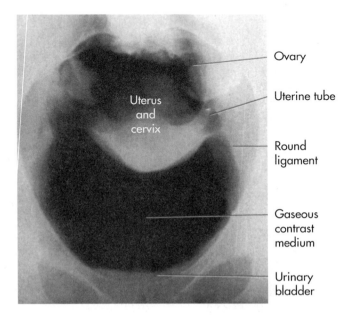

Ovary

Uterine tube

Round ligament

Uterus and cervix

Gaseous contrast medium

Urinary bladder

Fig. 19-7 Radiograph of the female reproductive system.

iii. Fig. 19-8:
    a. Pelvimetry
    b. Vaginography
    c. Pelvic pneumography
    d. Hysterosalpingography

iv. Fig. 19-9:
    a. Pelvimetry
    b. Fetography
    c. Placentography
    d. Hysterosalpingography

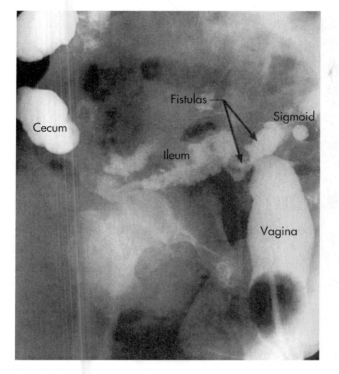

Fig. 19-8 Radiograph of the female reproductive system.

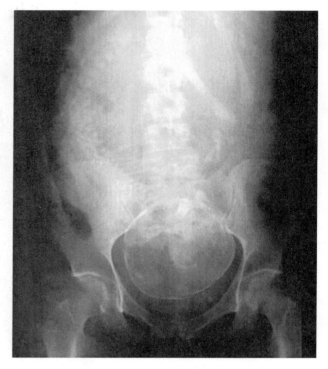

Fig. 19-9 Radiograph of the female reproductive system.

v. Fig. 19-10:
  a. Pelvimetry
  b. Fetography
  c. Placentography
  d. Pelvic pneumography

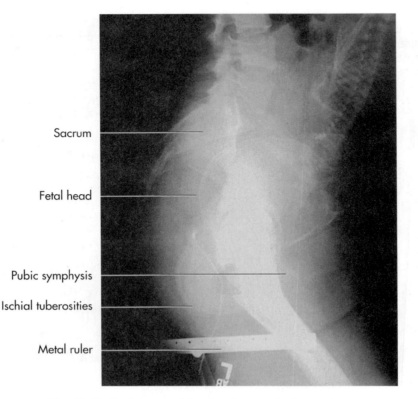

Fetal head

Sacrum

Pubic symphysis

Ischial tuberosities

Metal ruler

Fig. 19-10 Radiograph of the female reproductive system.

Exercise 2: Radiography of the Male Reproductive System

Although the demand for radiographic visualization of the male reproductive system has greatly decreased in recent years because of advances with diagnostic ultrasound, some facilities still radiographically demonstrate male reproductive structures. This exercise pertains to radiographic visualization of the male reproductive system. Provide a short answer for each question.

1. What type of contrast medium is used for radiographic examination of the seminal ducts?

   _____

2. Why might a radiolucent contrast medium be injected into the scrotum for epididymography?

3. What accessory organ of the male reproductive system can be radiographically examined?

   _____

4. Where is the image receptor centered for radiographic images of the male reproductive system?

5. Today, the prostate is primarily imaged via

   _____.

SELF-TEST: REPRODUCTIVE SYSTEM

Answer the following questions by selecting the best choice.

1. Which structures are parts of the female reproductive system?

   a. Ovaries, uterus, and fallopian tubes
   b. Ovaries, testes, and ductus deferens
   c. Epididymis, uterus, and fallopian tubes
   d. Epididymis, testes, and ductus deferens

2. Which part of the uterus is most superior?

   a. Body
   b. Cervix
   c. Fundus
   d. Isthmus

3. Which structure conveys female reproductive cells from a gonad to the uterus?

   a. Urethra
   b. Uterine tube
   c. Ductus deferens
   d. Ejaculatory duct

4. Which structure produces female reproductive cells?

   a. Ovary
   b. Uterus
   c. Testicle
   d. Epididymis

5. Which structure produces spermatozoa?

   a. Ovary
   b. Testicle
   c. Prostate
   d. Epididymis

6. Which structure conveys male reproductive cells from a gonad to the urethra?

   a. Uterine tube
   b. Fallopian tube
   c. Ductus deferens
   d. Ejaculatory duct

7. Which structure is attached to each male gonad?

   a. Urethra
   b. Prostate
   c. Epididymis
   d. Ejaculatory duct

8. Which examination can be performed on a pregnant patient?

   a. Fetography
   b. Prostatography
   c. Pelvic pneumography
   d. Hysterosalpingography

9. Which examination can be performed on a nongravid patient?

   a. Fetography
   b. Pelvimetry
   c. Placentography
   d. Hysterosalpingography

10. Which examination introduces contrast medium through a uterine cannula?

    a. Fetography
    b. Pelvimetry
    c. Vaginography
    d. Hysterosalpingography

11. Which examination is performed to verify the patency of uterine tubes?

    a. Fetography
    b. Pelvimetry
    c. Placentography
    d. Hysterosalpingography

12. Which examination determines pelvic diameters?

    a. Fetography
    b. Pelvimetry
    c. Placentography
    d. Hysterosalpingography

13. Which type of contrast medium is preferred for hysterosalpingography?

    a. Oily viscous
    b. Water-soluble
    c. Barium sulfate

14. When should a hysterosalpingographic examination be performed?

    a. After the first trimester
    b. During the first trimester
    c. 10 days after the onset of menstruation
    d. 10 days before the onset of menstruation

15. Which of the following conditions can be investigated by radiographic imaging of the male reproductive system?

    1. Inflammation
    2. Tumors
    3. Sterility
    a. 1 and 2 only
    b. 1 and 3 only
    c. 2 and 3 only
    d. 1, 2, and 3

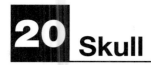

Skull

OSTEOLOGY OF THE SKULL

Exercise 1

This exercise pertains to the osteology of the skull. Identify structures for each illustration.

1. Identify each lettered structure shown in Fig. 20-1.

A. Parietal Bone

B. Glabella

C. greater wring of the sphenoid

D. nasal bone

E. temporal bone

F. zygomatic bone

G. perpendicular plate of the ethmoid

H. vomer

I. maxilla

J. frontal bone

K. sphenoid bone

L. lacrimal bone

M. ethmoid bone

N. middle nasal concha

O. infraorbital foramen

P. inferior nasal concha

Q. anterior nasal spine

R. mandible

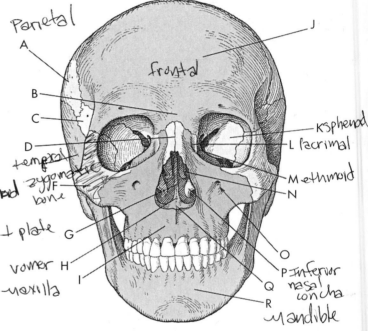

Fig. 20-1 Anterior aspect of the skull.

2. Identify each lettered structure shown in Fig. 20-2.

A. frontal bone

B. spenoid "

C. glabella

D. nasal bone

E. lacrimal "

F. ethmoid "

G. Anterior nasal spine (acanthion)

H. Zygomatic bone (zygoma)

I. temporal process

J. maxilla

K. mental foramen

L. mandible

M. bregma   (fontanel)

N. coronal   (suture)

O. parietal bone

P. squamosal   (suture)

Q. lamba   (fontanel)

R. lambdoidal   (suture)

S. occipatal bone

T. (inion) external occipatal protuberance

U. mastoid process

V. temporal bone

W. external accoustic meatus

X. styloid process

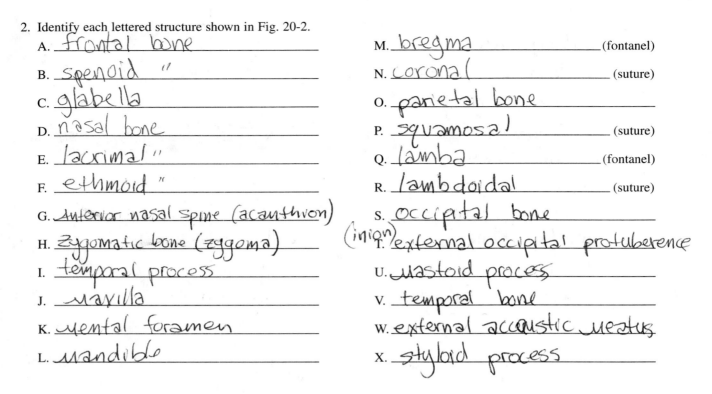

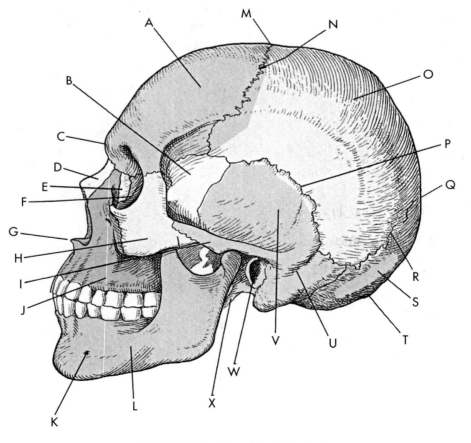

Fig. 20-2 Lateral aspect of the skull.

3. Identify each lettered structure shown in Fig. 20-3.

A. orbital plate
B. lesser wing
C. greater wing
D. optic groove
E. foramen ovale
F. foramen spinosum
G. temporal bone
H. petrous portion
I. clivous
J. occiptal bone
K. cristi gali

L. cribiform plate
M. optic canal and foramen
N. tuberculem sellae
O. anterior ctenoid process
P. sella turcica
Q. dorsum sellae
R. foramen lacerum
S. dorsum sellae
T. jugular foramen
U. hypoglossal canal
V. foramen magnum

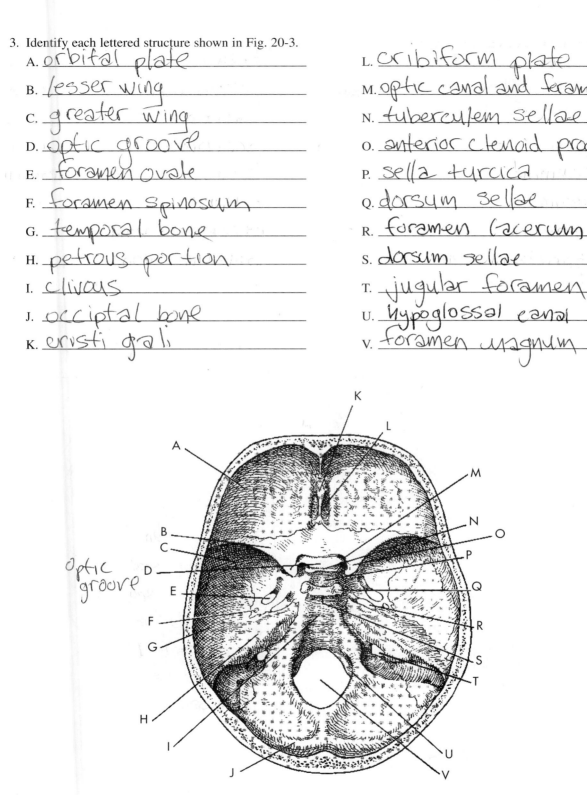

optic groove

Fig. 20-3 Superior aspect of the cranial base.

4. Identify each lettered structure shown in Fig. 20-4.

A. frontal bone
B. frontal sinus
C. cristi galli
D. nasal bone
E. ethmoid
F. vomer
G. maxilla
H. parietal bone

I. sphenoidal sinus
J. petrous portion
K. internal acoustic meatus
L. occipital bone
M. squamous portion of the temporal bone
N. clivus
O. pterygoid hamulus
P. palatine bone

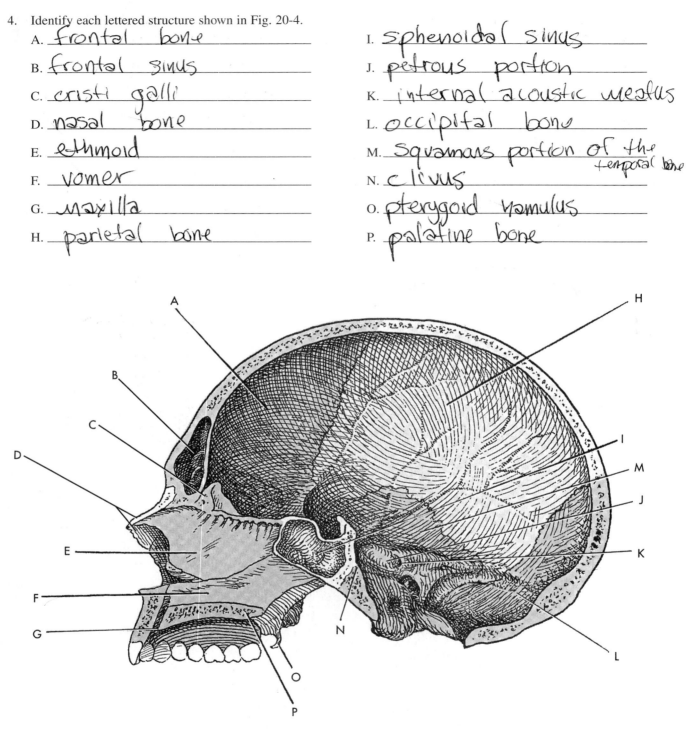

Fig. 20-4 Lateral aspect of the interior of the cranium.

5. Identify each lettered structure shown in Fig. 20-5.

A. Frontal squama

B. supraorbital foramen

C. supraorbital margin

D. glabella

E. nasal spine

F. supercilliary arch

G. frontal eminence

6. Identify each lettered structure shown in Fig. 20-6.

A. superior nasal concha

B. middle nasal concha

C. perpendicular plate

D. cristi galli

E. ethmoidal sinus

F. air cells in labyrinth

G. cribiform plate

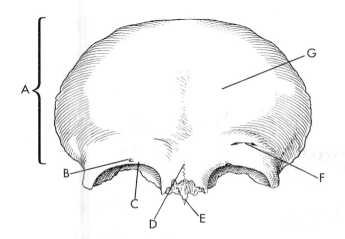

Fig. 20-5 Anterior aspect of the frontal bone.

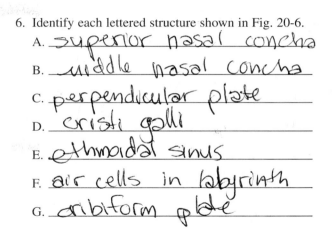

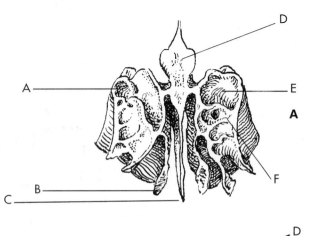

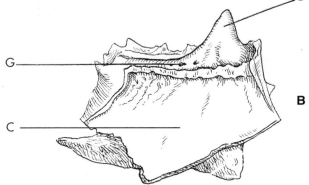

Fig. 20-6 Two illustrations of the ethmoid bone. **A,** The anterior aspect. **B,** The lateral aspect with the labyrinth removed.

7. Identify the four angles and the four articulating borders of the left parietal bone shown in Fig. 20-7.

A. Articulates with the _parietal_ bone

B. _occipital_ angle

C. Articulates with the _frontal_ bone

D. _mastoid_ angle

E. _frontal_ angle

F. Articulates with the _occipital_ bone

G. _sphenoid_ angle

H. Articulates with the _temporal_ bone

8. Identify each lettered structure shown in Fig. 20-8.

A. _Anterior Clinoid process_

B. _Posterior clinoid process_

C. _dorsum sellae_

D. _lateral pterygoid lamina_

E. _optic canal and foramen_

E. _↓ pterygoid hamulus_

G. _lesser wing_

H. _superior orbital fissure_

I. _greater wing_

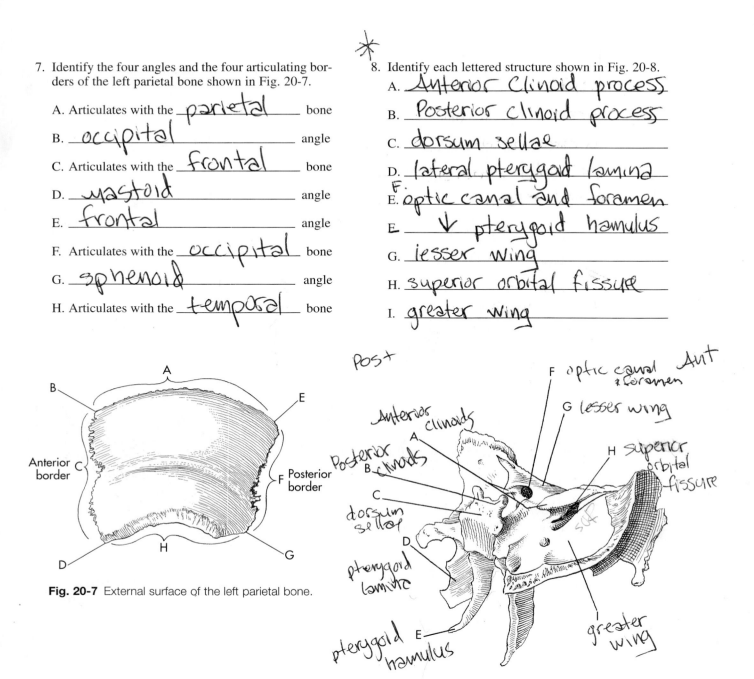

Fig. 20-7 External surface of the left parietal bone.

Fig. 20-8 Oblique view of the upper and lateroposterior aspects of the sphenoid bone.

9. Identify each lettered structure shown in Fig. 20-9.

A. _squama_

B. _foramen magnum_

C. _basilar portion_

D. _occipital condyle_

E. _EOP (Inion)_

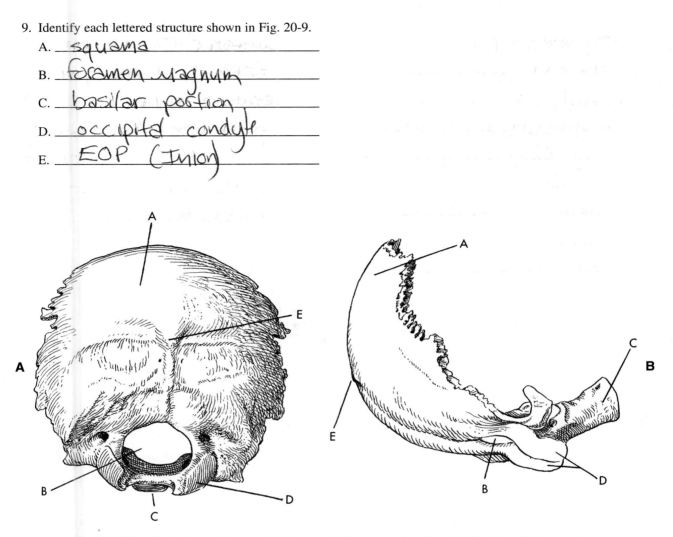

Fig. 20-9 Two illustrations of the occipital bone. **A,** The external surface. **B,** The lateroinferior surface.

10. Identify each lettered structure shown in Fig. 20-10.

A. Squamos portion
B. Mastoid portion
C. EAM
D. tympatic portion
E. Styloid process

F. Mandibular fossa
G. articular tubercle
H. zygomatic process
I. petrous portion

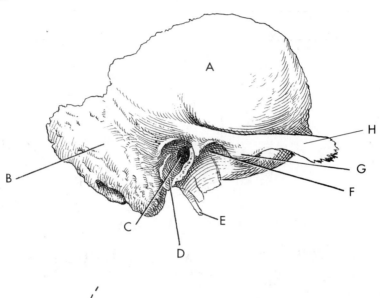

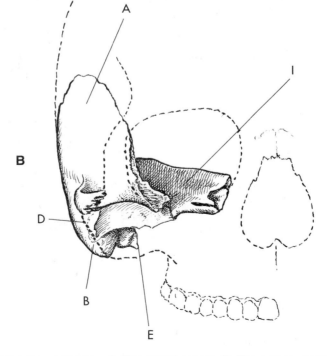

Fig. 20-10 Two illustrations of the temporal bone. **A,** The lateral aspect. **B,** The anterior aspect in relation to the surrounding structures.

11. Identify each lettered structure shown in Fig. 20-11.

A. External acoustic meatus

B. cartilage

C. tympanic portion membrane

D. auditory ossicles

E. semi-circular canals

F. stapes

G. internal acoustic meatus

H. cochlear nerve

I. cochlea

J. round window

K. auditory tube

L. nasopharynx

M. EAM

N. auditory tube

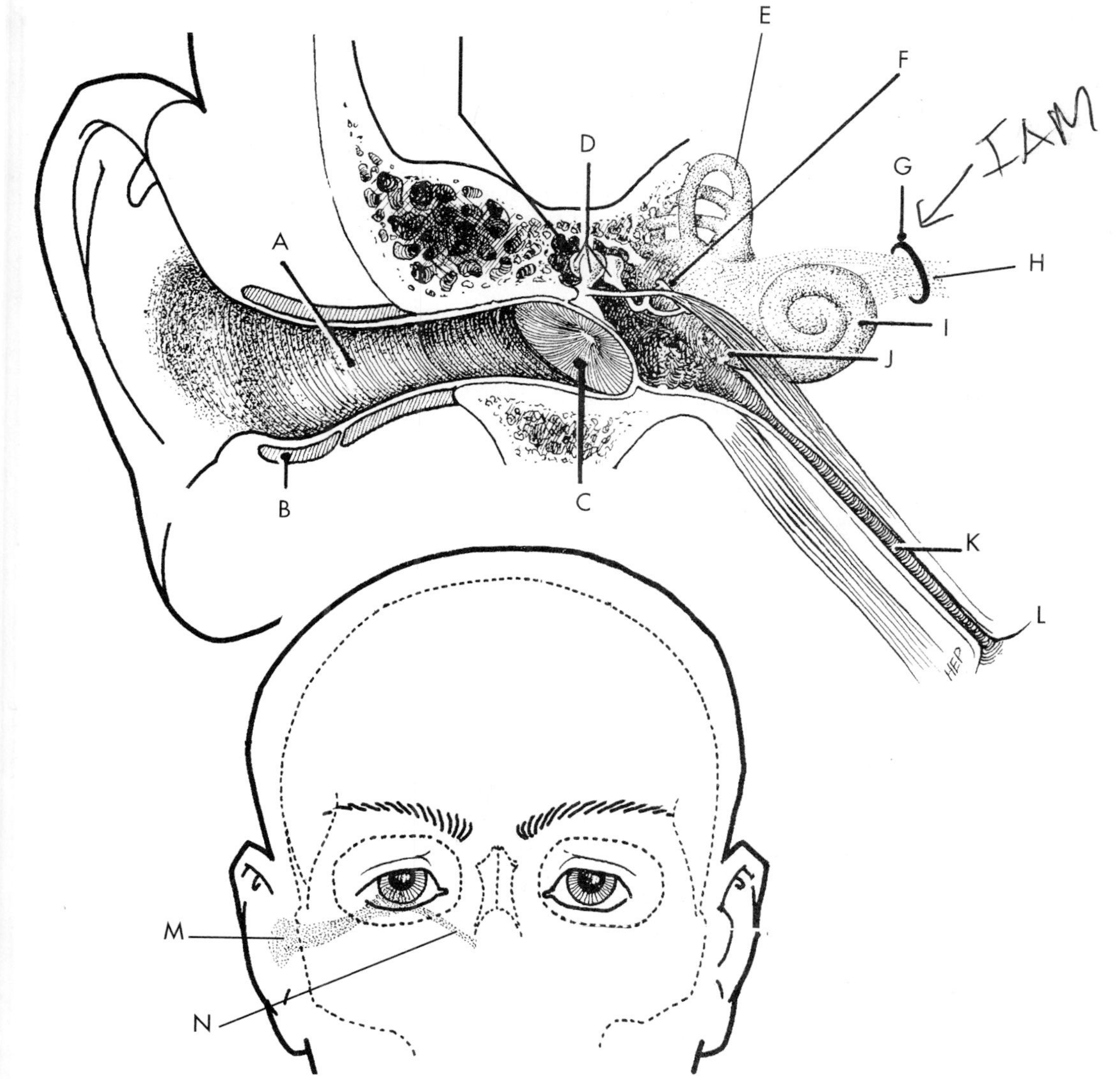

Fig. 20-11 Frontal section through the right ear showing the internal structures.

12. Identify each lettered structure shown in Fig. 20-12.

A. neck

B. condyle

C. alveolar portion

D. mental foramen

E. symphysis

F. coronoid process

G. ramus

H. body

I. mental protuberance

J. X

K. gonion

13. Identify each lettered structure shown in Fig. 20-13.

A. ~~symphysis~~ body

B. greater cornu

C. ~~coronoid process~~

lesser cornu

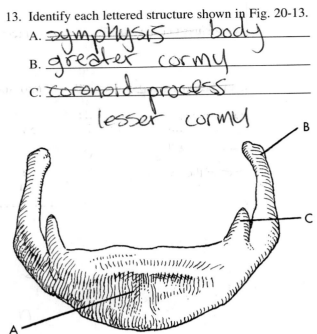

Fig. 20-13 Anterior aspect of the hyoid.

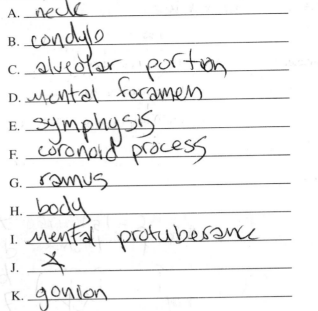

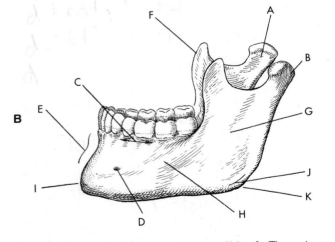

Fig. 20-12 Two illustrations of the mandible. **A,** The anterior aspect. **B,** The lateral aspect.

Exercise 2

Use the following clues to complete the crossword puzzle. All answers refer to the skull.

Across

1. Perpendicular _____
4. Midpoint of the frontonasal suturez
5. This bone has wings
7. Vertical part of the frontal bone
8. _____ galli
9. Number of cranial bones
12. Densest part of the cranial floor
13. Articulates frontal bone with parietals

16. Fibrous cranial joint
19. Anterior fontanel
20. Posterior fontanel
21. Forms top of the cranium
22. Posterior part of the skull
23. Eyebrow arches

Down

1. Inferior sphenoidal process
2. Sphenoidal endocrine
3. _____ turcica

5. Lateral suture
6. Long and narrow skull
10. Average skull
11. Smooth frontal elevation
14. Posterior to the nasal bones
15. Ear bone
17. Where occipital bone joins parietals
18. Forehead bone
19. Anteroinferior occipital part

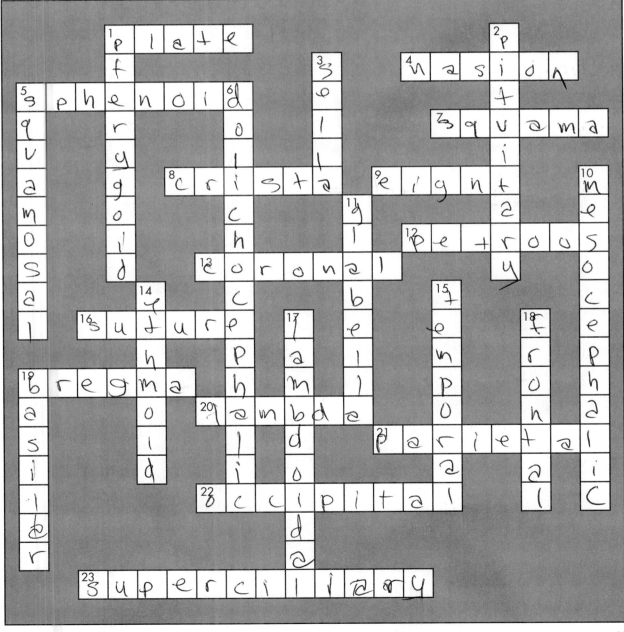

121

Exercise 3

Match the structures (Column A) with the cranial bones on which they are found (Column B).

Column A   **Column B**

_a_ 1. Nasion   a. Frontal

_a_ 2. Glabella   b. Ethmoid

_c_ 3. Four angles   c. Parietal

_d_ 4. Lesser wing   d. Sphenoid

_d_ 5. Greater wing   e. Temporal

_f_ 6. Two condyles   f. Occipital

_b_ 7. Crista galli

_d_ 8. Sella turcica

_f_ 9. Foramen magnum

_b_ 10. Cribriform plate

_e_ 11. Mastoid process

_f_ 12. Basilar portion

_e_ 13. Petrous portion

_d_ 14. Pterygoid hamulus

_e_ 15. Zygomatic process

_a_ 16. Supraorbital margin

_b_ 17. Perpendicular plate

_d_ 18. Lateral pterygoid process

_d_ 19. Anterior clinoid processes

_d_ 20. Posterior clinoid processes

Exercise 4

Match the statements (Column A) with the facial bone terms to which they refer (Column B). Only one selection from Column B applies to each statement in Column A. Not all terms from Column B should be used.

Column A   **Column B**

      a. Head

_m_ 1. Cheekbone   b. Body

_q_ 2. Largest facial bone   c. Nasal

_i_ 3. Number of facial bones   d. Hyoid

_c_ 4. Forms bridge of the nose   e. Ramus

_e_ 5. Vertical mandibular portion   f. Vomer

_n_ 6. Found in the roof of the mouth   g. Gonion

_r_ 7. Midpoint of the anterior nasal spine   h. Twelve

_l_ 8. Articulating process of the mandible   i. Fourteen

_k_ 9. Spongy processes that hold the teeth   j. Lacrimal

_p_ 10. Anterior part of the mandibular ramus   k. Alveolar

_g_ 11. Landmark at the angle of the mandible   l. Condyle

_j_ 12. Found in the medial walls of the orbits   m. Zygoma

_f_ 13. Forms the inferior portion of the nasal septum   n. Palatine

_b_ 14. Horseshoe-shaped mandibular portion   o. Maxillae

_s_ 15. Thin, scroll-like bones that extend horizontally inside nasal cavity   p. Coronoid

      q. Mandible

      r. Acanthion

      s. Inferior conchae

      t. Mental protuberance

Exercise 5

Match the pathology terms in Column A with the appropriate definition in Column B. Not all choices from Column B should be selected.

Column A

_i_ 1. Sinusitis

_g_ 2. Mastoiditis

_e_ 3. TMJ syndrome

_d_ 4. Basal fracture

_c_ 5. Linear fracture

_o_ 6. Tripod fracture

_f_ 7. LeFort fracture

_b_ 8. Blowout fracture

_n_ 9. Depressed fracture

_m_ 10. Contrecoup fracture

_a_ 11. Osteoma

_j_ 12. Metastases

_l_ 13. Acoustic neuroma

_k_ 14. Pituitary adenoma

_p_ 15. Multiple myeloma

Column B

a. Tumor composed of bony tissue

b. Fracture of the floor of the orbit

c. Irregular or jagged fracture of the skull

d. Fracture located at the base of the skull

e. Dysfunction of the temporomandibular joint

f. Bilateral horizontal fractures of the maxillae

g. Inflammation of the mastoid antrum and air cells

h. Inflammation of the bone due to a pyogenic infection

i. Inflammation of one or more of the paranasal sinuses

j. Transfer of a cancerous lesion from one area to another

k. Tumor arising from the pituitary gland, usually in the anterior lobe

l. Benign tumor arising from Schwann cells of the eighth cranial nerve

m. Fracture to one side of a structure caused by trauma to the other side

n. Fracture causing a portion of the skull to be pushed into the cranial cavity

o. Fracture of the zygomatic arch and orbital floor or rim and dislocation of the frontozygomatic suture

p. Malignant neoplasm of plasma cells involving the bone marrow and causing destruction of the bone

Exercise 6

This exercise is a comprehensive review of the osteology and arthrology of the skull. Fill in missing words or provide a short answer for each item.

1. The bones of the skull are divided into two major groups, the __crania__ bones and the __facial__ bones.

2. List the cranial bones by name and quantity.

frontal –1
ethmoidal –1
parietal –2
spenoid –1
temporal –2
occipital –1

3. List the facial bones by name and quantity.

nasal –2
lacrimal –2
maxilla –2
zygomatic –2
palantine –2

inferior nasal conchae –2
vomer –1
mandible –1

4. List the three classifications of fundamental skull shapes and indicate the number of degrees of angulation (formed by the petrous pyramids and the midsagittal plane) for each classification.

mesoceph – 47°
brady – 54°
doli – 40°

5. The bones of the cranial vault are classified as __flat__ bones.

6. The inner layer of spongy tissue found inside cranial bones is called __diploe__.

7. The two fontanels located on the midsagittal plane of the skull are the __bregma__ and the __lambda__.

8. The fontanel located at the junction of the coronal and sagittal sutures is the __frontal bregma__

9. The fontanel located at the junction of the lambdoidal and sagittal sutures is the __ethmoid lambda__

10. The bone that forms the anterior portion of the cranium is the __frontal__ bone.

11. The cranial bone located between the orbits and posterior to the nasal bones is the __ethmoid__ bone.

12. The cranial bones that form the vertex and most of the sides of the cranium are the __parietal__ bones.

13. The prominent bulge of a parietal bone is called the parietal __emenence__.

14. The two parietal bones join together to form the __sagittal__ suture.

15. The two parietal bones articulate with the frontal bone to form the __coronal__ suture.

16. The two parietal bones articulate posteriorly with the __occipital__ bone.

17. The two parietal bones and the occipital bone join together to form the __basilar__ __lambdoidal__ suture.

18. The cranial bone that provides a depression to house the pituitary gland is the __sphenoid__ bone.

19. The cranial bone that forms the posteroinferior portion of the cranium is the __occipital__ bone.

20. The portion of the occipital bone that projects anteriorly from the foramen magnum is the __basilar__ portion.

124

21. The large opening of the occipital bone through which part of the medulla oblongata passes is the

    foramen magnum .

22. The basilar portion of the occipital bone fuses anteriorly with the body of the _sphenoid_ bone.

23. The structure that articulates with the occipital condyles

    is the _C1 (atlas)_ .

24. The middle portion of the cranial base is formed by

    the _sphenoid_ bone.

25. The organs of hearing are located in the

    temporal bone.

26. The structure that separates the external acoustic meatus (EAM) from the auditory ossicles is the

    tympanic membrane.

27. The process of the temporal bone that encloses radiographically significant air cells is the

    mastoid process.

28. The thickest and densest portion of bone in the

    cranium is the _petrous portion (pars petrosa)_

29. The petrous portion is a part of the

    temporal bone.

30. The fibrocartilaginous, oval-shaped portion of the

    external ear is the _auricle_ .

31. The three auditory ossicles are the _malleus (hammer),_

    the _incus (anvil)_ , and the _stapes (stirrup)_

32. The zygomatic process projects anteriorly from the

    temporal bone.

33. The bone that forms part of the cranial base between the greater wings of the sphenoid bone and the occipital bone is the _temporal_ bone.

34. The facial bones that form the bridge of the nose are

    the _nasal_ bones.

35. The anterior portion of the medial walls of the orbits

    is formed by the _lacrimal_ bones.

36. The largest of the immovable bones of the face is the

    maxilla bone.

37. The body of each maxilla contains a large, pyramidal

    cavity called the _maxillary sinus_.

38. The thick ridge on the inferior border of the maxillary

    bone that supports the teeth is the _alveolar_

    process .

39. The anterior nasal spine projects superiorly from the

    maxillae .

40. The radiographically significant landmark that is the midpoint of the anterior nasal spine is the

    acanthion .

41. The facial bones that form the inferolateral portion of

    the orbital margin are the _zygomatic_ bones.

42. The facial bones that form the prominence of the

    cheeks are the _zygomatic_ bones.

43. The facial bones that form the posterior one fourth of

    the roof of the mouth are the _palatine_ bones.

44. The scroll-like bony tissues that extend along the lateral

    walls of the nasal cavity are the _inferior_

    nasal conchae .

45. The facial bone forming the inferior part of the nasal

    septum is the _vomer_ .

46. The largest and densest bone of the face is the

    _____mandible_____.

47. The portion of the mandible that extends superiorly from the posterior aspect of the mandibular body is

    the _____ramus_____.

48. The U-shaped bone located at the base of the tongue

    is the _____hyoid_____ bone.

49. The two processes that extend superiorly from a mandibular ramus are the _____condyle_____ and

    the _____coronoid_____ process.

50. The part of the mandible that articulates with the mandibular fossa of the temporal bone to form the

    temporomandibular joint is the _____condyle_____.

Hey Marianne —
This was a great year!
Lots a learning.

Exercise 7: Abbreviations

This exercise provides practice in the use of common abbreviations used in skull procedures. Write out the words beside each abbreviation.

1. AML: _acantheo meato Line_

2. TEA: _top of ear attatchment_

3. IAM: _internal acoustic meatus_

4. IPL: _interpupillary line_

5. GML: _glabellameato line_

RADIOGRAPHY OF THE SKULL

Exercise 1: Skull Topography

This exercise pertains to positioning landmarks used in skull radiography. Identify landmarks or provide a short answer for each item.

1. Identify each lettered positioning landmark shown in Fig. 20-14.

A. angle of the mandebe

B. infraorbital meatal Lin

C. outer canthus

D. mid-sagittal plane

E. glabella

F. interpupillary lin

G. inner canthus

H. nasion

I. acanthion

J. mental point

2. Identify each lettered positioning landmark shown in Fig. 20-15.

A. EAM

B. gonion (m. x)

C. glabellameatal line

D. orbitomeatal line

E. infraorbital meatal line

F. acanthiomeatal lin

G. glabelloalveolar lin

H. glabella

I. nasion

J. acanthion

K. mental point

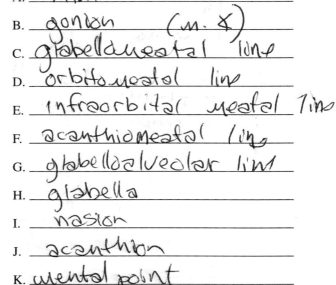

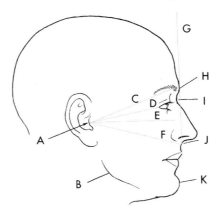

Fig. 20-15 Lateral aspect landmarks.

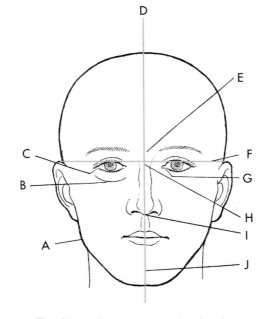

Fig. 20-14 Anterior aspect landmarks.

3. Match the definitions in Column A with the appropriate term from Column B. Each term may be used only once.

Column A

_c_ 1. Midpoint of the frontonasal suture

_f_ 2. Midpoint of the anterior nasal spine

_a_ 3. Posterior surface of the occipital bone

_e_ 4. Smooth elevation between the superciliary arches

_h_ 5. Lateral aspect of each orbit; where the two eyelids originate

_d_ 6. Angle of the mandible; lateroposterior aspect of the mandible

_b_ 7. Superior aspect of the cranium; where the parietal bones join together

_i_ 8. Raised prominence just above each orbit on the frontal bone; coincides with the eyebrows

_g_ 9. Midpoint of the mental protuberance; anterior aspect of the mandible; where the two mandibular bodies join together

Column B

a. Inion

b. Vertex

c. Nasion

d. Gonion

e. Glabella

f. Acanthion

g. Mental point

h. Outer canthus

i. Superciliary arch

4. Match the definitions in Column A with the appropriate terms in Column B. The terms represent skull topography lines or planes. Each term may be used once, more than once, or not at all.

Column A

_e_ 1. Line extending across the front through both eyes

_b_ 2. Plane dividing the skull into equal right and left halves

_h_ 3. Line extending from the glabella to the anterior aspect of the maxilla

_g_ 4. Line extending from the EAM to the outer canthus

_i_ 5. Line extending from the EAM to the inferior margin of the orbit

_g_ 6. Line extending from the EAM to the midpoint of the anterior nasal spine

_f_ 7. Line extending from the EAM to the smooth elevation between the superciliary arches

Column B

a. Sagittal

b. Midsagittal

c. Midcoronal

d. Orbitomeatal

e. Interpupillary

f. Glabellomeatal

g. Acanthiomeatal

h. Glabelloalveolar

i. Infraorbitomeatal

5. How many degrees exist in the angles formed by the following lines?

a. Orbitomeatal and infraorbitomeatal lines: _7°_

b. Orbitomeatal and glabellomeatal lines: _8°_

Exercise 2: Positioning for the Cranium

The typical radiographic evaluation of the skull, usually referred to as a skull series, involves a series of radiographs that may include a posteroanterior (PA) or anteroposterior (AP) projection, an AP axial projection, a full basal view, and one or two lateral views. This exercise pertains to those projections. Identify structures, fill in missing words, provide a short answer, select from a list, or choose true or false (explaining any statement you believe to be false) for each item.

Items 1 through 12 pertain to the *lateral projection*. Examine Fig. 20-16 as you answer the following questions.

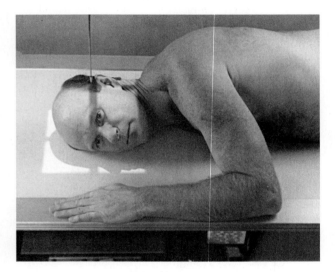

Fig. 20-16 Lateral skull.

1. Which size image receptor (IR) should be used for average-sized adult skulls, and how should it be placed in the IR holder?

   a. 18 × 24 cm; crosswise
   b. 18 × 24 cm; lengthwise
   c. 24 × 30 cm; crosswise
   d. 24 × 30 cm; lengthwise

2. Indicate how the midsagittal plane and the interpupillary line should be positioned—perpendicular or parallel—with reference to the plane of the IR.

   a. Midsagittal plane: __//__ *parellel*

   b. Interpupillary line: ___#___

3. Which positioning line of the head should be parallel with the plane of the IR?

   a. Interpupillary line
   b. Glabelloalveolar line
   c. Infraorbitomeatal line (IOML)

4. Which structure should be nearest to the center of the midline of the grid?

   a. Acanthion
   b. Zygomatic bone
   c. Outer canthus
   d. EAM

5. To what level of the patient should the IR be centered?

   2" above the EAM

6. Describe how and where the central ray should be directed. # to a point 2" above the EAM

7. For cross-table lateral projections with the patient supine, which procedure should be performed to ensure that the entire cranium is included in the image?

   a. Elevate the head on a radiolucent sponge.
   b. Increase the source–to–image-receptor distance (SID) to 72 inches.
   c. Use an 18- × 24-cm IR positioned lengthwise relative to the skull.

8. True or False. For cross-table lateral projections with the patient supine, the central ray should enter the side of the head at a point 2 inches (5 cm) anterior to the EAM. 2" ↑ EAM

9. True or False. For cross-table lateral projections with the patient supine, a vertically oriented grid IR should be placed against the side of interest.

   True

10. From the following list, circle the eight evaluation criteria that indicate the patient was properly positioned for a lateral projection.

a. The petrous ridges should be symmetric.

b. The sella turcica should be seen in profile.

c. The orbital roofs should be superimposed.

d. The mastoid regions should be superimposed.

e. The mandible should not overlap the cervical vertebrae.

f. The greater wings of sphenoid should be superimposed.

g. The temporomandibular joints should be superimposed.

h. The EAMs should be superimposed.

i. The dorsum sellae should be within the foramen magnum.

j. The entire cranium should be demonstrated without rotation or tilt.

k. The mental protuberance should be superimposed over the anterior frontal bone.

l. The distance from the lateral border of the skull to the lateral border of the orbit should be equal on both sides.

11. Fig. 20-17 shows two diagrams of a recumbent patient with the midsagittal plane improperly aligned. Examine the diagrams and explain how the position of the patient in each should be adjusted to properly align the midsagittal plane with the IR.

a. Diagram A: A support to be placed under the thorax so MSP // w/IR.

b. Diagram B: radiolucent sponge under head so MSP // w/IR

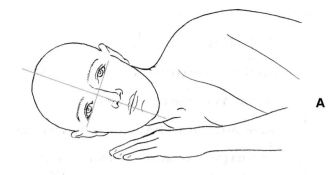

Asthenic or hyposthenic patient

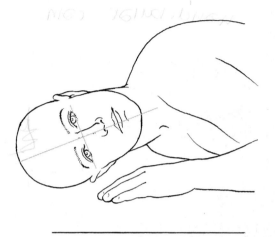

Hypersthenic patient

Fig. 20-17 Adjusting the midsagittal plane with the patient in the recumbent position. **A,** Asthenic or hyposthenic patient. **B,** Hypersthenic patient.

12. Identify each lettered structure shown in Fig. 20-18.

A. _orbital roof_

B. _sella turcica_

C. _sphenoidal sinus_

D. _petrous pt of temporal bones_

E. _tempo mandibular join_

F. _EAM_

G. _mandibular rami_

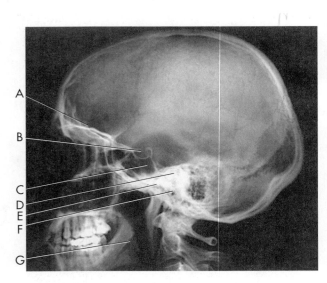

Fig. 20-18 Lateral skull.

Items 13 through 20 pertain to *PA and PA axial projections*. Examine Figs. 20-19 and 20-20 as you answer the following questions.

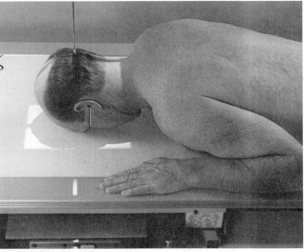

Fig. 20-19 PA skull.

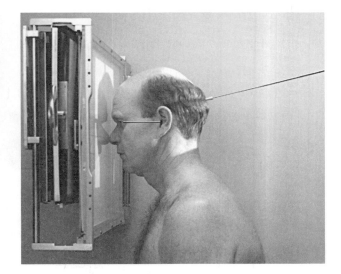

Fig. 20-20 PA axial skull.

13. Indicate how the midsagittal plane and the orbitomeatal line (OML) should be positioned—perpendicular or parallel—with reference to the plane of the IR.

a. Midsagittal plane: _____

b. Orbitomeatal line: _____

14. Which parts of the patient's facial area should be in contact with the table or vertical grid device?

a. Chin and nose
b. Chin and cheek
c. Forehead and nose
d. Forehead and cheek

15. To demonstrate each of the following structures (Column A), identify how the central ray should be directed (Column B) with the patient positioned for a PA projection of the skull.

Column A

___a___ 1. Frontal bone

___b___ 2. General survey

___d___ 3. Rotundum foramina

___c___ 4. Superior orbital fissures

Column B

a. Perpendicular

b. 15 degrees caudad

c. 20 to 25 degrees caudad

d. 25 to 30 degrees caudad

16. The central ray should exit the skull at the

_____nasion_____.

17. The IR should be centered to the skull at the level of

the _____nasion_____.

18. What breathing instructions should be given to the patient?

Stop breathing

19. From the following list, circle the five evaluation criteria that indicate the patient was properly positioned for either PA or PA axial projections.

(a) The petrous ridges should be symmetric.
b. The orbital roofs should be superimposed.
(c.) The entire cranial perimeter should be included.
d. The mandible should not overlap the cervical vertebrae.
e. The dorsum sellae should be within the foramen magnum.
f. The mental protuberance should be superimposed over the anterior frontal bone.
(g.) The frontal bone should be penetrated without excessive density at the lateral borders of the skull.
(h.) The distance from the lateral border of the skull to the lateral border of the orbit should be equal on both sides.
i. The petrous pyramids should lie in the lower third of the orbit with a central ray angulation of 15 degrees caudad and should fill the orbits with no central ray angulation.

20. Identify each lettered structure shown in Fig. 20-21.

A. ___dorsum sellae___

B. ___superior orbital margin___

C. ___sphenoid plane___

D. ___petrous ridge___

E. ___ethmoidal sinus___

F. ___inferior orbital margin___

G. ___cristi galli___

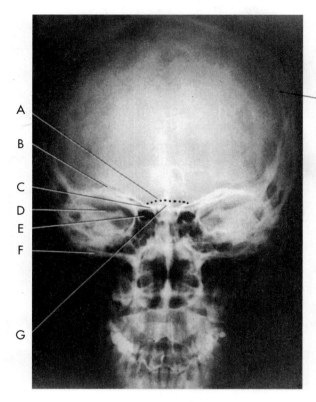

Fig. 20-21 PA skull.

Items 21 through 27 pertain to *AP and AP axial projections*. Examine Figs. 20-22 and 20-23 as you answer the following questions.

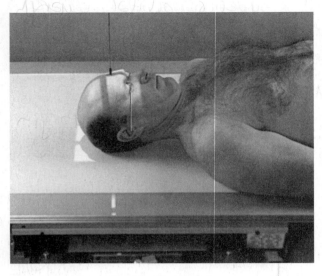

Fig. 20-22 AP skull.

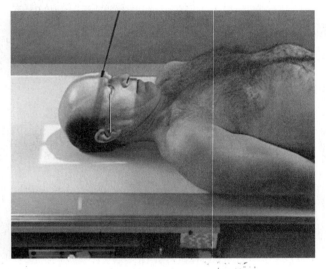

Fig. 20-23 AP axial skull.

21. Indicate how the midsagittal plane and the orbitomeatal line should be positioned—perpendicular or parallel—with reference to the plane of the IR.

    a. Midsagittal plane: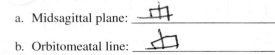

    b. Orbitomeatal line:

22. For the AP projection, the central ray should be directed _____ (caudally, cephalically, or perpendicularly).

23. For the AP axial projection, the central ray should be directed *cephallically* (caudally, cephalically, or perpendicularly).

24. When performing either the AP or AP axial projection for general surveys of the skull, where on the skull should the central ray be directed?

    a. Nasion
    b. Acanthion
    c. Tip of the nose

25. Which of the following image characteristics indicates that a general survey image of the skull is an AP projection instead of a PA projection?

    a. The petrous ridges are symmetric.
    b. The petrous pyramids fill the orbits.
    c. The orbits are considerably magnified.
    d. The entire cranial perimeter is demonstrated.

26. From the following list, circle the five evaluation criteria that indicate the patient was properly positioned for either the AP or AP axial projections.

    a. The petrous ridges should be symmetric.
    b. The orbital roofs should be superimposed.
    c. The entire cranial perimeter should be included.
    d. The mandible should not overlap the cervical vertebrae.
    e. The dorsum sellae should be within the foramen magnum.
    f. The mental protuberance should be superimposed over the anterior frontal bone.
    g. The frontal bone should be penetrated without excessive density at the lateral borders of the skull.
    h. The distance from the lateral border of the skull to the lateral border of the orbit should be equal on both sides.
    i. The petrous pyramids should lie in the lower third of the orbit, with a central ray angulation of 15 degrees caudad, and should fill the orbits with no central ray angulation.
    j. The petrous pyramids should lie in the lower third of the orbit, with a central ray angulation of 15 degrees cephalically, and should fill the orbits with no central ray angulation.

A   B

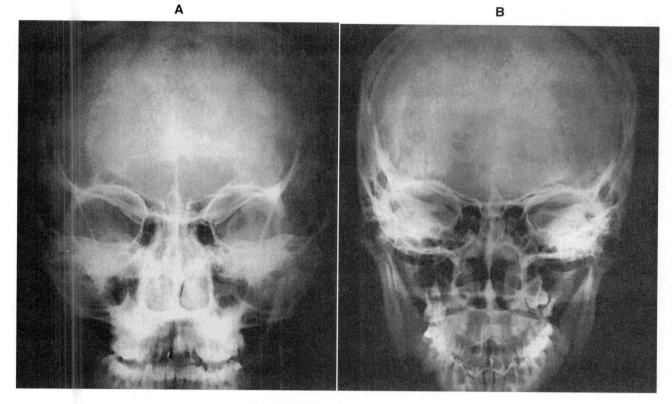

Fig. 20-24 Two views of the skull.

27. Fig. 20-24 shows two skull radiographs: one AP and one AP axial. Examine each image and state how the central ray was directed by indicating how specific structures appear in relation to the surrounding structures.

a. Figure A:

15° cephalad (petrous riges in lower 1/3).

b. Figure B:

0 - the petrous riges fill the entire orbits

Items 28 through 35 pertain to the *AP axial projection, Towne method*. Examine Fig. 20-25 as you answer the following questions.

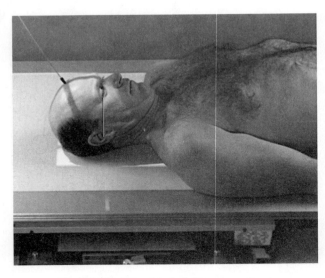

Fig. 20-25 AP axial skull, Towne method.

28. Which size IR should be used for average-sized adult skulls, and how should it be placed in the IR holder?

   a. 18 × 24 cm; crosswise
   b. 18 × 24 cm; lengthwise
   c. 24 × 30 cm; crosswise
   d. 24 × 30 cm; lengthwise

29. To what level of the patient should the upper border of the IR be aligned?

   a. Nasion
   b. Glabella
   c. Highest point of the vertex

30. In addition to the midsagittal plane, either the

   orbitalmeatal   line or the

   infraorbital meatal   line must be perpendicular to the plane of the IR.

31. Which two central ray angulations could be used to properly perform the AP axial projection?

   a. 30 degrees caudad and 37 degrees caudad
   b. 30 degrees caudad and 37 degrees cephalad
   c. 30 degrees cephalad and 37 degrees caudad
   d. 30 degrees cephalad and 37 degrees cephalad

32. Which positioning factor determines the number of degrees that the central ray should be angled?

   a. The type of skull being positioned
   b. Whether the patient is supine or seated upright
   c. How much SID is used
   d. Which positioning line is perpendicular to the IR

33. Where exactly on the patient's head should the central ray enter?

   a. 1 inch (2.5 cm) above the nasion
   b. 1 inch (2.5 cm) below the nasion
   c. 2 to 2½ inches (5 to 6.25 cm) above the glabella
   d. 2 to 2½ inches (5 to 6.25 cm) below the glabella

34. From the following list, circle the four evaluation criteria that indicate the patient was properly positioned for the AP axial projection, Towne method.

   a. The orbital roofs should be superimposed.
   b. The petrous pyramids should be symmetric.
   c. The mandible should not overlap the cervical vertebrae.
   d. The petrous pyramids should lie in the lower third of the orbits.
   e. The mental protuberance should be superimposed over the anterior frontal bone.
   f. The occipital bone should be penetrated without excessive density at the lateral borders of the skull.
   g. The dorsum sellae and posterior clinoid processes should be visualized within the foramen magnum.
   h. The distance from the lateral border of the skull to the lateral border of the orbit should be equal on both sides.
   i. The distance from the lateral border of the skull to the lateral margin of the foramen magnum should be equal on both sides.

35. Identify each lettered structure shown in Fig. 20-26.

A. _parietal_

B. _occipital_

C. _foramen magnum_

D. _petrous ridges_

E. _posterior clinoid process_

F. _dorsum sellae_

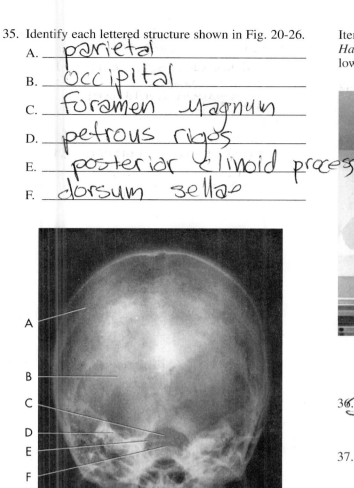

Fig. 20-26 AP axial skull, Towne method.

Items 36 through 43 pertain to the *PA axial projection, Haas method*. Examine Fig. 20-27 as you answer the following questions.

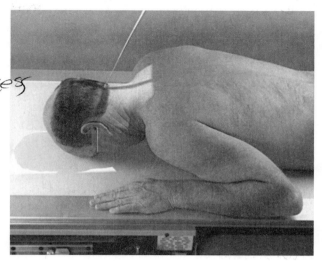

Fig. 20-27 PA axial skull, Haas method.

36. True or False. The PA axial projection, Haas method, demonstrates the occipital region of the cranium.

37. True or False. Hypersthenic patients should be positioned while recumbent in the supine position.

    Hyperstenic pts must be upright or prone

38. Which parts of the patient's head should be in contact with the table or vertical grid device?

    a. Chin and nose
    b. Chin and cheek
    c. Forehead and nose
    d. Forehead and cheek

39. In addition to the midsagittal plane, which positioning line of the skull should be perpendicular to the plane of the IR?

    a. Orbitomeatal
    b. Glabellomeatal
    c. Acanthiomeatal
    d. Infraorbitomeatal

40. How many degrees and in which direction should the central ray be directed?

    a. 25 degrees caudad
    b. 25 degrees cephalad
    c. 30 degrees caudad
    d. 30 degrees cephalad

41. Where on the midsagittal plane of the patient's skull should the central ray enter?

    a. At the vertex of the skull
    b. At a point approximately 1½ inches (3.8 cm) above the external occipital protuberance
    c. At a point approximately 1½ inches (3.8 cm) below the external occipital protuberance
    d. At a point approximately 3 inches (7.6 cm) below the external occipital protuberance

42. From the following list, circle the four evaluation criteria that indicate the patient was properly positioned for the PA axial projection, Haas method.

    a. The entire cranium should be included.
    b. The orbital roofs should be superimposed.
    c. The petrous pyramids should be symmetric.
    d. The mandible should not overlap the cervical vertebrae.
    e. The petrous pyramids should lie in the lower third of the orbits.
    f. The mental protuberance should be superimposed over the anterior frontal bone.
    g. The dorsum sellae and posterior clinoid processes should be seen within the foramen magnum.
    h. The distance from the lateral border of the skull to the lateral border of the orbit should be equal on both sides.
    i. The distance from the lateral border of the skull to the lateral border of the foramen magnum should be equal on both sides.

43. Identify each lettered structure shown in Fig. 20-28.

A. occipital bone

B. foramen magnum

C. petrous ridge

D. posterior clenoid process

E. dorsum sellae

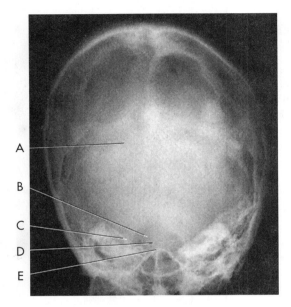

Fig. 20-28 PA axial skull, Haas method.

Items 44 through 50 pertain to the *submentovertical (SMV) projection, Schüller method*. Examine Fig. 20-29 as you answer the following questions.

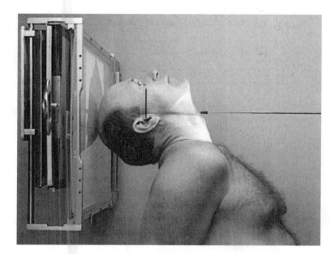

Fig. 20-29 SMV cranial base.

44. Indicate how the midsagittal plane and the infraorbitomeatal line should be positioned—perpendicular or parallel—with reference to the plane of the IR.

    a. Midsagittal plane: _____⊥_____

    b. Infraorbitomeatal: _____//_____

45. To what positioning line of the skull should the perpendicular central ray be directed?

    ___Ifraorbital meatal___

46. Describe where the central ray should enter the patient.

    MSP of the throat between the angles of the mandible passing through a point 3/4" anterior to the level of the EAM.

47. Through which cranial structure should the central ray pass?

    a. Sella turcica
    b. Ethmoidal air cells
    c. EAM

48. From the following list, select the two positioning factors on which the success of SMV projections most depend.

    a. Directing the central ray perpendicular to the OML
    b. Directing the central ray perpendicular to the IOML
    c. Directing the central ray perpendicular to the midsagittal plane
    d. Placing the OML as near as possible to parallel with the plane of the IR
    e. Placing the IOML as near as possible to parallel with the plane of the IR
    f. Placing the midsagittal plane as near as possible to parallel with the plane of the IR

49. From the following list, circle the five evaluation criteria that indicate the patient was properly positioned for an SMV projection.

    a. The petrosae should be symmetric.
    b. The orbital roofs should be superimposed.
    c. The mandibular rami should be superimposed.
    d. The mental protuberance should superimpose the anterior frontal bone.
    e. The petrous pyramids should lie in the lower third of the orbits.
    f. The mandibular condyles should be anterior to the petrous pyramids.
    g. The dorsum sellae should be seen and projected within the foramen magnum.
    h. The structures of the cranial base should be clearly visible as indicated by adequate penetration.
    i. The distance from the lateral border of the skull to the mandibular condyles should be equal on both sides.

50. Identify each lettered structure shown in Fig. 20-30.

A. maxillary sinus
B. ethmoidal air cells
C. mandible
D. sphenoidal sinus
E. foramen spinosum

F. mandibular condyle
G. dens (odontoid process)
H. petrosa
I. mastoid process

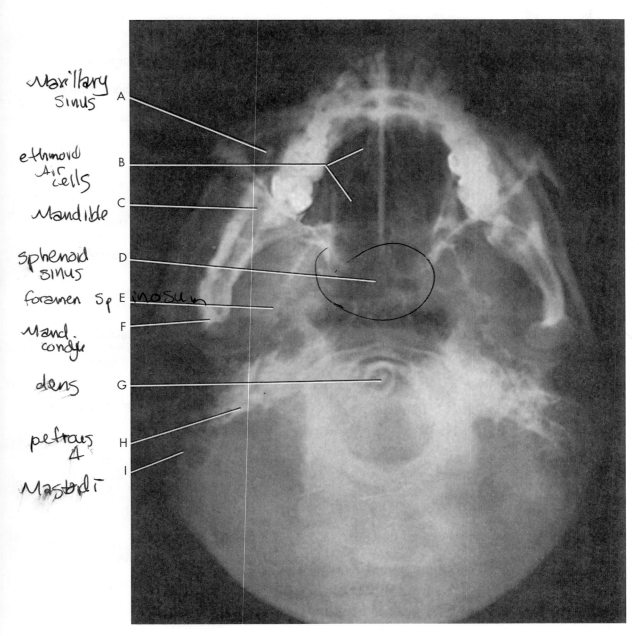

Fig. 20-30 SMV cranial base.

Exercise 3: Positioning for the Temporal Bone

Although computed tomography (CT) is often used to image internal cranial structures, small medical facilities still use standard radiography to demonstrate the mastoid processes and petrous portions. The axiolateral projections (modified Law method, single-tube angulation) can be used to image mastoid air cells, and both axiolateral oblique projections (Stenvers method, posterior profile, and Arcelin method, anterior profile) can be used to demonstrate petrous portions. This exercise pertains to those types of projections. Identify structures, provide a short answer, select from a list, or choose true or false (explaining any statement you believe to be false) for each item.

Items 1 through 11 pertain to the *axiolateral projection (modified Law method, single-tube angulation).* Examine Fig. 20-31 as you answer the following questions.

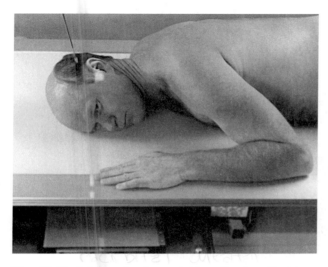

Fig. 20-31 Axiolateral petromastoid portion (modified Law method, single-tube angulation).

1. Describe how the patient's head should be positioned.

   From a true lateral, rotate the Head 15° ✗ to the IR Affected side centered to IR

2. Which procedure should be performed to prevent soft tissue structures from overlapping the mastoid process of interest?

   a. Tape the auricle of the ear forward.
   b. Angle the central ray 25 degrees caudad.
   c. Angle the central ray 25 degrees cephalad.
   d. Rotate the patient's head until the midsagittal plane forms an angle of 30 degrees with the plane of the IR.

3. If the patient is rotated 15 degrees from the right lateral position, which mastoid—right or left—is of interest? Is it the side closer to or farther from the IR?

   a. Left side; closer to
   b. Left side; farther from
   c. Right side; closer to
   d. Right side; farther from

4. Where should the IR be centered to the patient?

   a. 2 inches (5 cm) above the EAM
   b. 2 inches (5 cm) below the EAM
   c. 1 inch (2.5 cm) anterior to the EAM of the side adjacent to the IR
   d. 1 inch (2.5 cm) posterior to the EAM of the side adjacent to the IR

5. How many degrees and in what direction should the central ray be directed?

   15° caudad

6. Where should the central ray enter the patient?

   2" posterior & 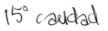 2" above the uppermost EAM

7. True or False. The patient's head should be placed and kept in the true lateral position.

   pt's head rotated 15° from true lat.

8. True or False. The midsagittal plane of the patient's head should be rotated from perpendicular to the IR until this line forms an angle of 15 degrees from vertical. The head should be rotated 15° from true lateral

9. True or False. The interpupillary line should remain perpendicular to the IR throughout the positioning procedure.

   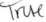 True

10. From the following list, circle the six evaluation criteria that indicate the patient was properly positioned for an axiolateral projection (modified Law method, single-tube angulation).

a. Close beam restriction of the mastoid region is needed.

b. The auricle of the ear should not superimpose the mastoid.

c. The entire side of the cranium should be clearly demonstrated.

d. The petrous ridges should superimpose the mastoid of interest.

e. The mastoid process should be in profile below the margin of the cranium.

f. The internal and external acoustic meatuses should be superimposed.

g. The temporomandibular joint should be visualized anterior to the mastoid.

h. The temporomandibular joint should be visualized posterior to the mastoid.

i. The opposite mastoid should not superimpose but should lie inferior and slightly anterior to the mastoid of interest.

j. The mastoid closer to the IR should be included, and the air cells should be demonstrated and centered to the IR.

11. Identify each lettered structure shown in Fig. 20-32.

A. _internal & external acoustic meatus_

B. _mastoid air cells_

C. _mastoid process_

D. _mandibular condyles_

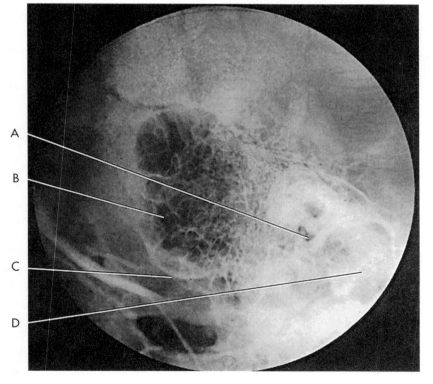

Fig. 20-32 Axiolateral petromastoid portion (modified Law method).

Items 12 through 18 pertain to the *axiolateral oblique projection (Stenvers method, posterior profile)*. Examine Fig. 20-33 as you answer the following questions.

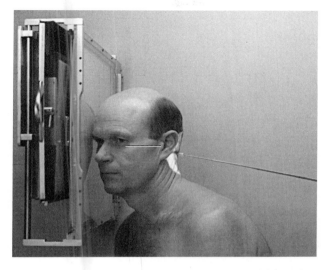

Fig. 20-33 Axiolateral oblique petromastoid portion (Stenvers method), posterior profile.

12. What three points of the face should be in contact with the x-ray table or vertical grid device?

    forehead, nose & cheek.

13. How many degrees and in what direction should the central ray be directed?

    12° cephalad

14. Where on the head should the central ray enter the patient?
    a. 2 inches (5 cm) above the EAM
    b. 2 inches (5 cm) below the EAM
    c. 3 to 4 inches (7.6 to 10 cm) anterior and ½ inch (1.2 cm) superior to the upside EAM
    d. 3 to 4 inches (7.6 to 10 cm) posterior and ½ inch (1.2 cm) inferior to the upside EAM

15. The midsagittal plane with the plane of the IR should form an angle of how many degrees?
    a. 15 degrees
    b. 37 degrees
    c. 45 degrees
    d. 53 degrees

16. Which positioning line of the head should be parallel with the transverse axis of the IR?
    a. Orbitomeatal
    b. Interpupillary
    c. Acanthiomeatal
    d. Infraorbitomeatal

17. Which petrous pyramid is demonstrated in profile when the patient is facing toward the left shoulder, as shown in Fig. 20-33? Is it the petrous pyramid closer to or farther from the IR?
    a. Left side; closer to
    b. Left side; farther from
    c. Right side; closer to
    d. Right side; farther from

18. Identify each lettered structure shown in Fig. 20-34.

A. _internal acoustic canal_

B. _arcuate eminence_

C. _mastoid air cells_

D. _EAM + canal_

E. _mandibular condyle_

F. _mastoid process_

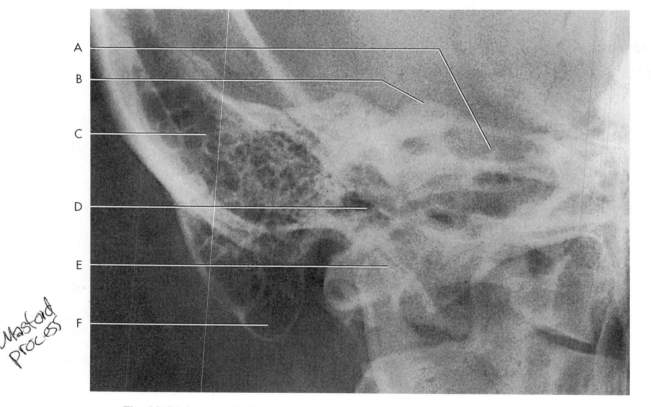

Mastoid Process

Fig. 20-34 Axiolateral oblique petromastoid portion (Stenvers method), posterior profile.

Items 19 through 25 pertain to the *axiolateral oblique projection (Arcelin method, anterior profile)*. Examine Fig. 20-35 as you answer the following questions.

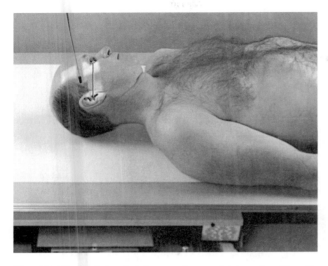

Fig. 20-35 Axiolateral oblique petromastoid portion (Arcelin method), anterior profile.

19. *True* or False. The patient should be placed in the supine position.

20. True or *False.* The midsagittal plane should be perpendicular to the IR.

$$MSP \ is \ 45° \ to \ IR$$

21. *True* or False. The infraorbitomeatal line should be perpendicular to the IR.

22. How many degrees and in what direction should the central ray be directed?

10° caudad

23. Where should the central ray enter the patient?

On the zygomatic bone approx. 1" anterior to & 3/4" above the EAM

24. Which petrous pyramid—right or left—is demonstrated in profile when the patient is facing toward the left shoulder, as shown in Fig. 20-35? Is it the petrous pyramid closer to or farther from the IR?

a. Left side; closer to
b. Left side; farther from
c. Right side; closer to
d. Right side; farther from

25. From the following list, circle the six evaluation criteria that indicate the patient was properly positioned for either a posterior profile projection (Stenvers method) or an anterior profile projection (Arcelin method).

a. The petrous ridges should completely fill the orbits.
b. The petromastoid portion should be demonstrated in profile.
c. The entire side of the cranium should be clearly demonstrated.
d. The internal and external acoustic meatuses should be superimposed.
e. The lateral border of the skull to the lateral border of the orbit should be included.
f. The mastoid should be demonstrated in profile below the margin of the cranium.
g. The mandibular condyle should be projected over the first cervical vertebra near the petrosa.
h. The posterior surface of the ramus should parallel or superimpose the lateral surface of the cervical vertebrae.
i. The opposite mastoid should not superimpose, but should lie inferior and slightly anterior to the mastoid of interest.
j. The petrous ridge should lie horizontally and at a point approximately two thirds of the way up the lateral border of the orbit.
k. The mastoid closer to the IR should be included, with the air cells demonstrated and centered to the IR.

Exercise 4: Positioning for the Optic Canal and Foramen

Parietoorbital oblique projections are standard radiographic procedures used to demonstrate the orbital region, specifically the optic canal and foramen. This exercise pertains to those projections. Identify structures, select from a list, provide a short answer, or choose true or false (explaining any statement you believe to be false) for each item.

Items 1 through 10 pertain to the *parietoorbital oblique projection, Rhese method.* Examine Fig. 20-36 as you answer the following questions.

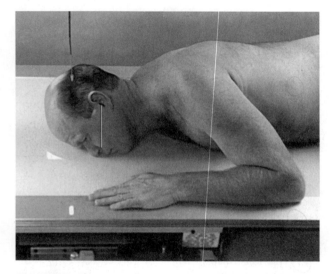

Fig. 20-36 Parietoorbital oblique projection, Rhese method.

1. In addition to the zygoma and nose, which other structure should be in contact with the x-ray table or vertical grid device?

   a. Ear
   b. Chin
   c. Forehead

2. Which positioning line of the head should be perpendicular to the plane of the IR?

   a. Interpupillary
   b. Acanthiomeatal
   c. Infraorbitomeatal

3. Which body plane or positioning line should form an angle of 53 degrees with the plane of the IR?

   a. Midsagittal plane
   b. Midcoronal plane
   c. Interpupillary line
   d. Acanthiomeatal line

4. True or False. Of the two orbits, the affected orbit should be placed closest to the IR.

5. True or False. The patient should suspend respiration for the exposure.

6. True or False. The central ray should be directed caudally 15 degrees. # to the orbit closest to IR.

7. True or False. The parietoorbital oblique projection demonstrates a cross-sectional view of the optic canal.

8. True or False. Incorrect angulation of the acanthiomeatal line will cause lateral deviation from the preferred location of the optic canal in the imaged orbit. Lateral = incorrect rotation AML — optic canal deviation

9. From the following list, circle the four evaluation criteria that indicate the patient was properly positioned for a parietoorbital oblique projection.

   a. The petrous ridges should be symmetric.
   b. The entire orbital rim should be included.
   c. The orbital roofs should be superimposed.
   d. The dorsum sellae should be within the foramen magnum.
   e. The supraorbital margins should lie in the same horizontal line.
   f. The optic canal and foramen should be seen at the end of the sphenoid ridge.
   g. The optic canal and foramen should lie in the inferior and lateral quadrant of the orbit.
   h. The optic canal and foramen should lie in the superior and medial quadrant of the orbit.

10. Identify each lettered structure shown in Fig. 20-37.

A. superior orbital margin

B. lateral orbital margin

C. optic canal and foramen

D. medial orbital margin

E. lesser wing of the sphenoid

F. ethmoidal sinus

G. inferior orbital margin

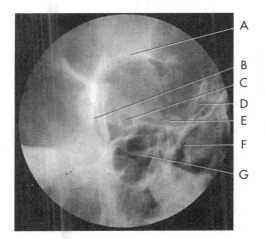

Fig. 20-37 Parietoorbital oblique projection.

Exercise 5: Evaluating Radiographs of the Skull

This exercise consists of radiographs of the skull, most of which show at least one positioning error, to give you some practice evaluating skull positioning. These images are not from Merrill's Atlas of Radiographic Positioning and Procedures. Examine each image and answer the questions that follow by providing a short answer.

1. Figs. 20-38 through 20-40 are lateral projection radiographs of a phantom skull. Only one image demonstrates acceptable positioning. Examine the images and answer the questions that follow. Refer to specific evaluation criteria for this projection when explaining your answers.

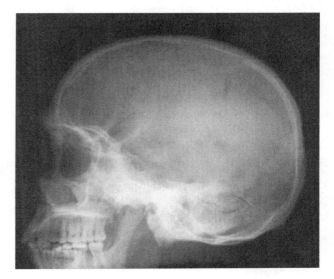

Fig. 20-38 Lateral skull.

certain structures are
S.I.

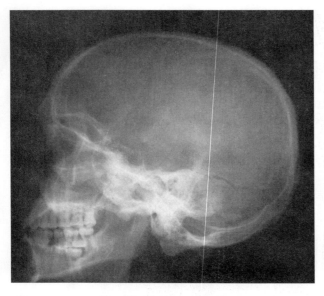

Fig. 20-39 Lateral skull.

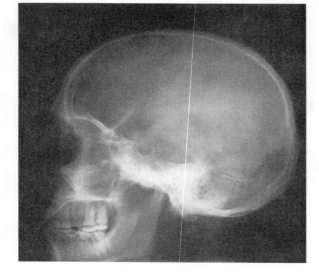

Fig. 20-40 Lateral skull.

a. Which image best demonstrates an optimally positioned skull? Explain.

EAM's seperated. 20-40
longitudillay

b. Which image shows the skull incorrectly positioned because the vertex and midsagittal plane are tilted toward the plane of the IR? Explain.

Laterally 20-39

c. Which image shows the skull incorrectly positioned because the face and midsagittal plane are rotated toward the x-ray table and IR? Explain.

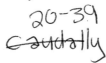

~~20-39~~ 20-38

d. Which image shows the skull positioned similarly to that seen in Fig. 20-17, Diagram B?

20-39
~~caudally~~

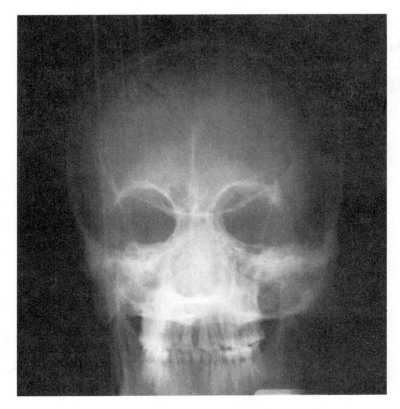

Fig. 20-41 PA skull showing incorrect positioning.

2. Fig. 20-41 shows a PA projection radiograph of a phantom skull with incorrect positioning. Examine the image and answer the questions that follow.

a. Assuming that the OML was perpendicular to the plane of the IR, describe how the central ray most likely was directed.

In the lower third of the orbits

b. Describe where the petrous ridges should appear in the image when the central ray is directed caudally 15 degrees.

Not symetrical from MSP

c. What image characteristic most likely prevents this image from meeting all the evaluation criteria for this projection?

MSP is not ⊥ to IR

d. Describe the positioning error that most likely caused the image to appear as it does.

⊥ to the nasion

3. Fig. 20-42 shows a PA projection radiograph of a phantom skull with incorrect positioning. Examine the image and answer the questions that follow.

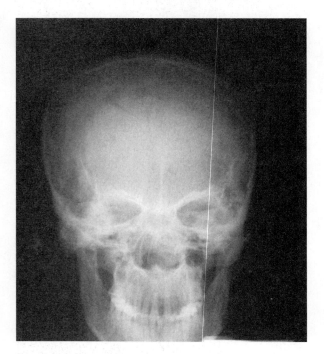

Fig. 20-42 PA skull showing incorrect positioning.

a. Assuming that the OML was perpendicular to the plane of the IR, describe how the central ray most likely was directed.

caudal 15°

b. Describe where the petrous ridges should appear in the image when the central ray is directed caudally 15 degrees.

not equal MSP

lower 1/3 orbits

c. Do the petrous ridges nearly fill the orbits?

yes

d. What image characteristic most likely prevents this image from meeting all evaluation criteria for this projection?

head toward left shoulder

e. Describe the positioning error that most likely caused the image to appear as it does.

not equal sides

4. Figs. 20-43 and 20-44 show AP projection radiographs of a phantom skull. Only one image demonstrates acceptable positioning. Examine the images and answer the questions that follow.

a. Is the positioning quality for Fig. 20-43 acceptable or unacceptable?

Acceptable

b. Is the positioning quality for Fig. 20-44 acceptable or unacceptable?

Unacceptable

c. Describe the positioning error that probably caused the unacceptable image.

MSP not ⊥
(rotation)

d. Assuming that the OML was perpendicular for both images, in which way does the central ray appear to have been directed?

⊥

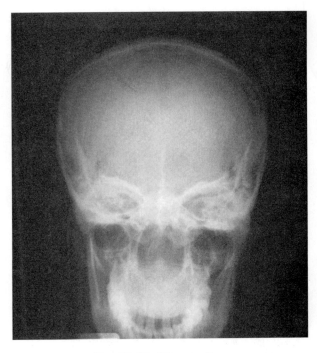

Fig. 20-43 AP projection.

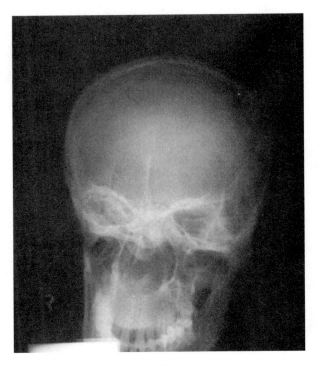

Fig. 20-44 AP projection.

5. Examine Fig. 20-45 and state why it does not meet the evaluation criteria for this type of projection.

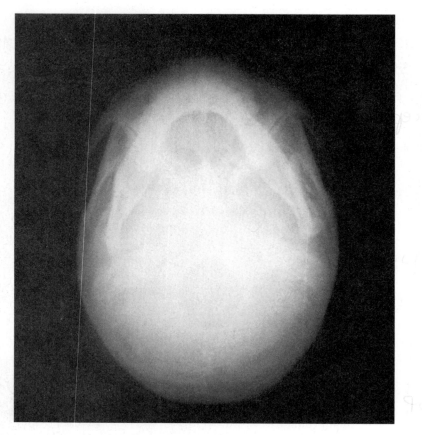

Fig. 20-45 SMV projection showing incorrect positioning.

The mandibular symphysis doesn't ~~show~~ superimpose the anterior frontal bone.

6. Figs. 20-46 through 20-48 are parietoorbital oblique projection radiographs of a phantom skull. Only one image demonstrates the correct rotation of the head. Examine the images and answer the questions that follow. Refer to specific evaluation criteria for this projection when explaining your answers.

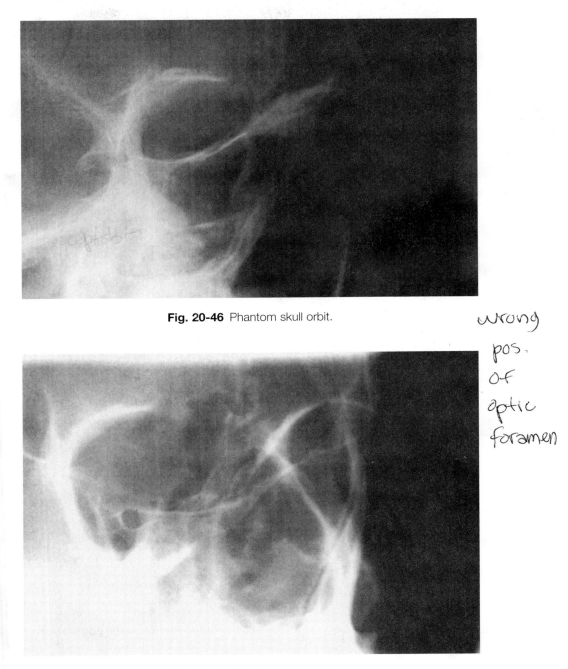

Fig. 20-46 Phantom skull orbit.

wrong
pos.
of
optic
foramen

Fig. 20-47 Phantom skull orbit.

20-47

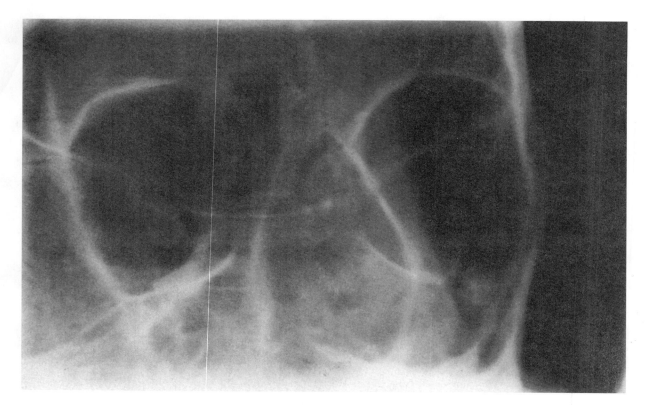

Fig. 20-48 Phantom skull orbit.

a. Which image best demonstrates ideal positioning of the phantom skull? Explain.

20-46

b. In which image does the midsagittal plane form an angle with the IR that is considerably less than the required amount? Explain.

20~

c. In which image does the midsagittal plane form an angle with the IR that is somewhat greater than the required amount? Explain.

20-48

Note to Students: Additional exercises referenced from Chapters 20 through 22 are found in the appendix (Supplemental Exercises for Skull Positioning), which is located in this workbook. Students should complete the review exercises for those chapters before completing the appendix exercises.

SELF-TEST: OSTEOLOGY AND RADIOGRAPHY OF THE SKULL

Answer the following questions by selecting the best choice.

1. Which positioning line extends from the EAM to the outer canthus?

    a. Orbitomeatal
    b. Glabellomeatal
    c. Acanthiomeatal
    d. Infraorbitomeatal

2. Which positioning landmark is located at the base of the nasal spine?

    a. Nasion
    b. Gonion
    c. Glabella
    d. Acanthion

3. Which positioning landmark is located at the most superior point of the nasal bones?

    a. Nasion
    b. Canthus
    c. Glabella
    d. Acanthion

4. Which positioning landmark is the smooth elevation that is located between the superciliary arches?

    a. Nasion
    b. Glabella
    c. Acanthion
    d. Mental point

5. Which positioning landmark is most superior?

    a. Nasion
    b. Gonion
    c. Glabella
    d. Acanthion

6. Where on the skull is the gonion located?

    a. Between the orbits
    b. On the anterior frontal bone
    c. On the posterior occipital bone
    d. On the lateroposterior part of the mandible

7. Where on the skull is the outer canthus located?

    a. Between the orbits
    b. At the mandibular angle
    c. Along each parietal eminence
    d. On the lateral border of each orbit

8. Which positioning landmark is located at the anterior portion of the mandible?

    a. Nasion
    b. Gonion
    c. Acanthion
    d. Mental point

9. Which suture articulates the frontal bone with both parietal bones?

    a. Sagittal
    b. Coronal
    c. Squamosal
    d. Lambdoidal

10. Which suture joins both parietal bones at the vertex of the skull?

    a. Sagittal
    b. Coronal
    c. Squamosal
    d. Lambdoidal

11. Which suture joins a parietal bone with both a sphenoid bone and a temporal bone?

    a. Sagittal
    b. Coronal
    c. Squamosal
    d. Lambdoidal

12. Which suture joins both parietal bones with the occipital bone?

    a. Sagittal
    b. Coronal
    c. Squamosal
    d. Lambdoidal

13. The bregma fontanel is located at the junction of which two sutures?

    a. Coronal and sagittal
    b. Coronal and squamosal
    c. Lambdoidal and sagittal
    d. Lambdoidal and squamosal

14. The lambda fontanel is located at the junction of which two sutures?

    a. Coronal and sagittal
    b. Coronal and squamosal
    c. Lambdoidal and sagittal
    d. Lambdoidal and squamosal

15. The bregma fontanel is located at the junction of which cranial bones?

    a. Frontal and both parietals
    b. Occipital and both parietals
    c. Frontal and sphenoid
    d. Occipital and sphenoid

16. The lambda fontanel is located at the junction of which cranial bones?

    a. Frontal and both parietals
    b. Occipital and both parietals
    c. Frontal and temporal
    d. Occipital and temporal

17. Which skull classification refers to a typical skull (in terms of width and length)?

    a. Mesocephalic
    b. Brachycephalic
    c. Dolichocephalic

18. Which skull classification refers to a long, narrow skull?

    a. Mesocephalic
    b. Brachycephalic
    c. Dolichocephalic

19. Which skull classification refers to a short, wide skull?

    a. Mesocephalic
    b. Brachycephalic
    c. Dolichocephalic

20. How many degrees are in the angle formed between the midsagittal plane and the petrous pyramids in the mesocephalic skull?

    a. 36 degrees
    b. 40 degrees
    c. 47 degrees
    d. 54 degrees

21. How many degrees are in the angle formed between the midsagittal plane and the petrous pyramids in the brachycephalic skull?

    a. 36 degrees
    b. 40 degrees
    c. 47 degrees
    d. 54 degrees

22. How many degrees are in the angle formed between the midsagittal plane and the petrous pyramids in the dolichocephalic skull?

    a. 36 degrees
    b. 40 degrees
    c. 47 degrees
    d. 54 degrees

23. On which cranial bone are the superciliary arches located?

    a. Frontal
    b. Parietal
    c. Ethmoid
    d. Occipital

24. On which cranial bone is the cribriform plate located?

    a. Frontal
    b. Ethmoid
    c. Temporal
    d. Sphenoid

25. On which cranial bone is the crista galli located?

    a. Ethmoid
    b. Occipital
    c. Temporal
    d. Sphenoid

26. Which cranial bone has a petrous pyramid?

    a. Parietal
    b. Ethmoid
    c. Temporal
    d. Sphenoid

27. On which cranial bone is the sella turcica located?

    a. Frontal
    b. Ethmoid
    c. Temporal
    d. Sphenoid

28. Which cranial bone has the mastoid process?

    a. Parietal
    b. Ethmoid
    c. Temporal
    d. Sphenoid

29. On which cranial bone is the perpendicular plate located?

    a. Parietal
    b. Ethmoid
    c. Temporal
    d. Sphenoid

30. Which cranial bone has both greater and lesser wings?

    a. Ethmoid
    b. Occipital
    c. Temporal
    d. Sphenoid

31. With which cranial bone does the first cervical vertebra articulate?

    a. Ethmoid
    b. Occipital
    c. Temporal
    d. Sphenoid

32. The pterygoid processes project inferiorly from which cranial bone?

    a. Frontal
    b. Ethmoid
    c. Temporal
    d. Sphenoid

33. The foramen magnum is a part of which cranial bone?

    a. Frontal
    b. Occipital
    c. Temporal
    d. Sphenoid

34. From which cranial bone does the zygomatic process arise?

    a. Frontal
    b. Parietal
    c. Temporal
    d. Sphenoid

35. The EAM is a part of which cranial bone?

    a. Frontal
    b. Parietal
    c. Temporal
    d. Sphenoid

36. The temporal process projects posteriorly from which facial bone?

    a. Vomer
    b. Maxilla
    c. Zygoma
    d. Temporal

37. Which bones comprise the bridge of the nose?

    a. Nasal
    b. Lacrimal
    c. Palatine
    d. Maxillae

38. With which bone does the mandible articulate?

    a. Hyoid
    b. Maxilla
    c. Zygoma
    d. Temporal

39. Where are the lacrimal bones located?

    a. Inside the nasal cavity
    b. On the lateral wall of each orbit
    c. On the medial wall of each orbit
    d. Inferior to the maxillary sinuses

40. Where is the vomer bone found?

    a. Posterior to the nasal bones
    b. On the floor of the nasal cavity
    c. On the lateral wall of the orbits
    d. In the posterior one fourth of the roof of the mouth

41. Which bone comprises most of the lateral wall of the orbital cavities?

    a. Maxilla
    b. Lacrimal
    c. Palatine
    d. Zygomatic

42. Which term refers to the anterior process of the mandibular ramus?

    a. Cornu
    b. Condyle
    c. Coracoid
    d. Coronoid

43. Which term refers to the posterior process of the mandibular ramus?

    a. Cornu
    b. Condyle
    c. Coracoid
    d. Coronoid

44. Which facial bones have alveolar processes?

    a. Vomer and mandible
    b. Vomer and zygomatic
    c. Maxillae and mandible
    d. Maxillae and zygomatic

45. Which bones form the posterior one fourth of the roof of the mouth?

    a. Maxillae
    b. Palatine
    c. Zygomatic
    d. Inferior nasal conchae

46. Which positioning landmark is located on the maxillae?

    a. Gonion
    b. Nasion
    c. Acanthion
    d. Mental point

47. Which two positioning lines or planes should be perpendicular to the IR for the PA projection of the skull?

    a. Orbitomeatal line and midsagittal plane
    b. Orbitomeatal line and interpupillary line
    c. Infraorbitomeatal line and midsagittal plane
    d. Infraorbitomeatal line and interpupillary line

48. With reference to the patient, where should the IR be centered for the PA projection of the skull?

    a. Nasion
    b. Glabella
    c. Acanthion
    d. Mental point

49. With reference to the patient, where should the IR be centered for the lateral projection of the skull?

   a. Nasion
   b. EAM
   c. 2 inches (5 cm) above the EAM
   d. 2 inches (5 cm) below the EAM

50. With reference to the IR, how should the interpupillary line and the midsagittal plane be positioned for the lateral projection of the skull?

   a. Interpupillary line: parallel; midsagittal plane: parallel
   b. Interpupillary line: parallel; midsagittal plane: perpendicular
   c. Interpupillary line: perpendicular; midsagittal plane: parallel
   d. Interpupillary line: perpendicular; midsagittal plane: perpendicular

51. For the AP axial projection, Towne method, of the skull, how many degrees and in which direction should the central ray be directed when the OML is perpendicular to the IR?

   a. 30 degrees caudad
   b. 30 degrees cephalad
   c. 37 degrees caudad
   d. 37 degrees cephalad

52. For the AP axial projection, Towne method, of the skull, how many degrees and in which direction should the central ray be directed when the IOML is perpendicular to the IR?

   a. 30 degrees caudad
   b. 30 degrees cephalad
   c. 37 degrees caudad
   d. 37 degrees cephalad

53. Which positioning line should be parallel with the IR for the SMV projection of the skull?

   a. Orbitomeatal line
   b. Glabellomeatal line
   c. Acanthiomeatal line
   d. Infraorbitomeatal line

54. Which projection of the skull can be correctly performed with the central ray angled 37 degrees?

   a. AP axial, Towne method
   b. PA axial, Haas method
   c. PA axial, Caldwell method
   d. Parietoorbital oblique, Rhese method

55. Which projection of the skull can be correctly performed with the central ray angled 15 degrees?

   a. SMV
   b. AP axial, Towne method
   c. PA axial, Haas method
   d. PA axial, Caldwell method

56. Which projection of the skull produces a full basal image of the cranium?

   a. Lateral
   b. AP axial, Towne method
   c. PA with perpendicular central ray
   d. SMV, Schüller method

57. Which projection of the skull projects the petrous bones in the lower third of the orbits?

   a. PA axial, Haas method
   b. AP axial, Towne method
   c. PA axial, Caldwell method
   d. PA with perpendicular central ray

58. Which projection of the skull should be obtained when the frontal bone is of primary interest?

   a. PA axial, Haas method
   b. AP axial, Towne method
   c. PA axial, Caldwell method
   d. PA with perpendicular central ray

59. Which evaluation criterion pertains to the AP axial projection, Towne method, of the skull?

   a. The orbital roofs should be superimposed.
   b. The mental protuberance should superimpose the anterior frontal bone.
   c. Part of the sella turcica should be seen within the foramen magnum.
   d. The distance from the lateral border of the skull to the lateral border of the orbit should be the same on both sides.

60. Which evaluation criterion pertains to the PA projection of the skull?

   a. The orbital roofs should be superimposed.
   b. The mental protuberance should superimpose the anterior frontal bone.
   c. Part of the sella turcica should be seen within the foramen magnum.
   d. The distance from the lateral border of the skull to the lateral border of the orbit should be the same on both sides.

61. Which evaluation criterion pertains to the lateral projection of the skull?

   a. The orbital roofs should be superimposed.
   b. The mental protuberance should superimpose the anterior frontal bone.
   c. Part of the sella turcica should be seen within the foramen magnum.
   d. The distance from the lateral border of the skull to the lateral border of the orbit should be the same on both sides.

62. Which evaluation criterion pertains to the SMV projection of the skull?

    a. The orbital roofs should be superimposed.
    b. The mental protuberance should superimpose the anterior frontal bone.
    c. Part of the sella turcica should be seen within the foramen magnum.
    d. The distance from the lateral border of the skull to the lateral border of the orbit should be the same on both sides.

63. For the PA axial projection, Haas method, of the skull, where should the central ray enter the patient's head?

    a. Nasion
    b. Acanthion
    c. 1½ inches (3.8 cm) above the external occipital protuberance
    d. 1½ inches (3.8 cm) below the external occipital protuberance

64. How many degrees and in which direction should the central ray be directed for the PA axial projection, Haas method, of the skull?

    a. 15 degrees caudad
    b. 15 degrees cephalad
    c. 25 degrees caudad
    d. 25 degrees cephalad

65. For the parietoorbital oblique projection, Rhese method, of the skull, which positioning line should be perpendicular to the IR?

    a. Orbitomeatal
    b. Glabellomeatal
    c. Acanthiomeatal
    d. Infraorbitomeatal

66. With reference to the orbit, where should the optic foramen be imaged on the radiograph to indicate correct positioning of the patient for the parietoorbital oblique projection, Rhese method, of the skull?

    a. Within the lower inner quadrant
    b. Within the lower outer quadrant
    c. Within the upper inner quadrant
    d. Within the upper outer quadrant

67. For the parietoorbital oblique projection, Rhese method, of the skull, how many degrees of angle should be formed between the midsagittal plane and the IR?

    a. 25 degrees
    b. 37 degrees
    c. 53 degrees
    d. 55 degrees

68. Which structure is best demonstrated when midsagittal plane of the patient's head is rotated from perpendicular to the IR to a 45 degree angle with the plane of the IR, positioning the face toward the right shoulder, and the central ray is directed to enter the side of the face about 1 inch (2.5 cm) anterior and ¾ inch (1.9 cm) superior to the EAM?

    a. Left petrous portion
    b. Right petrous portion
    c. Left mastoid air cells
    d. Right mastoid air cells

69. How many degrees and in which direction should the central ray be directed for axiolateral oblique projections (Arcelin method, anterior profile)?

    a. 10 degrees caudad
    b. 10 degrees cephalad
    c. 12 degrees caudad
    d. 12 degrees cephalad

70. Which projection requires that the patient's head be rotated from true lateral, moving the face closer to the IR, until the midsagittal plane forms an angle of 15 degrees with the IR?

    a. Parietoacanthial (Waters method)
    b. Axiolateral oblique (Arcelin method, anterior profile)
    c. Axiolateral oblique (Stenvers method, posterior profile)
    d. Axiolateral (modified Law method, single-tube angulation)

21 | Facial Bones

RADIOGRAPHY OF THE FACIAL BONES

Note to Students: For a review of facial bone anatomy, see Chapter 20.

Exercise 1: Positioning for Facial Bones and Nasal Bones

A standard radiographic series to demonstrate facial bones includes various projections that examine facial structures from different perspectives. Some projections commonly used are the lateral, the parietoacanthial (Waters method), and the acanthioparietal (reverse Waters method). Additionally, a lateral projection of the nasal bones is sometimes added to a facial bones series because nasal bones are sometimes affected when other facial bones are damaged by trauma. This exercise pertains to the projections of the facial bones and nasal bones. Identify structures, fill in missing words, select from a list, or provide a short answer for each item.

Items 1 through 9 pertain to *lateral projections of the facial bones.* Examine Fig. 21-1 as you answer the following questions.

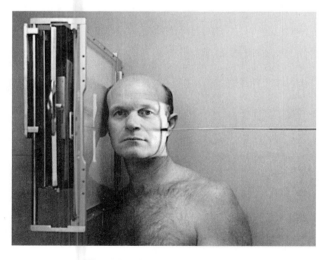

Fig. 21-1 Lateral facial bones.

1. The image receptor (IR) should be placed in the IR holder _lengthwise_ (crosswise or lengthwise).

2. The plane of the head that should be parallel with the plane of the IR is the _Midsaggital_ (midsagittal or midcoronal) plane.

3. Which positioning line of the head should be perpendicular to the IR?
   a. Orbitomeatal
   b. Interpupillary
   c. Acanthiomeatal
   d. Infraorbitomeatal

4. Which positioning line of the head should be parallel with the transverse axis of the IR?
   a. Orbitomeatal
   b. Interpupillary
   c. Acanthiomeatal
   d. Infraorbitomeatal

5. Which facial bone should be centered to the IR?
   a. Nasal
   b. Maxilla
   c. Mandible
   d. Zygomatic

6. How should the central ray be directed to the patient—perpendicularly, angled cephalically, or angled caudally?

   _⊥_

7. Where on the patient's face should the central ray be directed?

   ½ way between the outer canthus & EAM

8. From the following list, circle the four evaluation criteria that indicate the patient was properly positioned for a lateral projection of the facial bones.

(a.) The sella turcica should not be rotated.
(b.) The orbital roofs should be superimposed.
c. The sella turcica should be seen within the foramen magnum.
(d.) The mandibular rami should be almost perfectly superimposed.
e. The petrous bones should lie in the lower third of the orbit.
f. The mental protuberance should be superimposed over anterior frontal bone.
(g.) All facial bones should be completely included with the zygomatic bone in the center.
h. The distance from the lateral border of the skull to the lateral border of the orbit should be equal on both sides.

9. Identify each lettered structure shown in Fig. 21-2.

A. frontal sinus

B. nasal bones

C. sella turcica

D. maxillary sinus

E. EAM

F. maxilla

G. mandible

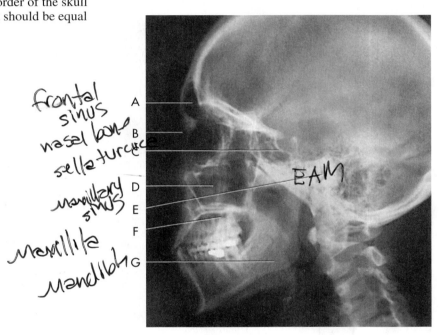

Fig. 21-2 Lateral facial bones.

Items 10 through 15 pertain to the *parietoacanthial projection, Waters method*. Examine Fig. 21-3 as you answer the following questions.

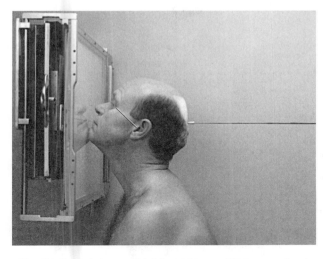

Fig. 21-3 Parietoacanthial facial bones, Waters method.

10. Indicate how the orbitomeatal line (OML) and the midsagittal plane should be positioned with reference to the IR.

   a. OML: _____ 37° ⊀ _____

   b. Midsagittal plane: _____ 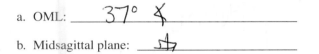 _____

11. To which landmark of the head should the IR be centered?

   a. Nasion
   b. Acanthion
   c. Mental point
   d. Outer canthus

12. How should the central ray be directed relative to the IR?

   a. Perpendicularly
   b. 37 degrees caudally
   c. 37 degrees cephalically

13. Describe where the petrous ridges most likely will appear in the image if the OML creates the following angles with the IR:

   a. 25 degrees:

   too far below maxilla

   b. 37 degrees:

   just below maxilla

   c. 55 degrees:

   SI maxillary sinuses

14. From the following list, circle the two evaluation criteria that indicate the patient was properly positioned for a parietoacanthial projection.

   a. The orbital roofs should be superimposed.
   b. The petrous ridges should nearly fill the orbits.
   c. The entire cranium should be demonstrated without rotation or tilt.
   d. The petrous ridges should be projected immediately below the maxillary sinuses.
   e. The distance between the lateral border of the skull and orbit should be equal on both sides.

15. Identify each lettered structure shown in Fig. 21-4.

A. orbit

B. zygomatic arch

C. Maxillary sinus

D. Maxilla

E. mandibular ×
    gonion

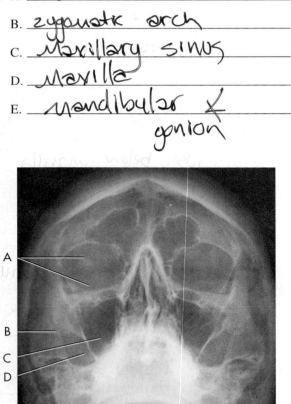

Fig. 21-4 Parietoacanthial facial bones, Waters method.

Items 16 through 24 pertain to the *acanthioparietal projection, reverse Waters method*. Examine Fig. 21-5 as you answer the following questions.

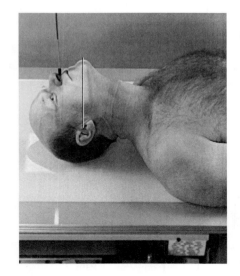

Fig. 21-5 Acanthioparietal facial bones, reverse Waters method.

16. The acanthioparietal projection can be used to demonstrate facial bones when the patient is lying in the __supine__ (prone or supine) position.

17. The image of the acanthioparietal projection is similar to the image of the __parietal__ __acanthio__ projection (__waters__ method).

18. Which plane and positioning line of the head should be perpendicular to the IR?
    a. Midsagittal plane and OML
    b. Midsagittal plane and mentomeatal line
    c. Midcoronal plane and OML
    d. Midcoronal plane and mentomeatal line

19. Where should the midpoint of the IR be centered to the patient?
    a. Nasion
    b. Glabella
    c. Acanthion
    d. 1 inch (2.5 cm) inferior to the acanthion

20. Which breathing instructions should be given to the patient?

   a. Stop breathing.
   b. Breathe slowly.
   c. Breathe rapidly.

21. How should the central ray be directed?

   a. Perpendicularly
   b. 15 degrees caudally
   c. 15 degrees cephalically
   d. 30 degrees cephalically

22. To which positioning landmark should the central ray be directed?

   a. Nasion
   b. Glabella
   c. Acanthion
   d. Mental point

23. From the following list, circle the two evaluation criteria that indicate the patient was properly positioned for an acanthioparietal projection, reverse Waters method.

   a. The orbital roofs should be superimposed.
   b. The petrous ridges should nearly fill the orbits.
   c. The petrous ridges should be projected in the maxillary sinuses.
   d. The petrous ridges should be projected immediately below the maxillary sinuses.
   e. The distance between the lateral border of the skull and orbit should be equal on both sides.

24. Identify each lettered structure shown in Fig. 21-6.

   A. orbit
   B. zygomatic bone
   C. maxillary sinus

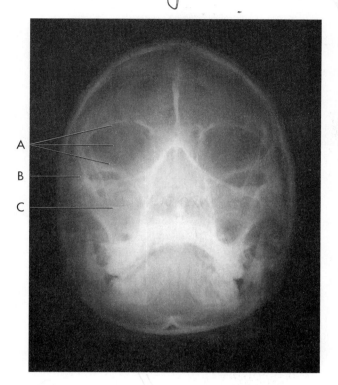

Fig. 21-6 Acanthioparietal facial bones, reverse Waters method.

Items 25 through 30 pertain to the *lateral projection of the nasal bones*. Examine Fig. 21-7 as you answer the following questions.

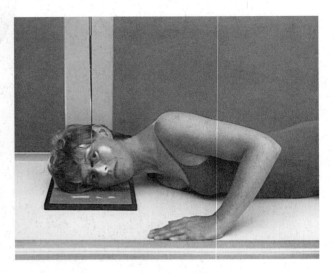

Fig. 21-7 Lateral nasal bones.

25. Indicate how the interpupillary line and midsagittal plane should be positioned with reference to the IR—perpendicular or parallel.

    a. Interpupillary line: _____⊣_____

    b. Midsagittal plane: ___//_____

26. How many exposures should be made on one IR?

    _____two_____

27. To which facial landmark—the nasion or acanthion—should the unmasked portion of the IR be centered?

    ___Superimposed w/the_____
    _____Maxillary sinuses

28. Describe how and where the central ray should be directed.

    foreshortened
    ⊥ to the bridge of
    the nose

    ½" distal to the nason

29. From the following list, circle the two evaluation criteria that indicate the patient was properly positioned for a lateral projection.

    a. All facial bones should be demonstrated.
    b. The zygomatic processes should be seen superimposed.
    (c.) The anterior nasal spine and frontonasal suture should be visualized.
    (d.) The nasal bone and soft tissue should be demonstrated without rotation.

30. Identify each lettered structure shown in Fig. 21-8.

    A. __frontonaso_____ (suture)
    B. __nasal bone_____
    C. __anterior nasal sprhe____

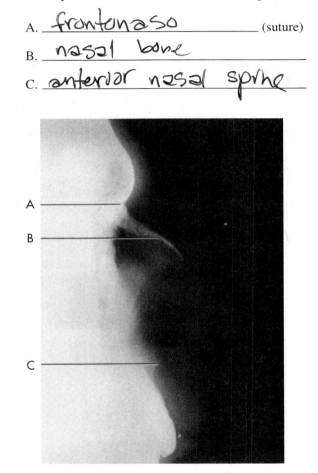

Fig. 21-8 Lateral nasal bones.

Exercise 2: Positioning for Zygomatic Arches

Zygomatic arches are commonly demonstrated with three projections: a submentovertical (SMV) projection, a tangential projection, and an anteroposterior (AP) axial projection. This exercise pertains to those projections. Identify structures, fill in missing words, provide a short answer, select from a list, or choose true or false (explaining any statement you believe to be false) for each item.

Items 1 through 9 pertain to the *SMV projection for bilateral zygomatic arches.* Examine Fig. 21-9 as you answer the following questions.

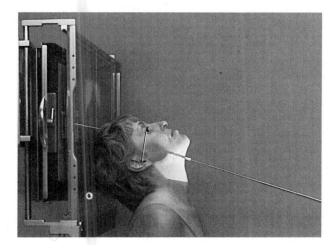

Fig. 21-9 SMV zygomatic arches.

1. True or False. The SMV projection should demonstrate both zygomatic arches with one exposure.

2. True or False. Zygomatic arches should be demonstrated superimposed with the anterior frontal bone.

   clearly dem

3. True or False. The entire cranial base should be demonstrated.

   not needed

4. True or False. The midsagittal plane should be parallel with the IR.

   MSP ⊥ to IR

5. Which positioning line of the head should be parallel with the IR?

   a. Orbitomeatal
   b. Acanthiomeatal
   c. Infraorbitomeatal

6. Which part of the patient should be in contact with the grid device?

   a. Forehead
   b. Mandible
   c. Vertex of the skull

7. Which statement best describes how the central ray should be directed?

   a. Angled cephalically and centered to the glabella
   b. Angled caudally and centered to the zygomatic arch of interest
   c. Perpendicular to the infraorbitomeatal line and centered on the midsagittal plane of the throat

8. For the SMV projection, what causes the zygomatic arches to be projected beyond the parietal eminences?

   a. The divergent x-ray beam
   b. The head tilted 15 degrees
   c. The head rotated 15 degrees

9. From the following list, circle the three evaluation criteria that indicate the patient was properly positioned for the SMV projection.

   a. No rotation of the head should occur.
   b. The zygomatic arches should be free from overlying structures.
   c. The entire cranium should be demonstrated without rotation or tilt.
   d. The zygomatic arches should be symmetric and without foreshortening.
   e. The structures of the cranial base should be clearly visible as indicated by adequate penetration.
   f. The distance from the lateral border of the skull to the lateral border of the orbit should be equal on both sides.

Items 10 through 14 pertain to the *tangential projection.* Examine Fig. 21-10 as you answer the following questions.

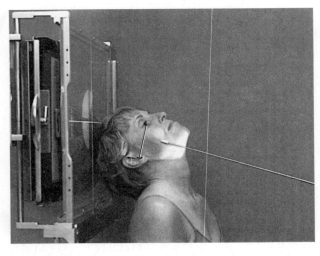

Fig. 21-10 Tangential zygomatic arch.

10. True or False. The patient should hyperextend the neck and rest the head on the vertex.

11. True or False. The midsagittal plane should be perpendicular to the IR.

12. What positioning line of the head should be as parallel as possible with the IR?

    IOML

13. Describe how the central ray should be directed.

    ⊥ to IOML
    centered to zyg. Arch
    apprx 1" post to outer-
    canthus

14. From the following list, circle the evaluation criterion that indicates the patient was properly positioned for a tangential projection.

    a. No rotation of the head should occur.
    b. The zygomatic arch should be free from overlying structures.
    c. The entire cranium should be demonstrated without rotation or tilt.

Items 15 through 20 pertain to the *AP axial projection, modified Towne method.* Examine Fig. 21-11 as you answer the following questions.

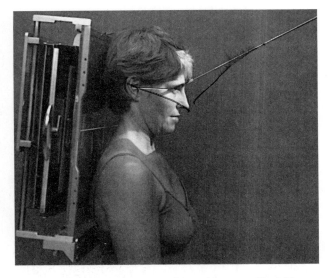

Fig. 21-11 AP axial zygomatic arches, modified Towne method.

15. Indicate how the OML and midsagittal plane should be positioned with reference to the IR—perpendicular or parallel.

    a. OML: ⊥

    b. Midsagittal plane: ⊥

16. How many degrees and in which direction should the central ray be directed when each of the following positioning lines is placed perpendicular to the plane of the IR?

    a. OML: 30° ↙ caudad

    b. Infraorbitomeatal line: 22 35 ↗

17. The central ray should enter 1 inch (2.5 cm) above

    the landmark nasion .

18. True or False. Both zygomatic arches should be demonstrated on the radiograph with a single exposure.

19. True or False. The entire vertex should be included on the radiograph. Close beam attenuation

20. Identify each lettered structure shown in Fig. 21-12.

A. _____occipital_____

B. _____mandible_____

C. _____zygomatic arches_____

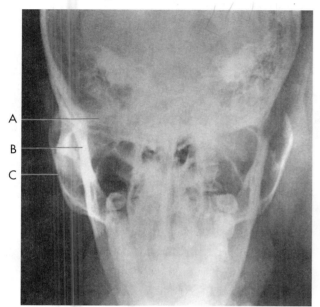

Fig. 21-12 AP axial zygomatic arches, modified Towne method.

PA   — full

Caldwell   lower ½

Mod Wat   Maxillary

Wat.   ↓ maxillary

Exercise 3: Positioning for the Mandible

Usually three or four projections are needed to demonstrate the mandible. Posteroanterior (PA), PA axial, and axiolateral oblique projections are often included in the typical mandible examination. This exercise pertains to those projections. Identify structures, provide a short answer, select from a list, or choose true or false (explaining any statement you believe to be false) for each item.

Items 1 through 10 pertain to the *PA projection demonstrating the mandibular rami.* Examine Fig. 21-13 as you answer the following questions.

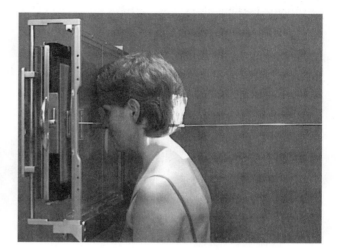

Fig. 21-13 PA mandibular rami.

1. To demonstrate the mandibular rami with the PA projection, which two facial structures should be touching the vertical grid device?
   a. Nose and chin
   b. Forehead and nose
   c. Forehead and cheek

2. Which positioning line should be perpendicular to the plane of the IR?
   a. Orbitomeatal
   b. Glabellomeatal
   c. Acanthiomeatal
   d. Infraorbitomeatal

3. How should the midsagittal plane be positioned with reference to the IR—parallel or perpendicular?

   _____

4. What breathing instructions should be given to the patient?

Stop respiration

5. Through which positioning landmark of the face should the central ray exit?

a. Nasion
ⓑ Acanthion
c. Mental point

6. How does the vertebral column affect the image?

a. It superimposes mandibular rami.
ⓑ It superimposes the central part of the mandibular body.
c. It increases the object–to–image-receptor distance (OID) of the mandible.

7. Ⓣrue or False. The central ray should be directed perpendicularly to the midpoint of the IR.

8. True or ~~False~~. The PA projection demonstrates the mandibular body without bony superimpositioning.

central portion is SI.

9. From the following list, circle the two evaluation criteria that indicate the patient was properly positioned for the PA projection of the mandibular rami.

ⓐ The entire mandible should be included.
b. The mandibular rami should be superimposed.
ⓒ The mandibular body and rami should be symmetric on both sides.
d. The temporomandibular articulation should be seen lying anterior to the external acoustic meatus (EAM).

10. Identify each lettered structure and fracture shown in Fig. 21-14.

A. _condyle_
B. _mastoid process_
C. _fx of mandibular ramus_
D. _body_

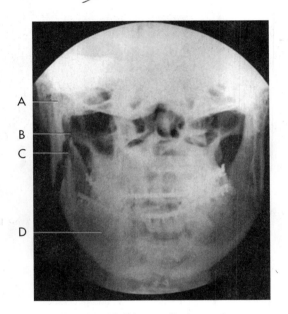

Fig. 21-14 PA mandibular rami.

Items 11 through 17 pertain to the *PA axial projection of the mandibular rami*. Examine Fig. 21-15 as you answer the following questions.

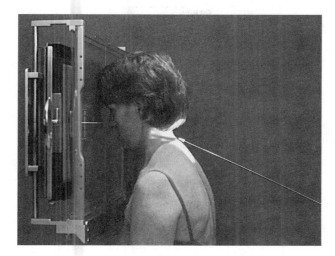

Fig. 21-15 PA axial mandibular rami.

11. Which two facial structures should be touching the vertical grid device?

    a. Nose and chin
    b. Forehead and nose
    c. Forehead and cheek

12. Which body plane and positioning line should be perpendicular to the plane of the IR?

    a. Midcoronal plane and OML
    b. Midcoronal plane and acanthiomeatal line
    c. Midsagittal plane and OML
    d. Midsagittal plane and acanthiomeatal line

13. Which breathing instructions should be given to the patient?

    a. Stop breathing.
    b. Breathe slowly.
    c. Breathe rapidly.

14. Which positioning landmark should be centered to the IR?

    a. Nasion
    b. Glabella
    c. Acanthion
    d. Mental point

15. How many degrees and in which direction should the central ray be directed?

    a. 10 to 15 degrees caudad
    b. 10 to 15 degrees cephalad
    c. 20 to 25 degrees caudad
    d. 20 to 25 degrees cephalad

16. What prevents the central part of the mandibular body from being clearly demonstrated?

    a. Superimposition with the spine
    b. Caudal angulation of the central ray
    c. Increased OID

17. From the following list, circle the three evaluation criteria that indicate the patient was properly positioned for a PA axial projection.

    a. The entire mandible should be demonstrated.
    b. The mandibular rami should be superimposed.
    c. The condylar processes should be clearly demonstrated.
    d. The mandibular body and rami should be symmetric on both sides.
    e. The temporomandibular articulation should be seen lying anterior to the EAM.

Items 18 through 31 pertain to axiolateral oblique projections of the mandible (with the patient either prone or upright). Figs. 21-16, 21-17, and 21-18 represent three upright axiolateral oblique projections that demonstrate parts of the mandible. Match each of the following positioning statements to one or more of these figures by writing the appropriate figure number in the space provided. Some statements may have more than one figure (projection) associated with them. Some statements do not relate to any of the three projections; answer "NA" for "not applicable" for these items.

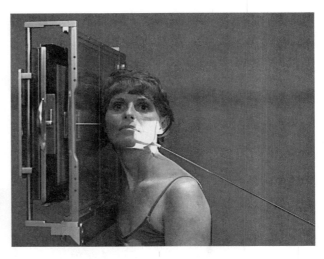

Fig. 21-18 Upright axiolateral oblique projection.

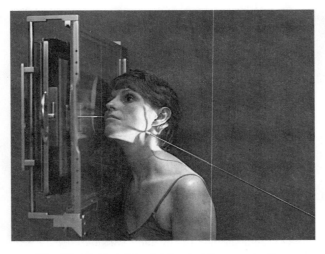

Fig. 21-16 Upright axiolateral oblique projection.

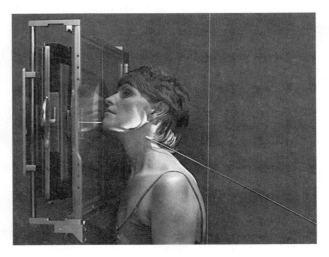

Fig. 21-17 Upright axiolateral oblique projection.

_NA_ 18. Keep the head in a true lateral position.

_16_ 19. Used for demonstrating the mandibular body

_18_ 20. Used for demonstrating the mandibular ramus

_17_ 21. Used for demonstrating the mental protuberance

_16_ 22. Rotate the head 30 degrees toward the IR.

_17_ 23. Rotate the head 45 degrees toward the IR.

_17_ 24. The central ray should exit the mental protuberance.

_N/A_ 25. The central ray should be directed 15 degrees cephalad.

_16, 17, 18_ 26. The central ray should be directed 25 degrees.

_N/A_ 27. The central ray should be directed perpendicular to the IR.

_N/A_ 28. The OML should be perpendicular to the plane of the IR.

_16, 17, 18_ 29. The interpupillary line should be perpendicular to the plane of the IR.

_18_ 30. The broad surface of the ramus should be parallel with the plane of the IR.

_16_ 31. The broad surface of the mandibular body should be parallel with the plane of the IR.

32. True or False. The mouth should be closed with the teeth held together.

33. True or False. The neck should be flexed to pull the chin downward.

neck extended

34. True or False. The area of interest should be parallel with the IR.

so mand body ∥

35. Identify each lettered structure shown in Fig. 21-19.

A. coronoid process

B. ramus

C. body

D. hyoid bone

E. X

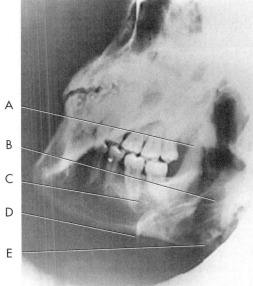

Fig. 21-19 Axiolateral oblique mandibular body.

Exercise 4: Positioning for the Temporomandibular Joints (TMJs)

Two projections often performed to demonstrate TMJs are the AP axial projection and the axiolateral oblique projection. This exercise pertains to those projections. Identify structures, provide a short answer, select from a list, or choose true or false (explaining any statement you believe to be false) for each question.

Items 1 through 10 pertain to the *AP axial projection.* Examine Fig. 21-20 as you answer the following questions.

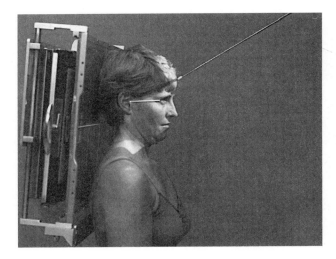

Fig. 21-20 AP axial TMJs.

1. True or False. For the AP axial projection in the closed-mouth position, the upper posterior teeth should be in contact with the lower posterior teeth.

2. True or False. The long axis of the mandibular body should be parallel with the transverse axis of the IR.

3. Why should the incisors not contact when the patient is positioned for the closed-mouth AP axial projection?

occlusion

4. Identify a typical situation in which the patient should not be asked to open his or her mouth wide for an AP axial projection. Explain why.

5. Which plane and positioning line of the head should be perpendicular to the IR?

   a. Midcoronal plane and OML
   b. Midcoronal plane and infraorbitomeatal line
   c. Midsagittal plane and OML
   d. Midsagittal plane and infraorbitomeatal line

6. How many degrees and in which direction should the central ray be directed?

   a. 25 degrees caudad
   b. 25 degrees cephalad
   c. 35 degrees caudad
   d. 35 degrees cephalad

7. Where should the central ray enter the patient?

   a. Glabella
   b. Acanthion
   c. 3 inches (7.6 cm) above the nasion
   d. 3 inches (7.6 cm) below the nasion

8. To which landmark should the IR be centered?

   a. Nasion
   b. Glabella
   c. Central ray
   d. Mental protuberance

9. From the following list, circle the two evaluation criteria that indicate the patient was properly positioned for an AP axial projection with the mouth closed.

   a. The head should not be rotated.
   b. The condyle should be seen anterior to the EAM.
   c. Only minimal superimposition by the petrosa on the condyle should be seen.
   d. The condyle and temporomandibular articulation should be seen below the pars petrosa.

10. From the following list, circle the two evaluation criteria that indicate the patient was properly positioned for an AP axial projection with the mouth open.

    a. The head should not be rotated.
    b. The condyle should be seen anterior to the EAM.
    c. Only minimal superimposition by the petrosa on the condyle should be seen.
    d. The condyle and temporomandibular articulation should be demonstrated below the petrosa.

Items 11 through 20 pertain to *axiolateral oblique projections*. Examine Fig. 21-21 as you answer the following questions.

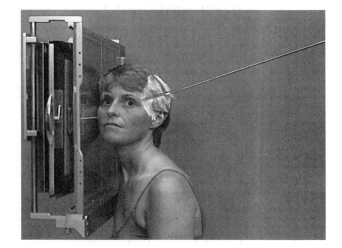

Fig. 21-21 Axiolateral oblique TMJ.

11. Where on the patient should the IR be centered?

    a. 2 inches (5 cm) inferior to the TMJs
    b. 2 inches (5 cm) superior to the TMJs
    c. ½ inch (1.2 cm) anterior to the EAM
    d. ½ inch (1.2 cm) posterior to the EAM

12. How should the midsagittal plane be positioned with reference to the IR?

    a. Parallel
    b. Perpendicular
    c. Form an angle of 15 degrees
    d. Form an angle of 37 degrees

13. Which positioning line of the head should be parallel with the transverse axis of the IR?

    a. Orbitomeatal
    b. Interpupillary
    c. Acanthiomeatal
    d. Infraorbitomeatal

14. How many degrees and in what direction should the central ray be directed?

_____

15. Through what structure should the central ray exit the patient?

_____

16. In relation to surrounding structures, where in the image should the mandibular condyle be seen for axiolateral oblique projections with the patient holding the mouth closed?

_____

17. True or False. The central ray should enter the patient at the TMJ farther from the IR.

18. True or False. Both open- and closed-mouth positions should be performed with the axiolateral oblique projection unless contraindicated.

19. True or False. The entire side of the mandible from the condyle to the symphysis should be demonstrated.

20. Identify each lettered structure shown in Fig. 21-22.

A. _____

B. _____

C. _____

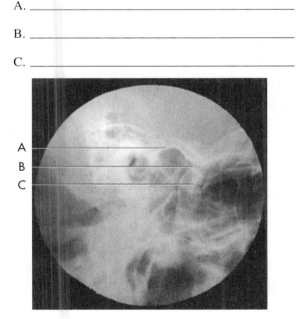

Fig. 21-22 Axiolateral oblique TMJ with the patient's mouth open.

Exercise 5: Evaluating Radiographs of Facial Bones

This exercise consists of facial bone radiographs to give you some practice evaluating facial bone positioning. These images are not from Merrill's Atlas of Radiographic Positioning and Procedures. *Most images show at least one positioning error. Examine each image and answer the questions that follow by providing a short answer.*

1. Fig. 21-23 shows a lateral projection radiograph of the facial bones with incorrect positioning of a phantom skull. Examine the image and state why it does not meet the evaluation criteria for this type of projection.

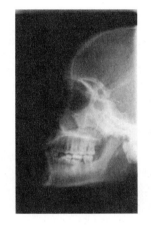

Fig. 21-23 Lateral facial bones showing incorrect positioning of a phantom skull.

2. Figs. 21-24 through 21-26 show parietoacanthial projection radiographs of the facial bones of a phantom skull. Only one image demonstrates acceptable positioning. Examine the images and answer the questions that follow.

   a. Which image demonstrates acceptable positioning?

   _____

   b. In which image does the phantom skull appear to be incorrectly positioned because the angle between the OML and the IR is greater than the required amount? (This error results when the patient is unable to extend the neck far enough.)

   _____

   c. In which image does the phantom skull appear to be incorrectly positioned because the angle between the OML and the IR is less than the required amount? (This error results when the patient extends the neck too much.)

   _____

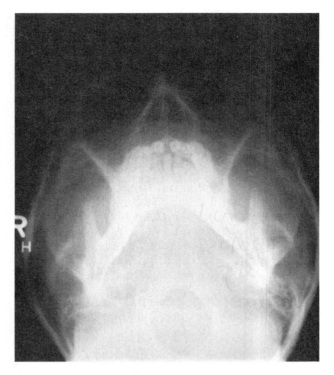

Fig. 21-25 Radiograph of a phantom skull positioned for the parietoacanthial projection.

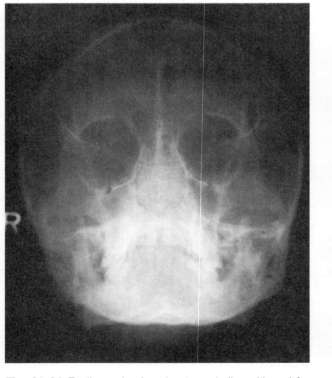

Fig. 21-24 Radiograph of a phantom skull positioned for the parietoacanthial projection.

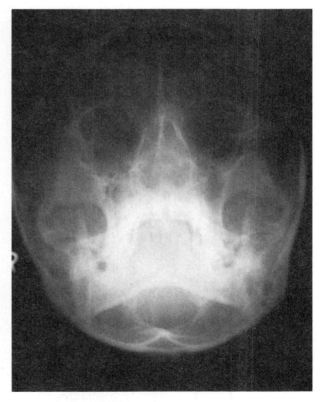

Fig. 21-26 Radiograph of a phantom skull positioned for the parietoacanthial projection.

Items 11 through 17 pertain to the *lateral projection*. Examine Fig. 22-2 as you answer the following questions.

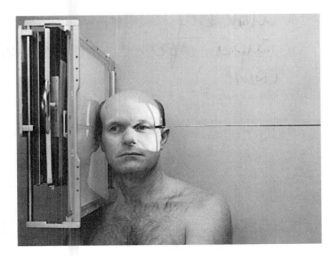

Fig. 22-2 Lateral sinuses.

11. State how the midsagittal plane and the interpupillary line should be placed with reference to the plane of the image receptor (IR)—perpendicular or parallel.

    a. Midsagittal plane: _____//_____

    b. Interpupillary line: _____⊥_____

12. Where on the patient's head should the central ray be directed?

    a. 2 inches (5 cm) above the external acoustic meatus

    b. 2 inches (5 cm) below the external acoustic meatus

    c. ½ to 1 inch (1.2 to 2.5 cm) anterior to the outer canthus

    d. ½ to 1 inch (1.2 to 2.5 cm) posterior to the outer canthus

13. How should the central ray be directed relative to the patient's head?

    a. Perpendicular

    b. 15 degrees caudad

    c. 15 degrees cephalad

14. Which sinus group is of primary importance?

    a. Frontal

    b. Maxillary

    c. Ethmoidal

    d. Sphenoidal

15. How many sinus groups should be clearly demonstrated with lateral projection radiographs?

    a. One

    b. Two

    c. Three

    d. Four

16. From the following list, circle the six evaluation criteria that indicate the patient was properly positioned for a lateral projection.

    a. The sella turcica should not be rotated.

    b. The sinuses should be visualized clearly.

    c. The orbital roofs should be superimposed.

    d. All four sinus groups should be included.

    e. The mandibular rami should be superimposed.

    f. Close beam restriction of the sinus area is needed.

    g. The petrous ridges should be lying in the lower third of the orbits.

    h. The anterior frontal bone should be superimposed by the mental protuberance.

    i. The petrous ridges should be lying just below the floor of the maxillary sinuses.

    j. The distance between the lateral border of the skull and the lateral border of the orbits should be equal.

    k. The distance from the lateral border of the skull to the mandibular condyles should be equal on both sides.

17. Identify each lettered structure shown in Fig. 22-3.

A. frontal sinus

B. sella turcica

C. sphenoidal sinus

D. ethmoid sinus

E. maxillary sinus

F. super-imposed mandibular ramo

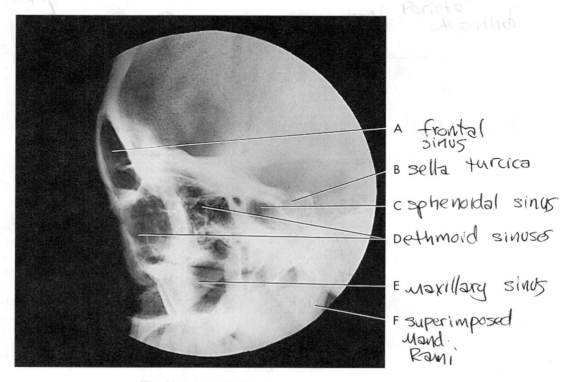

A frontal sinus
B sella turcica
c sphenoidal sinus
D ethmoid sinuses
E maxillary sinus
F superimposed Mand. Rami

Fig. 22-3 Lateral sinuses.

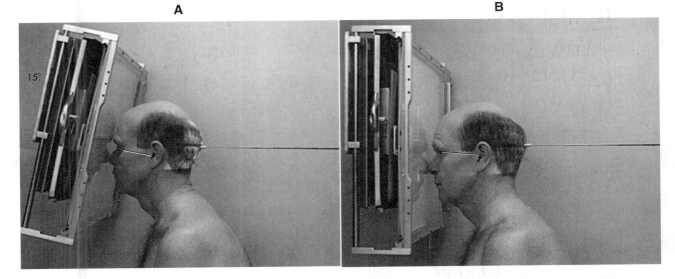

Fig. 22-4 PA axial sinuses, Caldwell method. **A,** IR tilted 15 degrees. **B,** Same projection with a vertical IR.

Items 18 through 25 pertain to the *PA axial projection, Caldwell method.* Examine Fig. 22-4 as you answer the following questions.

18. What are the two ways for performing PA axial projections, Caldwell method?

    a. Head tilt technique and vertical IR technique
    b. Head tilt technique and head rotation technique
    c. Angled IR technique and vertical IR technique
    d. Angled IR technique and head rotation technique

19. Regardless of which technique is used for performing the PA axial projection, Caldwell method, which of the following procedures is common for both techniques?

    a. Directing the central ray caudally
    b. Using a vertically placed IR
    c. Use of a horizontally directed central ray
    d. Centering the acanthion to the IR

20. How should the patient's head be positioned when the IR is not vertical?

    a. With the orbitomeatal line (OML) parallel with the central ray
    b. With the infraorbitomeatal line (IOML) parallel with the central ray
    c. With the OML perpendicular to the IR
    d. With the IOML perpendicular to the IR

21. To which positioning landmark of the skull should the IR be centered?

    a. Nasion
    b. Glabella
    c. Acanthion

22. Which sinus structures are primarily demonstrated?

    a. Frontal sinuses and anterior ethmoidal air cells
    b. Frontal sinuses and posterior ethmoidal air cells
    c. Maxillary sinuses and anterior ethmoidal air cells
    d. Maxillary sinuses and posterior ethmoidal air cells

23. Where should the petrous ridges be demonstrated in the image?

    a. Completely filling the orbits
    b. In the lower third of the orbits
    c. Just below the floor of the maxillary sinuses

24. From the following list, circle the eight evaluation criteria that indicate the patient was properly positioned for a PA axial projection, Caldwell method.

    a. The orbital roofs should be superimposed.
    b. The mandibular rami should be superimposed.
    c. The air-fluid levels, if present, are clearly visible.
    d. Close beam restriction of the sinus area is needed.
    e. The petrous ridges should be symmetric on both sides.
    f. All four sinus groups should be clearly demonstrated.
    g. The petrous ridges should lie in the lower one third of the orbits.
    h. The frontal and anterior ethmoidal sinuses should be visualized clearly.
    i. The anterior frontal bone should be superimposed by the mental protuberance.
    j. The petrous ridges should be lying just below the floor of the maxillary sinuses.
    k. The frontal sinuses should lie above the frontonasal suture and be clearly demonstrated.
    l. The anterior ethmoidal air cells above the petrous ridges should be clearly demonstrated.
    m. The distance between the lateral border of the skull and the lateral border of the orbits should be equal.

25. Identify each lettered structure shown in Fig. 22-5.
    A. _frontal sinus_
    B. _ethmoid sinus_
    C. _petrous ridge_
    D. _sphenoid sinus_
    E. _maxillary_

frontal
sinus   A
ethmoid
sella
turcica   B
sinus
Petrous C
ridge
Sphenoid
sinuses   D
              E
maxillary

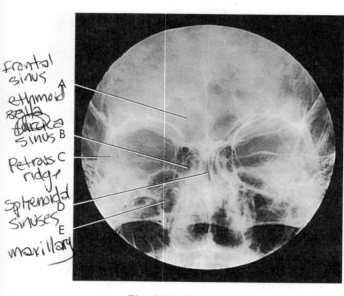

Fig. 22-5 PA axial sinuses.

Items 26 through 37 pertain to the *parietoacanthial projection, Waters method*. Examine Fig. 22-6 as you answer the following questions.

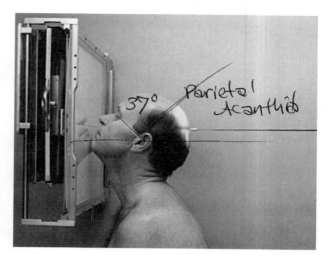

37°   Parietal
      Acanthid

Fig. 22-6 Parietoacanthial sinuses, Waters method.

26. Which paranasal sinuses are best demonstrated with the parietoacanthial projection, Waters method?

    maxillary

27. Where will the petrous ridges probably be demonstrated in the image if the patient does not sufficiently extend the neck?

    S.I with maxillary
    sinuses

28. How will the maxillary sinuses appear in the image—elongated or foreshortened—if the patient extends the neck too much?

foreshortened

29. What positioning line of the head should form an angle of 37 degrees with the plane of the IR?

orbitomeatal

30. What positioning line of the head should be approximately perpendicular to the plane of the IR?

mentomeatal

31. To what facial landmark should the IR be centered?

acanthion

32. With reference to the surrounding structures, where should petrous ridges be demonstrated in the image?

Immediately below the maxillary sinuses

33. Where on the image should the rotundum foramina be demonstrated? _One on each side, inferior 1. sup. to medial aspect of orbital floor 1. superior to the roof of the maxillary sinuses_

34. True or ~~False~~. The patient's nose and forehead should touch the vertical grid device.

35. ~~True~~ or False. The midsagittal plane should be perpendicular to the IR.

36. From the following list, circle the five evaluation criteria that indicate the patient was properly positioned for a parietoacanthial projection, Waters method.

a. The orbital roofs should be superimposed.
b. The mandibular rami should be superimposed.
(c.) The maxillary sinuses should be visualized clearly.
d. The petrous ridges should completely fill the orbits.
(e.) Close beam restriction of the sinus area is needed.
f. The petrous ridges should be lying in the lower third of the orbits.
(g.) The orbits and maxillary sinuses should be symmetric on both sides.
h. The sphenoidal sinuses should be seen projected through the open mouth.
i. The anterior frontal bone should be superimposed by the mental protuberance.
(j.) The petrous pyramids should lie immediately inferior to the floor of the maxillary sinuses.
(k.) The distance from the lateral border of the skull to the lateral border of the orbit should be equal on both sides.

37. Identify each lettered structure shown in Fig. 22-7.

A. _frontal sinus_
B. _ethmoid sinus_
C. _foramen rotundum_
D. _maxillary sinus_
E. _petrous Δ's_
F. _Mastoid air cells_

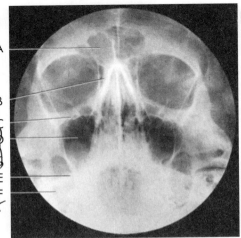

Fig. 22-7 Parietoacanthial sinuses, Waters method.

Items 38 through 42 pertain to the *parietoacanthial projection, open-mouth Waters method*. Examine Fig. 22-8 as you answer the following questions.

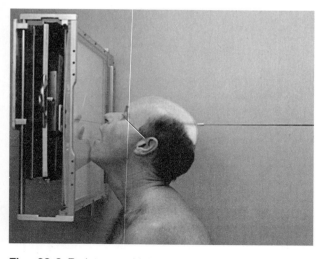

Fig. 22-8 Parietoacanthial sinuses, open-mouth Waters method.

38. To which landmark should the IR be centered?

   acanthion

39. What part of the patient's head should be resting on the vertical grid device?

   chin

40. What positioning line of the skull should form an angle of 37 degrees with the plane of the IR?

   Orbitomeatal

41. Which of the sinuses should be demonstrated in the image through the patient's open mouth?

   Sphenoidal

42. From the following list, circle the six evaluation criteria that indicate the patient was properly positioned for a parietoacanthial projection, open-mouth Waters method.
   a. The orbital roofs should be superimposed.
   b. The mandibular rami should be superimposed.
   c. The maxillary sinuses should be visualized clearly.
   d. The petrous ridges should completely fill the orbits.
   e. Close beam restriction of the sinus area is needed.
   f. The petrous ridges should be lying in the lower third of the orbits.
   g. The orbits and maxillary sinuses should be symmetric on both sides.
   h. The sphenoidal sinuses should be seen projected through the open mouth.
   i. The anterior frontal bone should be superimposed by the mental protuberance.
   j. The petrous pyramids should lie immediately inferior to the floor of the maxillary sinuses.
   k. The distance from the lateral border of the skull to the lateral border of the orbit should be equal on both sides.

Items 43 through 55 pertain to the *SMV projection*. Examine Fig. 22-9 as you answer the following questions.

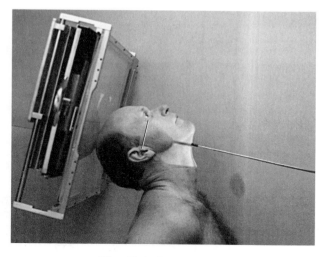

Fig. 22-9 SMV sinuses.

43. True or False. The patient should rest his or her head with the chin contacting the vertical grid device.

   false head on vertex is correct

44. True or False. The OML should be as close to parallel with the IR as possible.

   IOML close to // w/IR As Possvble.

45. True or False. The midsagittal plane should be perpendicular to the IR.

46. True or False. The central ray should be directed perpendicular to the IOML, entering the midline of the base of the skull so that it passes through the sella turcica.

47. True or False. The distance from the lateral border of the skull to the lateral border of the mandibular condyles should be the same on both sides.

48. True or False. The entire occipital bone should be included in the image of the SMV projection to demonstrate paranasal sinuses.

To dem paranasal sinuses close beam atten. to exclud occipital bone

49. What two sinus groups should be well demonstrated with the SMV projection?

sphenoidal & ethmoidal = SMV

50. Where in the image should the mental protuberance appear in relation to the frontal bone?

The mandibular symphysis should superimpose the anterior frontal bone

51. Where in the image should the mandibular condyles appear in relation to the surrounding structures?

Anterior to the petrous ridges

52. What positioning error most likely occurred if the mental protuberance is imaged posterior to, and separated from, the anterior frontal bone?

The IOML was not // to IR because the neck wasn't hyperextended far enough (If CR was correct)

53. What positioning error most likely occurred if the mental protuberance is imaged superior to the anterior frontal bone?

The vertical IR holder was too far tilted to pt or pt neck was extended too far

54. From the following list, circle the three evaluation criteria that indicate the patient was properly positioned for an SMV projection.

a. The orbital roofs should be superimposed.
b. The mandibular rami should be superimposed.
c. The maxillary sinuses should be visualized clearly.
d. The mental protuberance should superimpose the anterior frontal bone.
e. The mandibular condyles should be anterior to the petrous pyramids.
f. The distance from the lateral border of the skull to the mandibular condyles should be equal on both sides.

55. Identify each lettered structure shown in Fig. 22-10.

A. <u>Maxillary Sinus</u>

B. <u>ethmoid air cells</u>

C. <u>Mandible</u>

D. <u>Vomer</u>

E. <u>Sphenoidal Sinus</u>

F. <u>Mandibular condyle</u>

G. <u>Petrosa</u>

Note to Students: Additional exercises referenced from Chapters 20 through 22 are found in the appendix (Supplemental Exercises for Skull Positioning), which is located in this workbook. Students should complete the review exercises for those chapters before completing the appendix exercises.

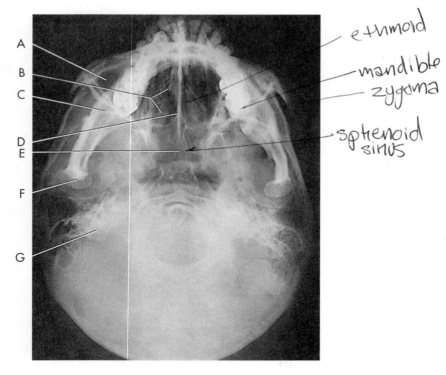

Fig. 22-10 SMV sinuses.

Answer the following questions by selecting the best choice.

1. Which structures should always be radiographed with the patient in an upright position?

   a. Orbits
   b. Mastoids
   c. Zygomatic arches
   d. Paranasal sinuses

2. Which of the following is the only projection for paranasal sinuses that adequately demonstrates all four sinus groups?

   a. Lateral
   b. SMV
   c. PA axial, Caldwell method
   d. Parietoacanthial, Waters method

3. With reference to the outer canthus, where should the central ray be directed for the lateral projections of the sinus?

   a. Inferior
   b. Superior
   c. Anterior
   d. Posterior

4. Which sinus group is of primary importance in the lateral projection of the sinuses?

   a. Frontal
   b. Maxillary
   c. Ethmoidal
   d. Sphenoidal *Sinus*

5. Which sinus groups are best demonstrated with the PA axial projection, Caldwell method?

   a. Frontal and sphenoidal
   b. Frontal and anterior ethmoidal
   c. Maxillary and sphenoidal
   d. Maxillary and anterior ethmoidal

6. For the PA axial projection, Caldwell method, of the sinuses, which positioning line, in addition to the midsagittal plane, should be perpendicular to the IR?

   a. Orbitomeatal
   b. Interpupillary
   c. Glabellomeatal
   d. Infraorbitomeatal

7. Where should petrous ridges be seen in the image of the PA axial projection, Caldwell method, of the sinuses?

   a. Superior to the orbits
   b. Lower third of the orbits
   c. Through the maxillary sinuses
   d. Below the maxillary sinuses

8. Which positioning line should form an angle of 37 degrees with the IR for the parietoacanthial projection, Waters method? *OML*

   a. Orbitomeatal
   b. Glabellomeatal
   c. Acanthiomeatal
   d. Infraorbitomeatal

9. With reference to the IR, how should the central ray be directed for the parietoacanthial projection, Waters method?

   a. Perpendicular
   b. 15 degrees caudad
   c. 23 degrees caudad
   d. 37 degrees caudad

10. Which paranasal sinus group is best demonstrated with the parietoacanthial projection, Waters method? *Waters for Maxillary sinus*

    a. Frontal
    b. Maxillary
    c. Ethmoidal
    d. Sphenoidal

11. Where should the petrous ridges be seen in the image of the parietoacanthial projection, Waters method, of the paranasal sinuses?

    a. Superior to the orbits
    b. Lower third of the orbits
    c. Through the maxillary sinuses
    d. Below the maxillary sinuses

12. Where should the central ray exit the head for the parietoacanthial projection, Waters method?

    a. Nasion
    b. Glabella
    c. Acanthion
    d. Mental point

13. Which sinus group is not well demonstrated in the image produced by the parietoacanthial projection, Waters method?

    a. Frontal
    b. Maxillary
    c. Ethmoidal
    d. Sphenoidal

14. Which two paranasal sinus groups are better demonstrated with the SMV projection than are the other sinuses? *SMV for ethmoidal sphenoidal*

    a. Frontal and maxillary
    b. Frontal and sphenoidal
    c. Ethmoidal and maxillary
    d. Ethmoidal and sphenoidal

15. Which projection of the sinuses demonstrates a symmetric image of the anterior portion of the base of the skull?

    a. Lateral
    b. SMV
    c. PA axial, Caldwell method
    d. Parietoacanthial, Waters method

16. In which projection of the sinuses is the IR centered to the nasion?

    a. Lateral
    b. SMV
    c. PA axial, Caldwell method
    d. Parietoacanthial, Waters method

CR @ Nasion = Caldwell

17. In which projection of the sinuses is the mentomeatal line approximately perpendicular to the plane of the IR?

    a. Lateral
    b. SMV
    c. PA axial, Caldwell method
    d. Parietoacanthial, Waters method

MML ⊥ to IR (Waters)

18. In which projection of the sinuses must the OML form an angle of 15 degrees with the plane of the IR?

    a. Lateral
    b. SMV
    c. PA axial, Caldwell method
    d. Parietoacanthial, Waters method

19. Which evaluation criterion pertains to the lateral projection of the paranasal sinuses?

    a. All four sinus groups should be included.
    b. The petrous pyramids should lie in the lower third of the orbits.
    c. The mental protuberance should superimpose the anterior frontal bone.
    d. The petrous pyramids should lie immediately below the floor of the maxillary sinuses.

20. Which evaluation criterion pertains to the lateral projection of the paranasal sinuses?

    a. The orbital roofs should be superimposed.
    b. The petrous ridges should lie in the lower third of the orbits.
    c. The mandibular condyles should be anterior to the petrous ridges.
    d. The mental protuberance should superimpose the anterior frontal bone.

21. Which evaluation criterion pertains to the PA axial projection, Caldwell method, of the sinuses?

    a. All four sinus groups should be included.
    b. The frontal and ethmoidal sinuses should be seen.
    c. The mandibular condyles should be anterior to the petrous ridges.
    d. The petrous ridges should lie immediately below the floor of the maxillary sinuses.

22. Which evaluation criterion pertains to the PA axial projection, Caldwell method, for sinuses?

    a. Orbital roofs should be superimposed.
    b. Mandibular rami should be superimposed.
    c. Petrous ridges should lie in the lower third of the orbits.
    d. Petrous ridges should lie immediately below the floor of the maxillary sinuses.

23. Which evaluation criterion pertains to the parietoacanthial projection, Waters method, for paranasal sinuses?

    a. Mandibular rami should be superimposed.
    b. Petrous ridges should lie in the lower third of the orbits.
    c. Mental protuberance should superimpose anterior frontal bone.
    d. Petrous ridges should lie immediately below the floor of the maxillary sinuses.

24. Which evaluation criterion pertains to the SMV projection for paranasal sinuses?

    a. Mandibular rami should be superimposed.
    b. Frontal and ethmoidal sinuses should be clearly seen.
    c. Mental protuberance should superimpose anterior frontal bone.
    d. Petrous ridges should lie immediately below the floor of the maxillary sinuses.

25. Which evaluation criterion pertains to the SMV projection for sinuses?

    a. Petrous ridges should lie in the lower third of the orbits.
    b. Mandibular condyles should be anterior to the petrous ridges.
    c. Mandibular condyles should be posterior to the petrous ridges.
    d. Petrous ridges should lie immediately below the floor of the maxillary sinuses.

ANATOMY AND PHYSIOLOGY OF THE BREAST

Exercise 1

This exercise pertains to the anatomy of the breast. Identify structures for each illustration.

1. Identify each lettered structure shown in Fig. 23-1.

A. _____

B. _____

C. _____

D. _____

2. Identify each lettered structure shown in Fig. 23-2.

A. _____

B. _____

C. _____

D. _____

E. _____

F. _____

G. _____

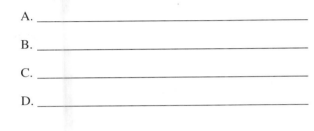

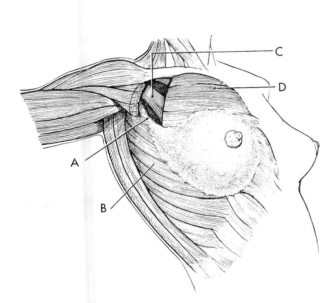

Fig. 23-1 Relationship of the breast to the chest wall.

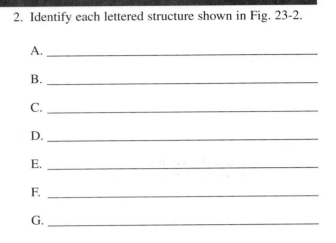

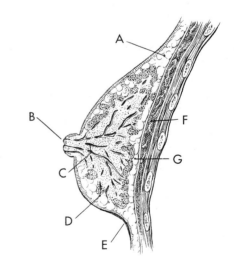

Fig. 23-2 Sagittal section through the breast illustrating structural anatomy.

Exercise 2

1. Another term for the female breast is the

   _____ gland.

2. The female breast functions as an accessory gland to the reproductive system by producing and secreting

   _____.

3. The axillary prolongation of the breast is also called

   the axillary _____.

4. The posterior surface of the breast overlying the

   muscles is the _____.

5. The female breast tapers anteriorly from the base,

   ending in the _____.

6. The circular area of pigmented skin that surrounds

   the nipple is the _____.

7. The adult female breast contains _____

   to _____ lobes.

8. The glandular elements found in the lobules of the

   female are the _____.

9. As a female gets older, the size of her breast lobules

   becomes _____.

10. The normal process of change in breast tissues that

    occurs as the patient ages is termed _____.

11. Normal involution replaces glandular and parenchymal

    tissues with increased amounts of _____.

12. The ducts that drain milk from the lobes are the

    _____ ducts.

13. Another term for the suspensory ligaments of the

    breast is _____ ligaments.

14. Approximately 75% of the lymph drainage is toward

    the _____.

15. The internal mammary lymph nodes are situated

    behind the _____.

Exercise 3

Match the pathology terms in Column A with the appropriate definition in Column B. Not all choices from Column B should be selected.

Column A

_____ 1. Cyst

_____ 2. Tumor

_____ 3. Fibrosis

_____ 4. Carcinoma

_____ 5. Calcification

_____ 6. Fibroadenoma

_____ 7. Intraductal papilloma

_____ 8. Epithelial hyperplasia

Column B

a. Narrowing or contraction of a passage

b. Formation of fibrous tissue in the breast

c. Proliferation of the epithelium of the breast

d. A benign, neoplastic papillary growth in a duct

e. Malignant new growth composed of epithelial cells

f. Benign tumor of the breast containing fibrous elements

g. New tissue growth in which cell proliferation is uncontrolled

h. Closed epithelial sac containing fluid or a semisolid substance

i. Deposit of calcium salt in tissue; characteristics may suggest either benign or malignant processes

RADIOGRAPHY OF THE BREAST

Exercise 1

Mammography is used to demonstrate diseases of the breast. This exercise pertains to mammographic procedures. Provide a short answer or select from a list for each question.

1. Why should the breast be bared for the examination?

2. Why should the patient remove deodorant and powder from the axilla?

3. Name the two standard projections routinely performed to demonstrate the breast.

4. What condition requires that a nipple marker be placed on the patient?

5. What procedure should a radiographer perform to help produce uniform breast thickness?

6. What procedure should a radiographer perform to identify the location of a palpable mass?

7. Why should the posterior nipple line be measured and compared between two projections?

8. Between what two structures should the posterior nipple line be measured in craniocaudal projections?

9. What is the maximum difference for the length of the posterior nipple line when comparing images of craniocaudal and mediolateral oblique projections?

10. Between examinations, what should a radiographer do to the image receptor (IR) surface and face guard?

Exercise 2

Identify each of the following four illustrations of mammography projections by selecting the best choice from the list provided for each illustration.

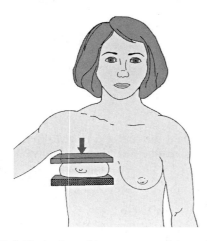

Fig. 23-3 Illustration of a mammographic projection.

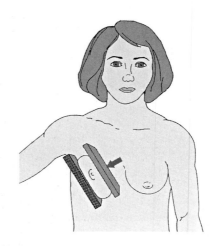

Fig. 23-5 Illustration of a mammographic projection.

1. Fig. 23-3

    a. Craniocaudal
    b. Mediolateral
    c. Mediolateral oblique
    d. Exaggerated craniocaudal

3. Fig. 23-5

    a. Craniocaudal
    b. Mediolateral
    c. Mediolateral oblique
    d. Exaggerated craniocaudal

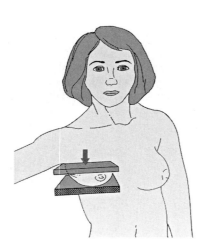

Fig. 23-4 Illustration of a mammographic projection.

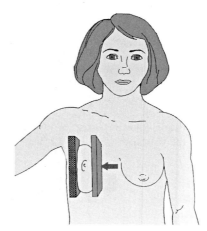

Fig. 23-6 Illustration of a mammographic projection.

2. Fig. 23-4

    a. Craniocaudal
    b. Mediolateral
    c. Mediolateral oblique
    d. Exaggerated craniocaudal

4. Fig. 23-6

    a. Craniocaudal
    b. Mediolateral
    c. Mediolateral oblique
    d. Exaggerated craniocaudal

Exercise 3

Items 1 through 10 are statements that refer to mammography positioning procedures. Examine each statement in Column A and identify the mammography projection from Column B that most closely relates to the statement. Some statements pertain to more than one projection.

Column A

_____ 1. The breast should be perpendicular to the chest wall.

_____ 2. Slowly apply compression until the breast feels taut.

_____ 3. Elevate the inframammary fold to its maximum height.

_____ 4. Direct the central ray perpendicular to the base of the breast.

_____ 5. Direct the central ray 5 degrees mediolaterally to the base of the breast.

_____ 6. Instruct the patient to stand or be seated facing the IR holder.

_____ 7. Rotate the C-arm to direct the central ray to the medial side of the breast.

_____ 8. Adjust the height of the IR to the level of the inferior surface of the breast.

_____ 9. Adjust the height of the IR so that the superior border is level with the axilla.

_____ 10. Pull the breast tissue superiorly and anteriorly, ensuring that the lateral rib margin is firmly pressed against the IR.

Column B

a. Mediolateral

b. Craniocaudal

c. Mediolateral oblique

d. Exaggerated craniocaudal

Exercise 4

Items 1 through 8 are statements that refer to structures that are demonstrated with various mammography projections. Examine each statement in Column A and identify the mammography projection from Column B that most closely relates to the statement.

Column A

_____ 1. Demonstrates air-fluid and fat-fluid levels in breast structures.

_____ 2. Resolves superimposed structures seen on the mediolateral oblique projection.

_____ 3. Demonstrates the pectoral muscle approximately 30% of the time.

_____ 4. Demonstrates all breast tissue with emphasis on the lateral aspect and axillary tail.

_____ 5. The central, subareolar, and medial fibroglandular breast tissue should be demonstrated.

_____ 6. Demonstrates lesions on the lateral aspect of the breast in the superior or inferior aspects.

_____ 7. Demonstrates a sagittal orientation of a lateral lesion located in the axillary tail of the breast.

_____ 8. Demonstrates a superoinferior projection of the lateral fibroglandular breast tissue and posterior aspect of the pectoral muscle.

Column B

a. Mediolateral

b. Craniocaudal

c. Mediolateral oblique

d. Exaggerated craniocaudal

Answer the following questions by selecting the best choice.

1. The lymphatic vessels of the breast drain laterally into which of the following lymph nodes?

   a. Axillary
   b. Thoracic
   c. Abdominal
   d. Internal mammary chain

2. Where is the tail of the breast located?

   a. Adjacent to the nipple
   b. Along the lateral side to the axilla
   c. Along the medial aspect of the breast
   d. In the glandular tissue against the chest wall

3. Which ducts drain milk from the lobes of the breast?

   a. Axillary
   b. Thoracic
   c. Lymphatic
   d. Lactiferous

4. How do breast tissues change after involution?

   a. Glandular tissues become dense and opaque.
   b. Parenchymal tissues become dense and opaque.
   c. Fatty tissues are replaced with glandular tissues.
   d. Glandular tissues are replaced with fatty tissues.

5. Which two projections comprise the standard examination for demonstrating the breasts?

   a. Craniocaudal and lateromedial
   b. Craniocaudal and mediolateral oblique
   c. Caudocranial and lateromedial
   d. Caudocranial and mediolateral oblique

6. Which projection requires that the central ray pass through the breast at an angle of 30 to 60 degrees?

   a. Axillary
   b. Caudocranial
   c. Craniocaudal
   d. Mediolateral oblique

7. Which muscle is often demonstrated with the craniocaudal projection?

   a. Pectoralis major
   b. Serratus anterior
   c. Rectus abdominis
   d. Lateral abdominal oblique

8. What is the primary objective of compressing the breast for mammography?

   a. To reduce exposure time
   b. To decrease geometric distortion
   c. To produce uniform breast thickness
   d. To produce uniform radiographic density

9. Where should the radiopaque marker, used to indicate which side is being examined, be seen on the image of craniocaudal projections?

   a. On the nipple
   b. On the chest wall
   c. Along the lateral side of the breast
   d. Along the medial side of the breast

10. How should a radiographer identify the location of a palpable mass?

    a. Draw a circle around the mass on the resultant mammogram.
    b. Use an ink marker to draw a circle on the skin overlying the mass.
    c. Place a radiopaque marker such as a BB on the breast overlying the mass.
    d. Place a radiopaque arrow marker alongside the breast to point to the mass.

11. What is the maximum difference for the length of the posterior nipple line when comparing images of craniocaudal and mediolateral oblique projections?

    a. 0.5 cm
    b. 1.0 cm
    c. 1.5 cm
    d. 2.0 cm

12. Between which two projections should the posterior nipple lines be measured and compared?

    a. Craniocaudal and mediolateral oblique
    b. Craniocaudal and 90-degree mediolateral
    c. Exaggerated craniocaudal and mediolateral oblique
    d. Exaggerated craniocaudal and 90-degree mediolateral

13. In which body position should the patient be placed for craniocaudal or mediolateral oblique projections?

    a. Prone
    b. Supine
    c. Upright
    d. Lateral recumbent

14. Which projection demonstrates all breast tissue with an emphasis on the lateral aspect and axillary tail?

    a. Mediolateral
    b. Craniocaudal
    c. Mediolateral oblique
    d. Exaggerated craniocaudal

15. Which projection requires that the central ray be moved to a horizontal position?

    a. Mediolateral
    b. Craniocaudal
    c. Mediolateral oblique
    d. Exaggerated craniocaudal

24 Central Nervous System

SECTION 1

ANATOMY OF THE CENTRAL NERVOUS SYSTEM

This exercise pertains to the anatomic structures of the central nervous system (CNS). Identify structures, fill in missing words, or provide a short answer for each item.

1. Identify each lettered structure shown in Fig. 24-1.

   A. _____

   B. _____

   C. _____

   D. _____

   E. _____

   F. _____

   G. _____

   H. _____

2. Identify each lettered structure shown in Fig. 24-2.

   A. _____

   B. _____

   C. _____

   D. _____

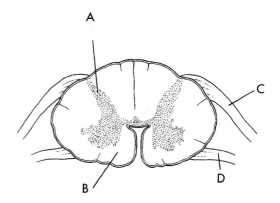

Fig. 24-2 Transverse section of the spinal cord.

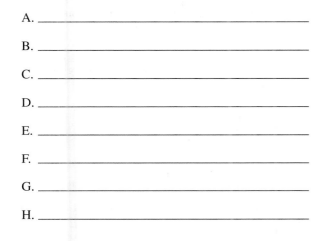

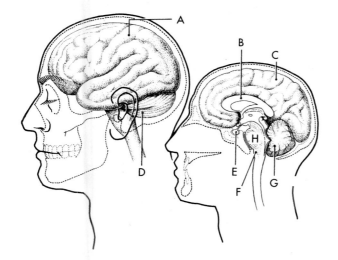

Fig. 24-1 Lateral surface and midsection of the brain.

201

3. Identify each lettered structure shown in Fig. 24-3.

A. _____

B. _____

C. _____

D. _____

4. Identify each lettered structure shown in Fig. 24-4.

A. _____

B. _____

C. _____

D. _____

E. _____

F. _____

G. _____

H. _____

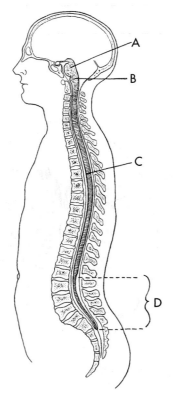

Fig. 24-3 Sagittal section showing the spinal cord.

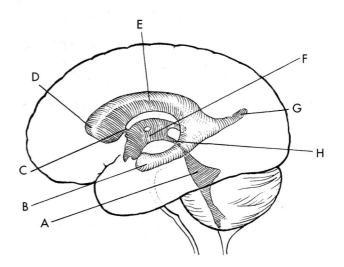

Fig. 24-4 Lateral aspect of the cerebral ventricles in relation to the surface of the brain.

5. Identify each lettered structure shown in Fig. 24-5.

A. _____

B. _____

C. _____

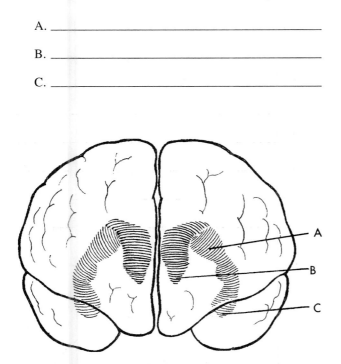

Fig. 24-5 Anterior aspect of the lateral cerebral ventricles in relation to the surface of the brain.

6. Identify each lettered structure shown in Fig. 24-6.

A. _____

B. _____

C. _____

D. _____

E. _____

F. _____

G. _____

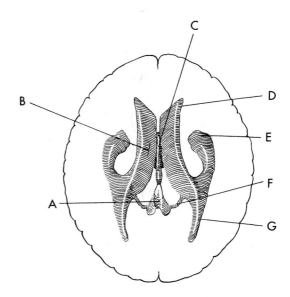

Fig. 24-6 Superior aspect of the cerebral ventricles in relation to the surface of the brain.

203

7. Name the two main parts of the CNS.

8. Name the three parts of the brain.

9. Name the four parts of the brain stem.

10. Name the three parts of the hindbrain.

11. The largest part of the brain is the _____.

12. Another name for the cerebrum is the

_____.

13. The stemlike portion of the brain that connects the

cerebrum to the hindbrain is the _____.

14. The deep cleft that separates the cerebrum into right

and left hemispheres is the _____

_____.

15. Another name for the hypophysis cerebri is

_____.

16. The largest part of the hindbrain is the

_____.

17. The portion of the hindbrain that connects the pons

to the spinal cord is the _____

_____.

18. The protective membranes that enclose the brain and

spinal cord are the _____.

19. The membrane that closely adheres to the brain and

spinal cord is the _____.

20. The outermost membrane that forms the tough
fibrous covering for the brain and spinal cord is the

_____.

21. The two uppermost ventricles are called the right and

left _____ventricles.

22. The lateral ventricles are located in the portion of the

brain called the _____.

23. Each lateral ventricle communicates with the third

ventricle by way of the _____
foramen.

24. Another name for the interventricular foramen is the

foramen of _____.

25. What are the two names for the passage between the
third and fourth ventricles?

RADIOGRAPHY OF THE CENTRAL NERVOUS SYSTEM

This exercise pertains to examinations that demonstrate CNS structures. Provide a short answer for each item.

1. Define *myelography*.

2. Identify three common sites for the injection of the contrast medium during myelography.

3. What abnormality is demonstrated using myelography?

4. What type or group of contrast media is preferred for myelography? Explain why.

5. When the exposure room is prepared for myelography, why should the spot-filming device be locked in place?

6. What should be done to reduce patient apprehension?

7. What are the two body positions most frequently used when the contrast medium is injected for myelography?

8. During myelography, what procedure is used to control the movement of the contrast medium after its injection?

9. During myelography, why should the patient hyperextend the neck?

10. When a traumatized patient with possible CNS involvement is radiographed, what radiograph should be the first one made?

205

Answer the following questions by selecting the best choice.

1. Which two structures comprise the CNS?

   a. Brain and cerebellum
   b. Brain and spinal cord
   c. Cerebrum and cerebellum
   d. Cerebrum and spinal cord

2. Which part of the brain is also referred to as the forebrain?

   a. Pons
   b. Cerebrum
   c. Cerebellum
   d. Diencephalon

3. Which three parts of the CNS comprise the hindbrain?

   a. Cerebrum, cerebellum, and spinal cord
   b. Cerebrum, pons, and medulla oblongata
   c. Pons, cerebellum, and medulla oblongata
   d. Pons, spinal cord, and medulla oblongata

4. Which cerebral structure is the largest part of the brain?

   a. Pons
   b. Cerebrum
   c. Cerebellum
   d. Medulla oblongata

5. Which structure is divided into right and left hemispheres by the longitudinal fissure?

   a. Pons
   b. Cerebrum
   c. Cerebellum
   d. Medulla oblongata

6. What other term refers to the hypophysis cerebri?

   a. Pituitary gland
   b. Medulla spinalis
   c. Corpus callosum
   d. Conus medullaris

7. Which membrane forms the tough, fibrous outer covering for the meninges?

   a. Pia mater
   b. Arachnoid
   c. Dura mater

8. Which vessel connects the lateral ventricles to the third ventricle?

   a. Cerebral aqueduct
   b. Foramen of Luschka
   c. Foramen of Magendie
   d. Interventricular foramen

9. In which part of the brain is the fourth ventricle found?

   a. Midbrain
   b. Forebrain
   c. Hindbrain

10. Which projection should be the first radiograph for a traumatized patient with possible CNS involvement?

    a. AP axial
    b. AP oblique
    c. Upright lateral
    d. Cross-table lateral

11. Which examination is performed to demonstrate the contour of the subarachnoid space?

    a. Diskography
    b. Myelography
    c. Ventriculography
    d. Pneumonography

12. For which examination is the contrast medium injected directly into the fibrous cartilage between two vertebral bodies?

    a. Diskography
    b. Myelography
    c. Ventriculography
    d. Pneumonography

13. Which examination can be used to evaluate the dynamic flow pattern of cerebral spinal fluid?

    a. Diskography
    b. Myelography
    c. Ventriculography
    d. Pneumonography

14. During myelography, which procedure should be performed to prevent contrast medium from entering the cerebral ventricles?

    a. Tilt the head of the table down.
    b. Instruct the patient to hyperflex the neck.
    c. Place the patient in the lateral recumbent position.
    d. Have the patient hyperextend the neck.

15. What is the purpose of tilting the table during myelography?

    a. To attach the footboard
    b. To facilitate patient comfort
    c. To control the flow of contrast medium
    d. To remove cerebral spinal fluid from the patient

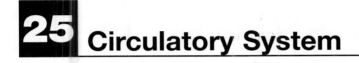

25 Circulatory System

ANATOMY OF THE CIRCULATORY SYSTEM

Exercise 1

This exercise pertains to the anatomy of the circulatory system. Identify structures for each item.

1 Identify each lettered structure shown in Fig. 25-1.

A. superior saggital sinus

B. transverse sinus

C. internal jugular vein

D. right subclavian artery & vein

E. superior vena cava

F. brachial artery and cephalic basilic vein

G. celiac axis

H. portal vein

I. renal artery and vein

J. superior mesenteric artery & vein

K. common illiac artery and vein

L. common femoral artery & vein

M. popiteal artery

N. anterior tibial artery

O. posterior tibial artery

P. anterior facial artery & vein

Q. common carotid artery

R. aortic arch

S. pulmonary artery & vein

T. aorta

U. inferior vena cava

V. inferior mesenteric vein

W. radial artery & cephalic vein

X. ulnar artery & basilic vein

Y. deep femoral artery

Z. superficial femoral artery

AA. popiteal vein

BB. large saphenous vein

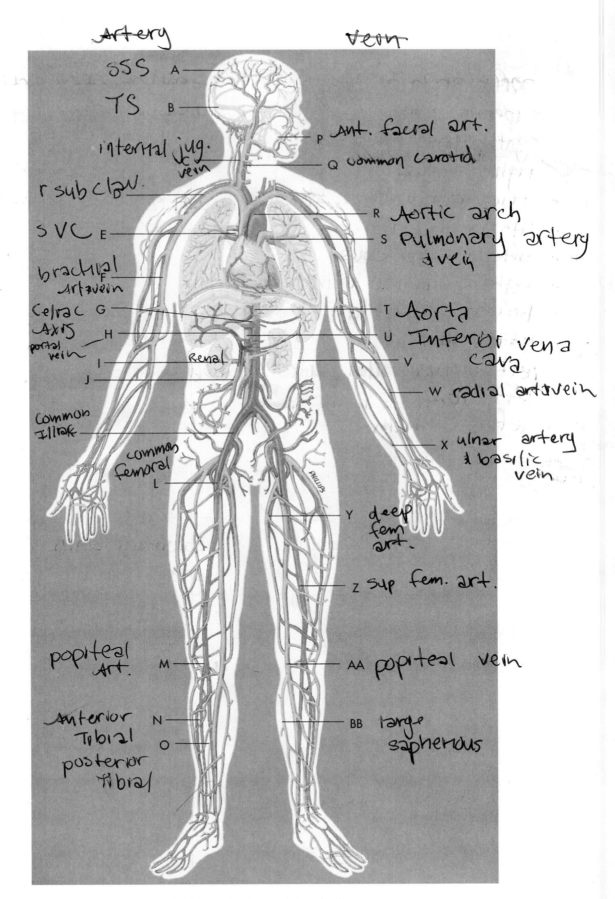

Artery   Vein

SSS   A

TS   B

                                                P Ant. facial art.

internal jug.   Q common carotid
vein

r subclav.

                                                R Aortic arch
SVC   E   S Pulmonary artery
                                                   & vein
brachial   F
art & vein
celiac   G   T Aorta
axis
                H   U Inferior vena
portal   cava
vein   I
        J   Renal   V

                                                W radial art & vein

common
iliac
                                                X ulnar artery
common   & basilic
femoral   vein
        L

                                                Y deep
                                                   fem
                                                   art.

                                                Z sup fem. art.

popiteal   AA popiteal vein
Art.   M

Anterior   N   BB large
Tibial   saphenous
        O
posterior
Tibial

Fig. 25-1 Major arteries and veins.

2. Identify each lettered structure shown in Fig. 25-2.

A. aortic arch

B. superior vena cava

C. right pulmonary artery

D. right antrum

E. tricuspid valve (r. atrioventricular)

F. right ventricle

G. inferior vena cava

H. right pulmonar veins

I. desending aorta

J. left ventricle

K. left atrioventricular (mitral/bicuspid)

L. left lung

M. left antrum

3. Identify each lettered structure shown in Fig. 25-3.

A. right coronary artery

B. left coronary artery

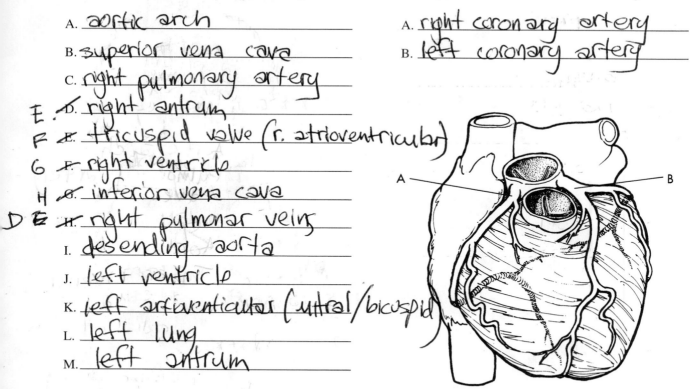

Fig. 25-3 Anterior view of the coronary arteries.

4. Identify each lettered structure shown in Fig. 25-4.

A. coronary sinus

B. great cardiac vein

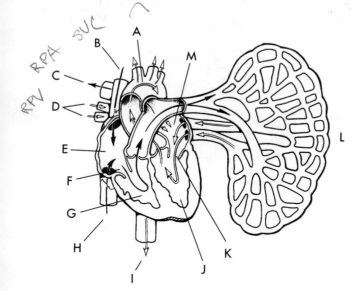

Fig. 25-2 The heart and greater vessels. Black arrows indicate deoxygenated blood flow. White arrows indicate oxygenated blood flow.

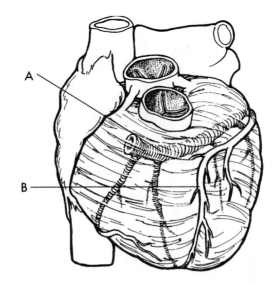

Fig. 25-4 Anterior view of the coronary veins.

5. Identify each lettered structure shown in Fig. 25-5.

A. capillaries

B. lungs

C. r. atrium

D. r. ventricle

E. liver

F. intestine

G. aorta

H. L. atrium

I. L. ventricle

J. stomach

K. spleen

L. pancreas

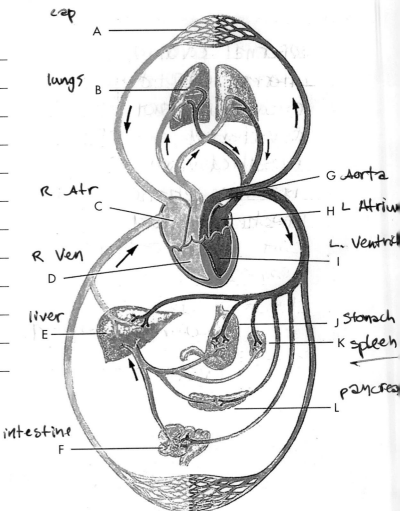

Fig. 25-5 The pulmonary, systemic, and portal circulation.

6. Identify each lettered structure shown in Fig. 25-6.

A. external carotid
B. internal carotid
C. r. common carotid
D. r. vertebral artery
E. r. subclavian
F. brachiocephalic artery
G. brachial artery

H. radial artery
I. ulnar artery
J. left subclavian artery
K. l. vertebral artery
L. l. common carotid artery
M. thyroid

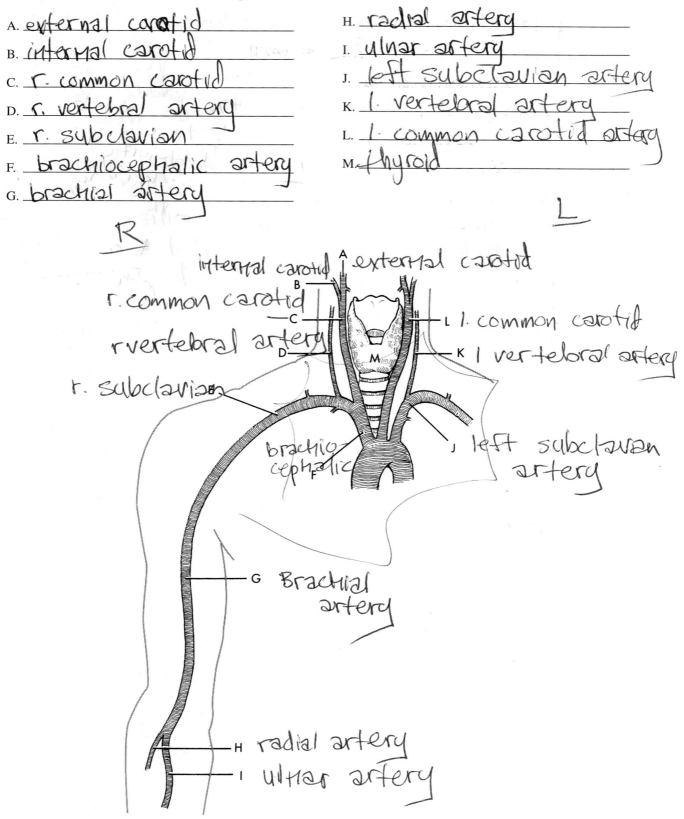

Fig. 25-6 Major arteries of the upper chest, neck, and arm.

7. Identify each lettered structure shown in Fig. 25-7.

A. _anterior communicating cerebral artery_

B. _posterior communicating artery_

C. _anterior cerebral artery_

D. _middle cerebral artery_

E. _internal carotid artery_

F. _posterior cerebral artery_

G. _basilar artery_

H. _vertebral artery_

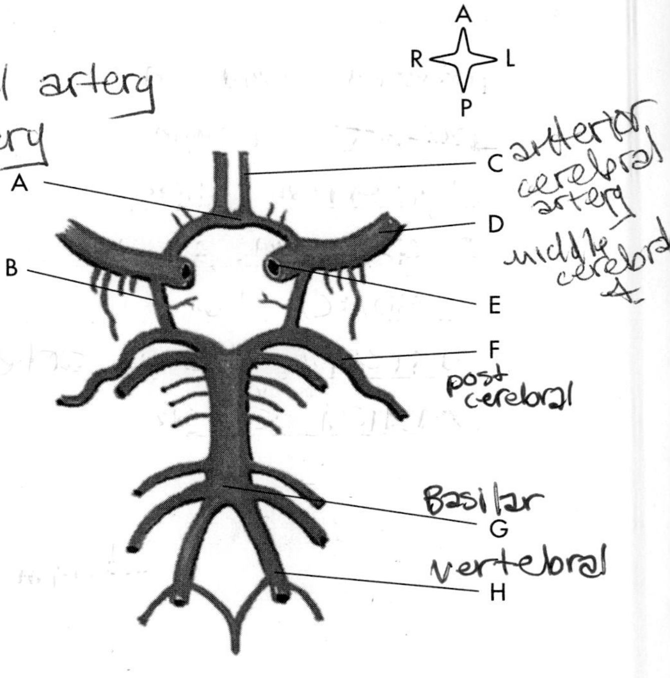

Fig. 25-7 Circle of Willis. (From Thibodeau GA, Patton KP: *Anatomy and physiology*, ed 6, St Louis, 2007, Mosby.)

8. Identify each lettered structure shown in Fig. 25-8.

A. inferior vena cava

B. posterior common illiac artery

C. external iliac artery

D. deep femoral artery

E. popliteal artery

F. anterior tibial artery

G. Abdominal aorta

H. Internal iliac artery

I. femoral artery

J. dorsalis pedis artery

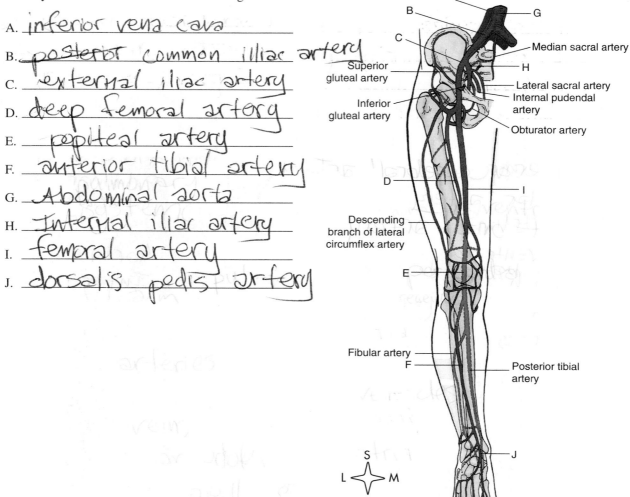

Fig. 25-8 Major arteries of the lower limb. (From Thibodeau GA, Patton KP: *Anatomy and physiology*, ed 6, St Louis, 2007, Mosby.)

9. Identify each lettered structure show in Fig. 25-9.

A. axillary nodes

B. common iliac artery

C. anterior

D. cervical nodes

E. thoracic ducts

F. lumbar nodes

G. superior inguinal nodes

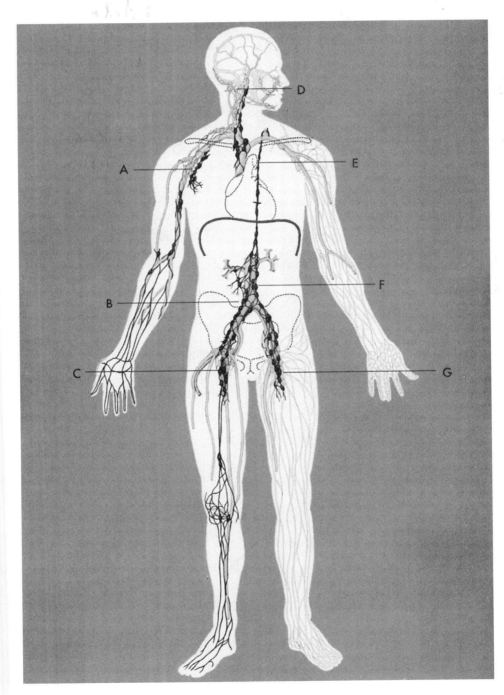

Fig. 25-9 The lymphatic system.

Exercise 2

This exercise is a comprehensive review of the circulatory system. Fill in missing words for each item.

1. The circulatory system comprises two systems of related vessels, the _blood vascular_ system and the _lymphatic_ system.

2. The two systems that comprise the blood-vascular system are _pulmonary_ circulation and _systemic_ circulation.

3. The system that traverses the lungs to discharge carbon dioxide and take up oxygen is _pulmon_ _____ circulation.

4. The vessels that carry blood away from the heart are collectively called _arteries_.

5. The vessels that carry blood back toward the heart are collectively called _veins_.

6. Arteries subdivide to form _arterioles_.

7. Arterioles subdivide to form _capillaries_

8. Capillaries unite to form _venules_.

9. The beginning branches for veins are _venules_.

10. Blood is transported to the left atrium by _pulmonary_ veins.

11. The major vein that returns blood from the upper parts of the body to the heart is the _superior vena cava_.

12. The major vein that returns blood from the lower parts of the body to the heart is the _inferior vena cava_.

13. The muscular wall of the heart is the _myocardium_.

14. The membrane that lines the chambers of the heart is the _endocardium_.

15. The membrane that covers the heart is the _epicardium_.

16. The chamber of the heart where the myocardium is the thickest is the _L. ventricle_.

17. The space between the two walls of the pericardial sac is the _pericardial cavity_.

18. The two upper chambers of the heart are the receiving _atria_.

19. The two lower chambers of the heart are the _ventricles_.

20. The receiving (upper) chambers of the heart are the _atria_.

21. The distributing chambers of the heart are the _ventricles_.

22. Another name for the right atrioventricular valve is the _tricuspid_ valve.

23. Two other terms that refer to the left atrioventricular valve are the _mitral_ valve and the _bicuspid_ valve.

24. The side of the heart that pumps venous (deoxygenated) blood is the _right_ (right or left) side.

25. The side of the heart that pumps arterial (oxygenated) blood is the _left_ (right or left) side.

26. The chamber of the heart that pumps blood through the aortic valve is the __l. ventricle__ .

27. The vessels that supply blood to the myocardium are the right and left __coronary__ arteries.

28. The coronary sinus receives blood from the __cardiac__ veins.

29. The coronary sinus empties blood into the __right__ (right or left) atrium.

30. The great vessel that arises from the left ventricle to transport blood to the body is the __aorta__ .

31. The abdominal aorta divides into the right and left common __iliac__ arteries.

32. The external iliac artery enters the lower limb and becomes the __femoral__ artery.

33. The femoral artery passes blood into the __popiteal__ artery.

34. The popliteal artery bifurcates into the anterior and posterior __tibial__ arteries.

35. The vessel that drains blood into the liver is the __portal__ vein.

36. The vessels that drain blood from the liver are the __hepatic__ veins.

37. Hepatic veins transport blood to the __inferior vena cava__ .

38. The large vessel that arises from the right atrium is the __pulmonary__ artery.

39. The only arteries of the body that transport deoxygenated blood are the __pulmonary__ arteries.

40. The only veins of the body that transport oxygenated blood are the __pulmonary__ veins.

41. The contraction phase of the heart is called the __systole__ .

42. The relaxation phase of the heart is called the __diastole__ .

43. The four arteries that supply the brain are the right and left __common carotid__ arteries and the right and left __vertebral__ arteries.

44. Of the four trunk arteries that supply the brain, the one that arises directly from the arch of the aorta is the __left common carotid__ artery.

45. The right and left vertebral arteries arise from the __subclavian__ arteries.

46. The right and left vertebral arteries unite to form the __basilar__ artery.

47. Each common carotid artery bifurcates into the __internal__ and __external__ carotid arteries.

48. Each internal carotid artery bifurcates into anterior and middle __cerebral__ arteries.

49. The basilar artery bifurcates into the right and left __posterior cerebral__ arteries.

50. Blood is drained from the head by the __jugular__ veins.

51. To reach the right subclavian artery, blood passes from the aorta through the _brachiocephalic_ artery.

52. Blood passes from the brachiocephalic artery to the right _subclavian_ artery.

53. A subclavian artery supplies blood to the axillary artery and then to the _brachial_ artery.

54. The brachial arteries bifurcate into the _radial_ and _ulnar_ arteries.

55. The part of the body in which the cephalic vein originates is the _forearm_.

56. The renal arteries arise from the _aorta_.

57. The circle of Willis is located within the _brain_.

58. The central organ of the blood–vascular system is the _heart_.

59. The main terminal trunk of the lymphatic system is the _thoracic_ duct.

60. The thoracic duct drains its contents at the junction of the left _subclavian_ vein and the internal _jugular._ vein.

RADIOGRAPHY OF THE CIRCULATORY SYSTEM

This exercise pertains to various radiographic examinations for the circulatory system. Because many of these procedures are dependent on the preferences of the radiologist, most of the following exercise items are general in content rather than emphasizing a specific procedure. Identify structures, fill in missing words, select from a list, or provide a short answer for each item.

1. List four reasons that catheterization is preferred over direct injection of the contrast medium through a needle.

   The risk of extravasion is reduced, most body parts can be reached for selective injection, pt can be pos. as needed, the catheter may be left in the body

2. The most widely used method of catheterization is

   the ___seldinger___ technique.

3. The preferred site for insertion of the catheter for most

   selective angiography is the ___femoral___
   artery.

4. What is the purpose of side holes near the tip of the catheter?

   a. To draw fluid into the catheter
   (b.) To reduce whiplash, stabilizing the catheter
   c. To maintain positive pressure inside the catheter

5. From the following list, circle the three symptoms of a vasovagal reaction that are caused by the injection of the contrast medium.

   a. Hives
   (b.) Nausea
   (c.) Sweating
   d. Difficult breathing
   e. Increase in pulse rate
   f. Increase in blood pressure
   (g.) Decrease in blood pressure

6. From the following list, circle the three symptoms of shock.

   a. Low pulse rate
   (b.) High pulse rate
   c. Rapid breathing
   (d.) Shallow breathing
   (e.) Loss of consciousness
   f. Rise in body temperature

7. What treatment should be given to patients experiencing low blood pressure because of a vasovagal reaction?

   1. elevate pt's legs
   2. give IV fluids

8. In preparation for angiography, why should the patient be instructed not to consume solid food?

   To reduce the pt's possibility for aspiration of vomitus

9. In preparation for angiography, why should the patient be allowed to drink clear liquids?

   To saturate the kidneys & minimize damage from ~~ionized~~ ionated contrast media

10. For thoracic aortography, to which vertebra should the perpendicular central ray be directed?

     T6

11. Identify each lettered structure shown in Fig. 25-10.

A. braciocephalic artery

B. ascending artery aorta

C. r coronary artery

D. intercostal artery

E. L common coratid artery

F. L subclavian artery

G. L coronary artery

H. descending thoracic aorta.

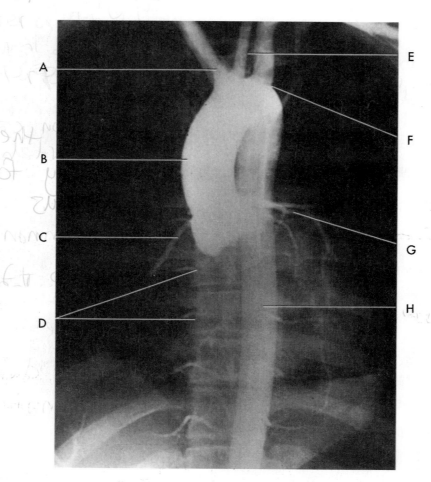

Fig. 25-10 AP thoracic aortogram.

12. How much of the aorta should be imaged for abdominal aortography?

from the diapragm to the aortic bifurcation

13. For abdominal aortography, which projection of the abdominal aorta—anteroposterior (AP) or lateral—best demonstrates the celiac and superior mesenteric artery origins?

lateral abdomen best dem superior mesenteric artery orgins

14. Identify each lettered structure shown in Fig. 25-11.

A. *hepatic*
B. *right renal*
C. *right common iliac artery*
D. *splenic artery*
E. *left renal artery*
F. *abdominal*

15. Identify each lettered structure shown in Fig. 25-12.

A. *celiac axis*
B. *superior mesenteric artery*
C. *abdominal aorta*

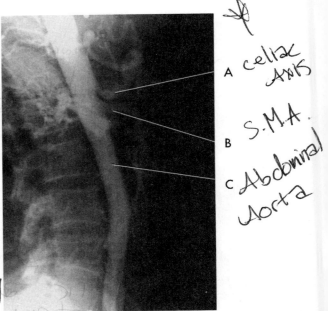

Fig. 25-12 Lateral abdominal aortogram.

A celiac Axis
B S.M.A.
C Abdominal Aorta

16. For pulmonary arteriography, which projection—AP or lateral—should use a compensating (trough) filter to obtain a radiograph with more uniform density between the vertebrae and the lungs?

AP

17. All radiographs for selective abdominal visceral arteriography should be exposed when the patient has suspended *expiration* (inspiration or expiration).

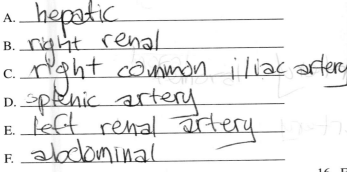

hepatic A
R renal B
r common iliac art. C
D splenic
E renal art
F abdominal

Fig. 25-11 AP abdominal aortogram.

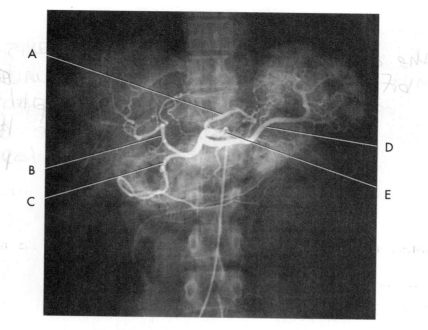

Fig. 25-13 Selective AP celiac arteriogram.

18. Identify each lettered structure shown in Fig. 25-13.

   A. _Left gastric artery_

   B. _Hepatic artery_

   C. _gastroduodenal artery_

   D. _splenic artery_

   E. _celiac axis_

19. What is the advantage of examining the patient's intravenous urography radiographs before positioning the patient for a renal arteriogram?

   To ensure proper position of the tub-part-film alignment and close collimation of the x-ray tube.

20. For demonstrating the portal venous system, the contrast medium should be injected into the

   splenic artery.

21. Blood in veins flows _proximal_ (proximally or distally).

22. For renal venography, the renal vein is most easily catheterized using the _upper_ (upper or lower) limb approach.

23. Into which vein should a catheter be positioned to best demonstrate the superior vena cava?

   a. Subclavian
   b. Common iliac
   c. Inferior vena cava

24. Into which vein should a catheter be positioned to best demonstrate the inferior vena cava?

   a. Portal
   b. Common iliac
   c. Superior vena cava

25. Into which artery should the catheter be positioned to best demonstrate the arteries of an entire upper limb with a single injection of contrast medium?

   a. Femoral
   b. Subclavian
   c. Common iliac

ulnar artery
~~radial~~

A   B   C   D

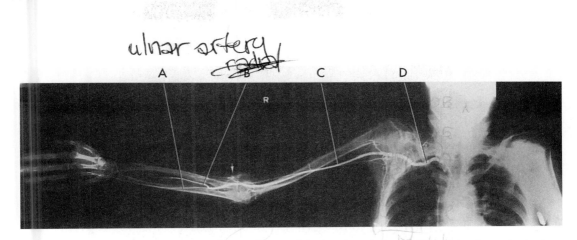

Fig. 25-14 Right upper-limb arteriogram. (The radial artery is not demonstrated due to occlusion.)

26. Identify each lettered structure shown in Fig. 25-14.

A. _ulnar artery_

B. _~~radial artery~~_ posterior interosseous artery

C. _brachial artery_

D. _r subclavian artery_

27. Where is the injection site for the introduction of contrast medium for upper-limb venography?

In the superficial vein (dem entire arm) or in the elbow (dem upper arm)

A   B   C

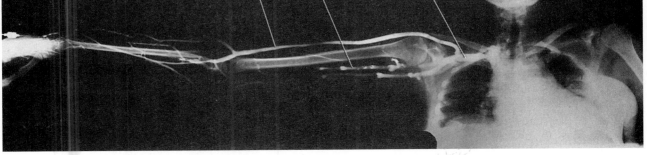

Fig. 25-15 Right upper-limb venogram.

28. Identify each lettered structure shown in Fig. 25-15.

A. _cephalic vein_

B. _basilic vein_

C. _subclavian vein_

29. For simultaneous bilateral femoral arteriograms, how should the patient's legs be positioned?

extended and internally rotated 30°

30. Identify each lettered structure shown in Fig. 25-16.

A. Common illiac artery

B. external iliac artery

C. profunda femoris artery

D. femoral artery

E. popliteal artery

F. anterior tibial

G. peroneal artery

H. posterior tibial artery

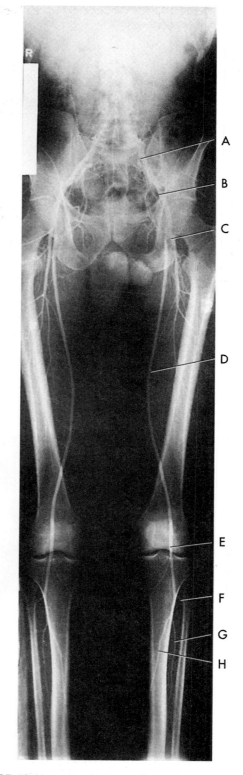

Fig. 25-16 Normal aortofemoral arteriogram in the late arterial phase.

31. At what area of the leg should radiographs begin for lower limb venography?

   a. Hip
   b. Knee
   c. Ankle

32. For lower limb venography, what is the purpose of applying tourniquets just proximal to the ankle and knee?

   a. To stop the pulse within the leg
   b. To prevent blood flow into the leg
   c. To force the filling of the deep veins of the leg

33. Approximately how many seconds does it take for blood to flow from the internal carotid artery to the jugular vein in cerebral angiography?

   a. 3 seconds
   b. 6 seconds
   c. 9 seconds

34. Why should the first radiograph of a cerebral arteriography series be made before the arrival of the contrast medium?

   a. To check exposure factors
   b. To confirm patient positioning
   c. To serve as a subtraction mask
   d. To demonstrate soft-tissue abnormalities

35. What is the visualization sequence for the three phases of blood flow that should be seen in cerebral angiography?

   a. Arterial, capillary, and venous
   b. Arterial, venous, and capillary
   c. Capillary, arterial, and venous
   d. Capillary, venous, and arterial
   e. Venous, arterial, and capillary
   f. Venous, capillary, and arterial

36. Figs. 25-17, 25-18, and 25-19 are cerebral angiograms, and each shows a phase of blood flow. Examine each image and identify which phase of blood flow—arterial, capillary, or venous—the image represents.

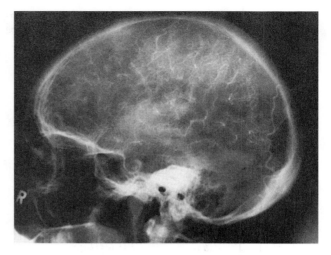

Fig. 25-17 Cerebral angiogram.

a. Fig. 25-17: capillary

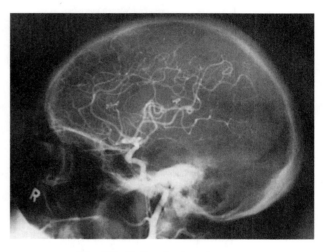

Fig. 25-18 Cerebral angiogram.

b. Fig. 25-18: arterial

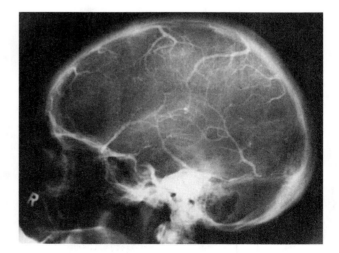

Fig. 25-19 Cerebral angiogram.

c. Fig. 25-19: venous

37. For the basic AP projection during cerebral angiography, what positioning line of the skull should be perpendicular to the horizontal plane?

Infraorbital meatal

38. For the AP axial oblique projection (transorbital) demonstrating anterior circulation during cerebral angiography, in which direction—toward the injected side or away from the injected side—should the head be rotated?

Away from the injected side

39. For the AP axial projection (supraorbital) demonstrating anterior circulation during cerebral angiography, how should the central ray be directed to project the vessels above the floor of the anterior cranial fossa?

a. Caudally
b. Cephalically
c. Perpendicularly

40. For the AP axial oblique projection (transorbital) demonstrating the internal carotid bifurcation and the anterior communicating and middle cerebral arteries within the orbital shadow, how should the central ray be directed?

a. Caudally
b. Cephalically
c. Perpendicularly

Answer the following questions by selecting the best choice.

1. Which vessels originate immediately because of the division of arteries?

   a. Veins
   b. Venules
   c. Arterioles
   d. Capillaries

2. In which part of the body is the basilic vein located?

   a. Head
   b. Abdomen
   c. Lower limb
   d. Upper limb

3. Which chamber of the heart receives deoxygenated blood?

   a. Left atrium
   b. Left ventricle
   c. Right atrium
   d. Right ventricle

4. Which chamber of the heart receives blood from the pulmonary veins?

   a. Left atrium
   b. Left ventricle
   c. Right atrium
   d. Right ventricle

5. What is the purpose of the septa of the heart?

   a. To separate atria from ventricles
   b. To provide openings into the atria
   c. To form the atrioventricular valves
   d. To divide the heart into right and left halves

6. The circuit for blood flow from the left ventricle to the right atrium is _____ circulation.

   a. Deep
   b. Systemic
   c. Superficial
   d. Pulmonary

7. Which arteries are the first to branch from the ascending aorta?

   a. Coronary
   b. Vertebral
   c. Subclavian
   d. Common carotid

8. Through which valve does blood pass when it exits the heart for systemic circulation?

   a. Aortic
   b. Mitral
   c. Bicuspid
   d. Tricuspid

9. Which of the following is a disadvantage of nonionic contrast agents compared with ionic contrast agents of lower iodine concentrations?

   a. Increased viscosity
   b. Increased cardiovascular side effects
   c. Increased exposure factor requirements
   d. Decreased radiographic contrast of opacified vessels

10. Why can exposures not occur in both planes at the same moment during simultaneous biplane imaging?

    a. X-ray tubes will overload.
    b. Scatter radiation will fog the images.
    c. Two injections of contrast medium are required.
    d. X-ray generators cannot be synchronized for multiple exposures.

11. Which procedure should be performed to reduce the magnification of structures for lateral projections during thoracic aortography?

    a. Use an image receptor (IR) changer.
    b. Use the smallest available focal spot.
    c. Increase the source–to–image-receptor distance (SID).
    d. Increase the object–to–image-receptor distance (OID).

12. Which arteriogram requires the use of a compensating (trough) filter to obtain a more uniform density between the vertebral structures and lungs?

    a. AP celiac axis
    b. AP pulmonary
    c. Lateral pulmonary
    d. AP superior mesenteric

13. To which level of the patient should the IR and central ray be centered for AP abdominal aortograms?

    a. T6
    b. T10
    c. L2
    d. Iliac crests

14. To which level of the patient should the IR and central ray be centered for celiac arteriograms?

    a. T2
    b. T6
    c. L2
    d. S1

15. Which area of the patient should be prepared for the injection of contrast medium for cephalic venography?

    a. Thigh
    b. Ankle
    c. Wrist
    d. Upper arm

16. Which area of the patient should be prepared for the injection of contrast medium for demonstration of the superior vena cava?

    a. Thigh
    b. Ankle
    c. Wrist
    d. Upper arm

17. Which area of the patient is the preferred site for insertion of the catheter through the skin for internal carotid arteriography?

    a. Neck
    b. Thigh
    c. Abdomen
    d. Upper arm

18. Why should a radiograph be taken before the arrival of contrast medium for cerebral angiography?

    a. To serve as a subtraction mask
    b. To ensure that collimation is adequate
    c. To check for proper positioning of the patient
    d. To verify that the correct exposure factors are used

19. Which phase of blood flow should have the most films exposed during cerebral angiography?

    a. Venous
    b. Arterial
    c. Capillary
    d. Parenchymal

20. Which positioning line of the skull should be perpendicular to the horizontal plane for basic AP projections during cerebral arteriography?

    a. Orbitomeatal
    b. Glabellomeatal
    c. Acanthiomeatal
    d. Infraorbitomeatal

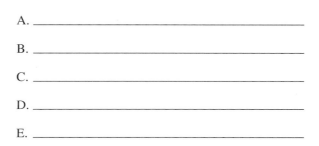

26 Sectional Anatomy for Radiographers

REVIEW

It is essential that the radiographer have an understanding of the relationships between organ and skeletal structures to perform computed tomography (CT), magnetic resonance imaging (MRI), and diagnostic ultrasound examinations because all three modalities create images of sectional anatomy. This exercise is a review of sectional anatomy. Identify structures for each item.

Fig. 26-1 shows a CT localizer, or scout, image of the skull. Figs. 26-2 through 26-5 pertain to the imaging planes shown in Fig. 26-1.

1. Identify each lettered structure shown in Fig. 26-2.

A. _____

B. _____

C. _____

D. _____

E. _____

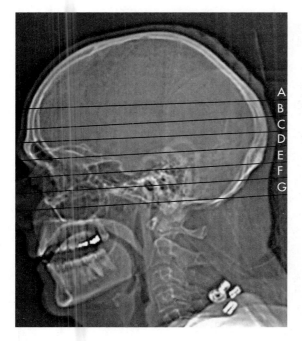

Fig. 26-1 CT localizer, or scout, image of the skull.

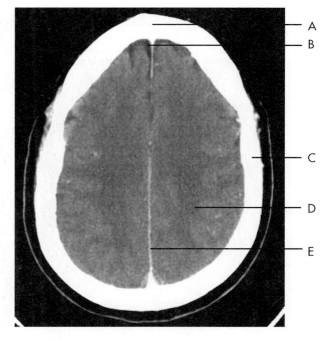

Fig. 26-2 CT image corresponding to level A in Fig. 26-1.

2. Identify each lettered structure shown in Fig. 26-3.

A. _____

B. _____

C. _____

D. _____

E. _____

F. _____

G. _____

H. _____

I. _____

J. _____

K. _____

3. Identify each lettered structure shown in Fig. 26-4.

A. _____

B. _____

C. _____

D. _____

E. _____

F. _____

G. _____

H. _____

I. _____

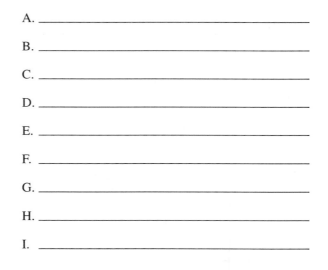

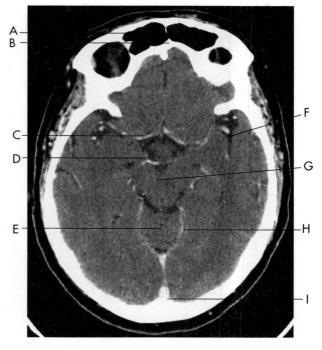

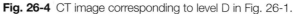

Fig. 26-4 CT image corresponding to level D in Fig. 26-1.

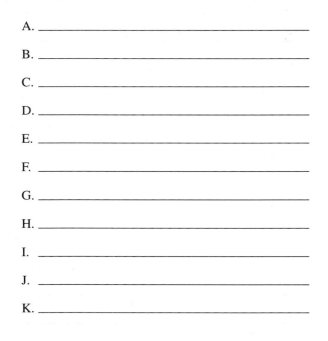

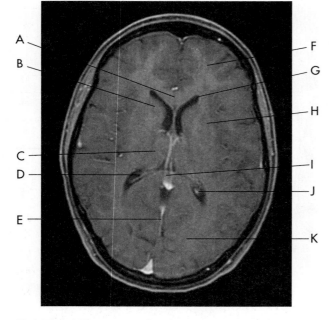

Fig. 26-3 MR image corresponding to level C in Fig. 26-1.

4. Identify each lettered structure shown in Fig. 26-5.

A. _____

B. _____

C. _____

D. _____

E. _____

F. _____

G. _____

H. _____

I. _____

J. _____

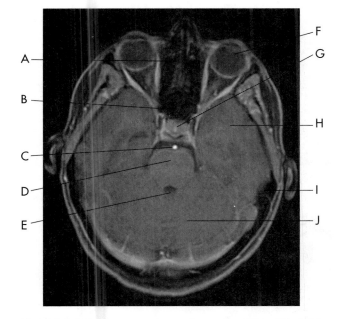

Fig. 26-5 MR image corresponding to level E in Fig. 26-1.

5. Identify each lettered structure shown in Fig. 26-6.

A. _____

B. _____

C. _____

D. _____

E. _____

F. _____

G. _____

H. _____

I. _____

J. _____

K. _____

L. _____

M. _____

N. _____

O. _____

P. _____

Q. _____

R. _____

S. _____

T. _____

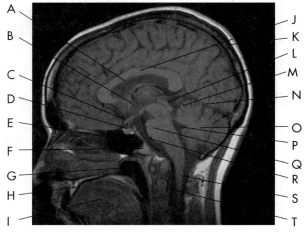

Fig. 26-6 Sagittal MR image of brain through the midsagittal plane.

233

Fig. 26-7 shows a CT localizer, or scout, image of the skull. Figs. 26-8, 26-9, and 26-10 pertain to the imaging planes shown in Fig. 26-7.

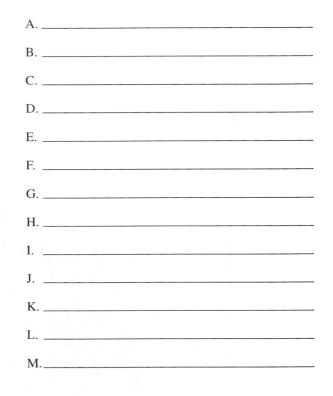

Fig. 26-7 CT localizer, or scout, image of the skull.

6. Identify each lettered structure shown in Fig. 26-8.

A. _____

B. _____

C. _____

D. _____

E. _____

F. _____

G. _____

H. _____

I. _____

J. _____

K. _____

L. _____

M. _____

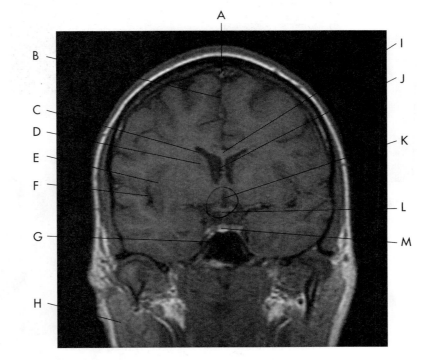

Fig. 26-8 MR image corresponding to level A in Fig. 26-7.

7. Identify each lettered structure shown in Fig. 26-9.

A. _____

B. _____

C. _____

D. _____

E. _____

F. _____

G. _____

H. _____

I. _____

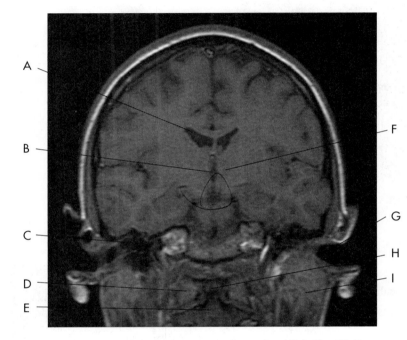

Fig. 26-9 MR image corresponding to level B in Fig. 26-7.

8. Identify each lettered structure shown in Fig. 26-10.

A. _____   D. _____

B. _____   E. _____

C. _____   F. _____

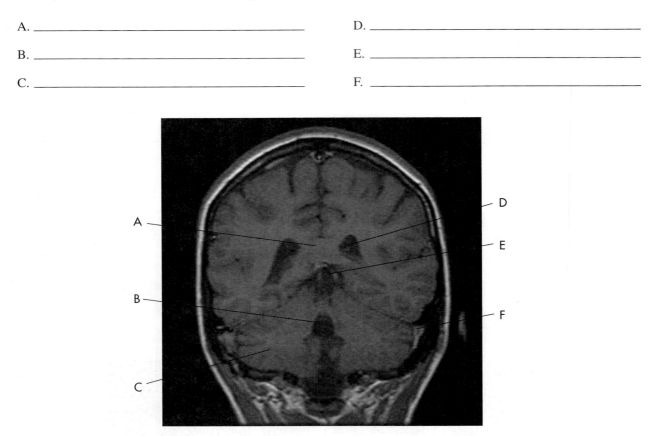

Fig. 26-10 MR image corresponding to level C in Fig. 26-7.

Fig. 26-11 shows a CT localizer, or scout, image of the thorax. Figs. 26-12, 26-13, and 26-14 pertain to the imaging planes shown in Fig. 26-11.

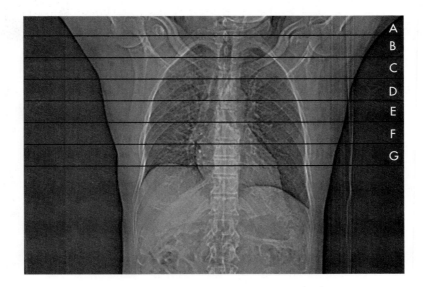

Fig. 26-11 CT localizer, or scout, image of the thorax.

236

Chapter **26 Sectional Anatomy for Radiographers**   Workbook for Merrill's Atlas of Radiographic Positioning and Procedures • Volume 2

9. Identify each lettered structure shown in Fig. 26-12.

A. _____

B. _____

C. _____

D. _____

E. _____

F. _____

G. _____

H. _____

I. _____

J. _____

K. _____

L. _____

M. _____

N. _____

O. _____

P. _____

Q. _____

R. _____

S. _____

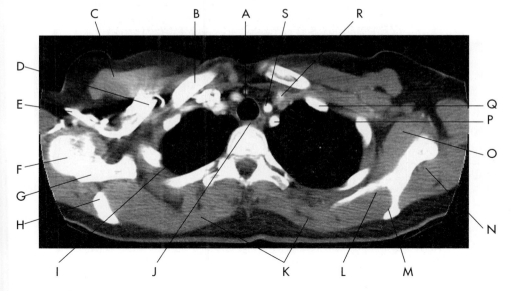

Fig. 26-12 CT image corresponding to level B in Fig. 26-11 through the jugular notch.

10. Identify each lettered structure shown in Fig. 26-13.

A. _____

B. _____

C. _____

D. _____

E. _____

F. _____

G. _____

H. _____

I. _____

J. _____

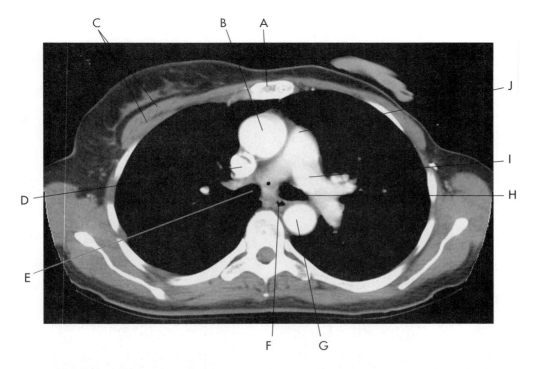

Fig. 26-13 CT image corresponding to level E of Fig. 26-11 through the pulmonary trunk.

11. Identify each lettered structure shown in Fig. 26-14.

A. _____

B. _____

C. _____

D. _____

E. _____

F. _____

G. _____

H. _____

I. _____

J. _____

K. _____

L. _____

M. _____

N. _____

O. _____

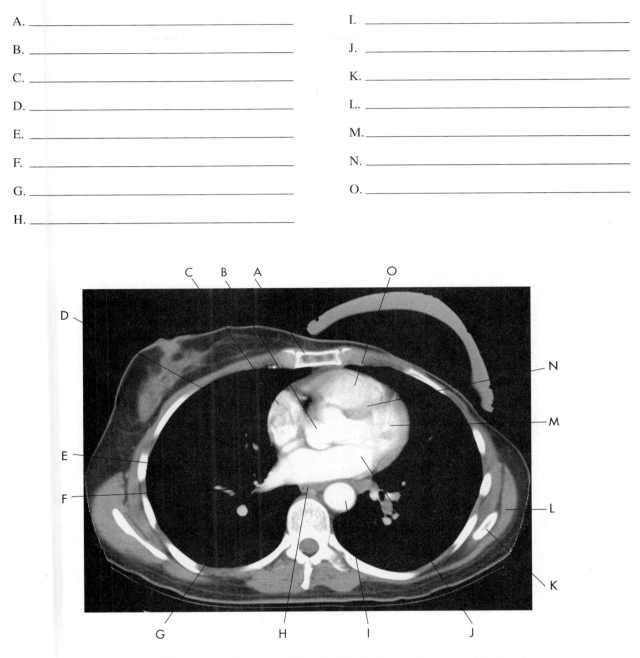

Fig. 26-14 CT corresponding to level F in Fig. 26-11 through the base of the heart.

12. Identify each lettered structure shown in Fig. 26-15.

A. _____

B. _____

C. _____

D. _____

E. _____

F. _____

G. _____

H. _____

I. _____

J. _____

K. _____

L. _____

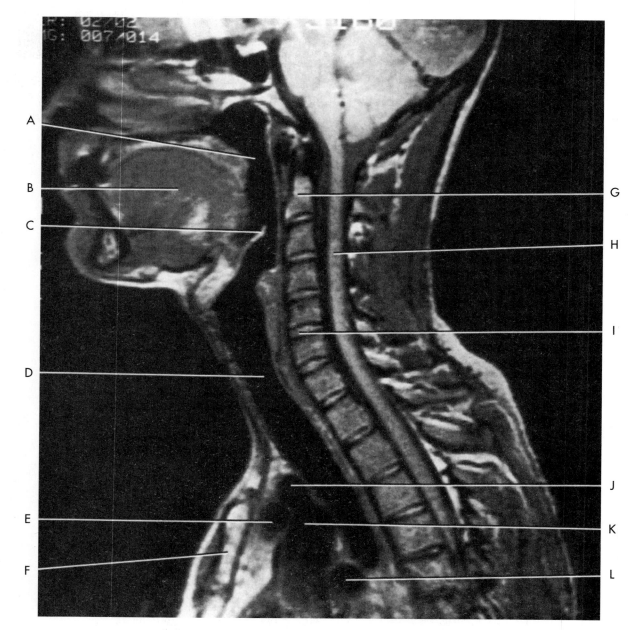

Fig. 26-15 Median sagittal MR image through the neck and upper thorax.

13. Identify each lettered structure shown in Fig. 26-16.

A. _____

B. _____

C. _____

D. _____

E. _____

F. _____

G. _____

H. _____

I. _____

J. _____

K. _____

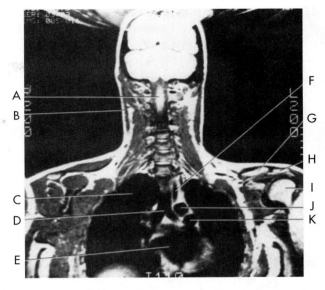

Fig. 26-16 MR image of the neck and thorax through the median coronal plane.

Fig. 26-17 shows a CT localizer, or scout, image of the abdominopelvic region. Figs. 26-18 through 26-23 pertain to the imaging planes shown in Fig. 26-17.

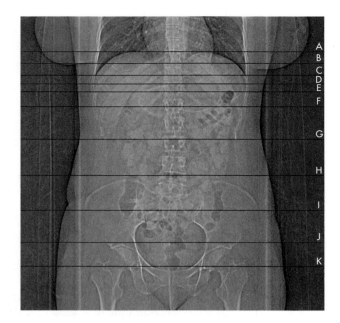

Fig. 26-17 CT localizer, or scout, image of the abdominopelvic region.

14. Identify each lettered structure shown in Fig. 26-18.

A. _____

B. _____

C. _____

D. _____

E. _____

F. _____

G. _____

H. _____

I. _____

J. _____

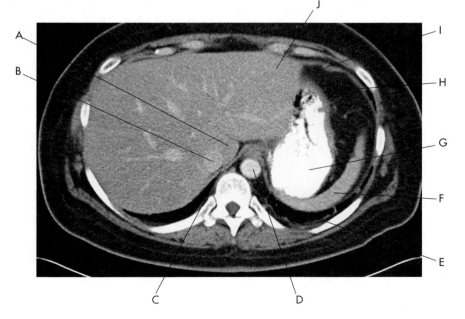

Fig. 26-18 CT corresponding to level B in Fig. 26-17.

15. Identify each lettered structure shown in Fig. 26-19.

A. _____   H. _____

B. _____   I. _____

C. _____   J. _____

D. _____   K. _____

E. _____   L. _____

F. _____   M. _____

G. _____   N. _____

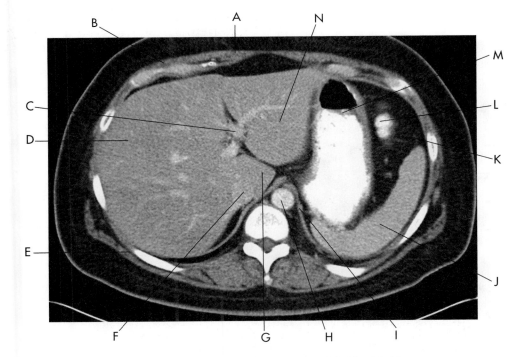

Fig. 26-19 CT corresponding to level C in Fig. 26-17.

16. Identify each lettered structure shown in Fig. 26-20.

A. _____   H. _____

B. _____   I. _____

C. _____   J. _____

D. _____   K. _____

E. _____   L. _____

F. _____   M. _____

G. _____

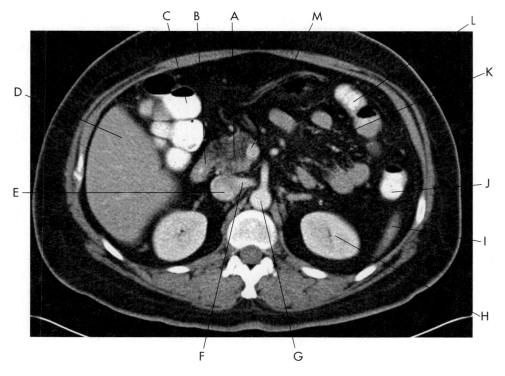

Fig. 26-20 CT corresponding to level F in Fig. 26-17.

244

Chapter **26 Sectional Anatomy for Radiographers**   Workbook for Merrill's Atlas of Radiographic Positioning and Procedures • Volume 2

17. Identify each lettered structure shown in Fig. 26-21.

A. _____

B. _____

C. _____

D. _____

E. _____

F. _____

G. _____

H. _____

I. _____

J. _____

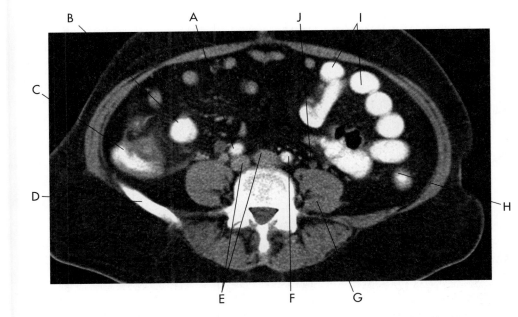

Fig. 26-21 CT image corresponding to level H in Fig. 26-17.

18. Identify each lettered structure shown in Fig. 26-22.

A. _____

B. _____

C. _____

D. _____

E. _____

F. _____

G. _____

H. _____

I. _____

J. _____

K. _____

L. _____

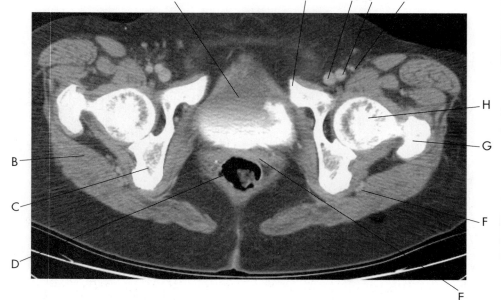

Fig. 26-22 CT image of female pelvis corresponding to level K in Fig. 26-17.

19. Identify each lettered structure shown in Fig. 26-23.

A. _____

B. _____

C. _____

D. _____

E. _____

F. _____

G. _____

H. _____

I. _____

J. _____

K. _____

L. _____

M. _____

N. _____

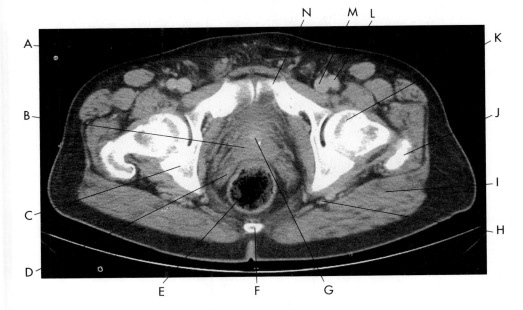

Fig. 26-23 CT image of male pelvis corresponding to level K in Fig. 26-17.

20. Identify each lettered structure shown in Fig. 26-24.

A. _____

B. _____

C. _____

D. _____

E. _____

F. _____

G. _____

H. _____

I. _____

J. _____

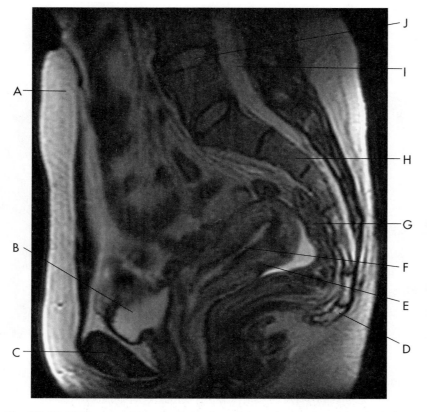

Fig. 26-24 MR image of female abdominopelvic region at the midsagittal plane.

21. Identify each lettered structure shown in Fig. 26-25.

A. _____

B. _____

C. _____

D. _____

E. _____

F. _____

G. _____

H. _____

I. _____

J. _____

K. _____

L. _____

M. _____

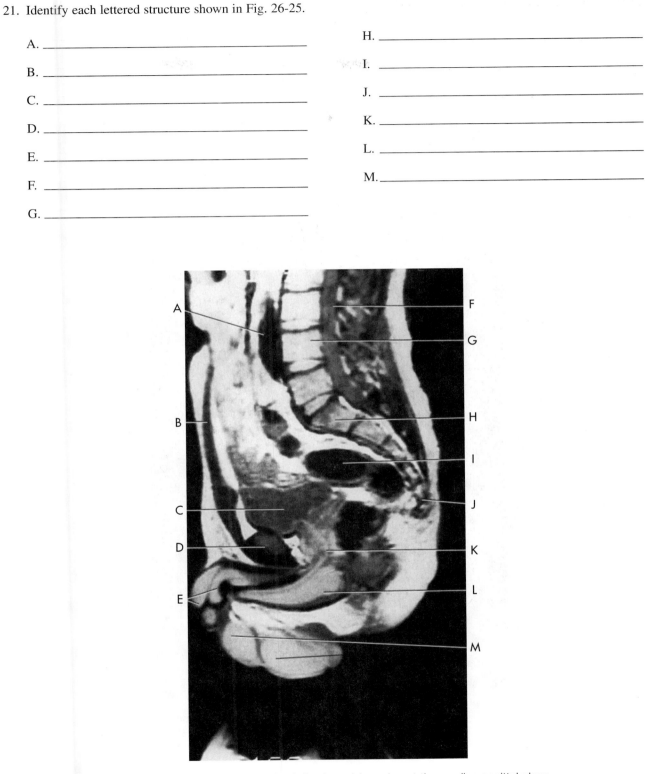

Fig. 26-25 MR image of the male abdominopelvic region at the median sagittal plane.

22. Identify each lettered structure shown in Fig. 26-26.

A. _____

B. _____

C. _____

D. _____

E. _____

F. _____

G. _____

H. _____

I. _____

J. `_____

K. _____

L. _____

M. _____

N. _____

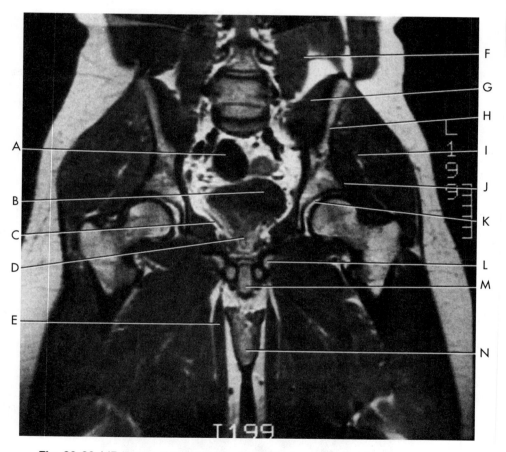

Fig. 26-26 MR image of the abdominopelvic region at the median coronal plane.

27 Pediatric Imaging

Students must be prepared to meet the challenges of specific patient populations. Children are not just smaller versions of adults, so unique and specific skills are required to successfully image pediatric patients. The following questions provide a review of necessary skills to successfully work with pediatric patients.

1. List two main areas in which radiographers lack confidence in pediatric radiography.

2. When communicating with a child, it is important to (circle all that apply):
   a. Use language that the child can understand.
   b. Bend down and talk to the child at the child's eye level.
   c. Provide plenty of options to allow child freedom of choice.
   d. Threaten the child to intimidate them to cooperate.
   e. Employ distraction techniques, such as talking to the child about school, TV shows, or siblings.
   f. Use sincere praise.

3. Which age group is eager to please, but is also modest and embarrasses easily?

4. Which pediatric patient is at high risk for hypothermia?

5. A congenital defect in which a portion of bowel herniates through a defect near the navel is called

   _____.

6. Which of the following is one of the most dangerous causes of acute upper airway obstruction in children and is treated as an emergency?
   a. Osteogenesis imperfecta
   b. Epiglottitis
   c. Omphalocele
   d. Hypothermia

7. Which pediatric disease makes children more prone to spontaneous fractures?

8. What is the first course of action for a radiographer who suspects child abuse of a pediatric patient?

9. The _____ is a commonly used immobilization device for pediatric chest radiography on patients from birth to age 3 years.

10. For skull radiography, the _____ immobilization technique is often employed.

11. True or False. The Pigg-O-Stat requires two persons to be used safely.

12. Which of the following is the most reliable method of detecting inspiration on chest radiography for patients from birth to age 3 years?

    a. Waiting for the end of a cry
    b. Watching the rise and fall of the sternum
    c. Watching the abdomen
    d. All of these methods

13. Which immobilizer should be used if there is not another adult available to assist throughout the procedure?

14. Which of the following are true regarding gonadal shielding during pelvis/hip radiography of pediatric patients? Check all that apply.

    _____ a. Always use on males.

    _____ b. Females may be shielded after the initial exam has ruled out sacral problems.

    _____ c. Always use on females.

    _____ d. Place shielding on males in midline at the level of the anterior superior iliac spine (ASIS).

    _____ e. Place shielding on females in midline at the level of the ASIS.

    _____ f. Place shielding on males level with the greater trochanters.

15. In imaging the limbs of a pediatric patient, it is often

    necessary to examine the _____

    side for _____.

16. What type of fracture occurs through the epiphysis?

17. What are the disadvantages of the octagonal infant immobilizer?

18. When examining a pediatric patient for a possible aspirated foreign body, the routine protocol should include the following:

    a. _____

    b. _____

    c. _____

19. Which of the following are important radiation protection practices for scoliosis images?

    1. Accurate collimation
    2. Breast shields
    3. Gonadal shield
       a. 1 and 2 only
       b. 1 and 3 only
       c. 2 and 3 only
       d. 1, 2, and 3

20. _____ is

    often required to perform an MRI exam on a pediatric patient, thus greatly increasing the

    _____ of the procedure.

Answer the following questions by selecting the best choice.

1. One of the ways to obtain a pediatric patient's cooperation is to:

   a. Make sure you explain everything to the parents.
   b. Talk to the child at their eye level.
   c. Talk to the child in "baby talk."
   d. Give the child plenty of options to choose from.

2. In communicating with the adolescent patient, it is important to assess their:

   a. Maturity level
   b. Intelligence level
   c. Sensitivity level
   d. Level of independence

3. One of the greatest dangers facing the premature infant is:

   a. Radiation exposure
   b. Exposure to contagions
   c. Hyperthermia
   d. Hypothermia

4. Whenever possible, the premature infant should be examined:

   a. Within the isolette or infant warmer
   b. In an upright position
   c. With the diaper in place
   d. Within the imaging department

5. Pediatric patients with a myelomeningocele must be examined in the _____ position.

   a. Upright
   b. Supine
   c. Prone
   d. Trendelenburg's

6. Which congenital anomaly resembles an enormous umbilical hernia?

   a. Myelomeningocele
   b. Omphalocele
   c. Osteogenesis imperfecta
   d. Spina bifida

7. The peak incidence of epiglottitis is ages:

   a. Birth to 2 years
   b. 3 to 6 years
   c. 7 to 9 years
   d. 10 to 13 years

8. Which pediatric pathology requires that a physician accompany the patient during imaging procedures?

   a. Myelomeningocele
   b. Child abuse
   c. Osteogenesis imperfecta
   e. Epiglottitis

9. Which of the following is characteristic of osteogenesis imperfecta?

   a. Acute respiratory distress
   b. Increased risk of hypothermia
   c. Increased susceptibility to fractures
   d. Increased dependency upon parents

10. In a case of suspected child abuse, the radiographer's first course of action is to:

    a. Talk with the parents.
    b. Call the police.
    c. Consult with a radiologist or other attending physician.
    d. Submit a written report to the social work department.

11. "Classic indicators" of physical abuse of a child include:

    1. Posterior rib fractures
    2. "Bucket-handle" limb fractures
    3. Corner fractures
       a. 1 and 2 only
       b. 1 and 3 only
       c. 2 and 3 only
       d. 1, 2, and 3

12. One of the most commonly used immobilizers for pediatric chest and abdominal radiography is the:

    a. Pigg-O-Stat
    b. Octagonal infant immobilizer
    c. "Bunny" wrap
    d. Conscious sedation

13. How many people are required to safely immobilize a pediatric patient using a Pigg-O-Stat?

    a. 1
    b. 2
    c. 3
    d. 4

14. The most reliable method to detect inspiration for chest radiography on patients from birth to age 3 years is:

    a. Watch the rise and fall of the sternum.
    b. Watch the chest wall.
    c. Watch the abdomen.
    d. Wait for the end of a cry.

15. What type of immobilization is recommended for skull radiography of pediatric patients age 3 years or younger?

    a. Pigg-O-Stat
    b. Conscious sedation
    c. "Bunny" wrap
    d. Velcro straps and adult physical restraint

253

16. Which of the following is the recommended method of limb radiography of preschool-age patients?

    a. Sitting on a parent's lap
    b. Modified "bunny" wrap immobilization
    c. Octagonal infant immobilizer
    d. Velcro straps and adult restraint

17. Which of the following is often required for limb radiography of a pediatric patient?

    a. Conscious sedation
    b. Examination of the contralateral limb
    c. Neurologic assessment
    d. Stress positions

18. Which type of fracture occurs through the epiphysis?

    a. Salter-Harris fractures
    b. "Bucket-handle" fractures
    c. Greenstick fractures
    d. Torus or buckle fractures

19. Hip examinations on children are most often ordered to assess for:

    a. Fractures
    b. Legg-Calvé-Perthes disease
    c. Osteogenesis imperfecta
    d. Osgood-Schlatter disease

20. Which of the following is true regarding shielding of female patients during hip and pelvic radiography?

    a. Female patients are always shielded.
    b. The top of the shield is placed at the level of the greater trochanters.
    c. Female patients can be shielded after the initial exam has ruled out sacral problems.
    d. Female patients can never be shielded for pelvis/hip radiographs.

21. Which of the following body parts may be imaged for bone age studies?

    1. Left hand and wrist
    2. Left knee
    3. Bilateral hips
        a. 1 and 2 only
        b. 1 and 3 only
        c. 2 and 3 only
        d. 1, 2, and 3

22. Which type of immobilization can be more uncomfortable and appear more traumatic?

    a. "Bunny" wrap technique
    b. Velcro straps
    c. Pigg-O-Stat
    d. Octagonal infant immobilizer

23. Which of the following should be part of the routine protocol when imaging a pediatric patient for a suspected aspirated foreign body?

    1. PA chest on inspiration
    2. PA chest on expiration
    3. Lateral chest
        a. 1 and 2 only
        b. 1 and 3 only
        c. 2 and 3 only
        d. 1, 2, and 3

24. Where is an aspirated foreign body more likely to lodge?

    a. The upper esophagus
    b. Just superior to the cricoid cartilage of the trachea
    c. The right primary bronchus
    d. The left primary bronchus

25. What is the primary hindrance for the use of MRI on pediatric patients?

    a. Length and nature of the exam requires general anesthesia to avoid patient motion, thus increasing the risk.
    b. Magnet strength has not been proven safe for persons with premature skeletons and organs.
    c. Pediatric patients do not have sufficient hydrogen atom content to provide quality, diagnostic MR images.
    d. Computer algorithms cannot compensate for smaller patients with less body mass, so image quality is compromised.

28 Geriatric Radiography

Students must be prepared to meet the challenges of specific patient populations. The rising number of elderly persons demands that radiographers be prepared to meet their unique needs. The following questions provide a review of necessary skills to successfully work with geriatric patients.

1. Define *geriatrics*.

2. To work successfully with elderly patients, the radiographer must be able to differentiate between:
   a. Age-related changes and disease processes
   b. Senility and dementia
   c. Senior citizens and elderly persons
   d. Cognitive impairments and dementia

3. List the top ten chronic conditions of people age 65 years and older.

4. What are the most common health complaints of the elderly?

5. Progressive cognitive impairment that eventually interferes with daily functioning is termed

   _____.

6. True or False. All elderly persons develop dementia.

7. What is the most common form of dementia?

255

8. Match the age-associated condition with the organ system in which it manifests or affects. Some systems may be used more than once and some conditions may be linked to more than one system.

Column A

_____ 1. Anemia system

_____ 2. Incontinence

_____ 3. Hearing loss

_____ 4. Postural hypotension

_____ 5. Difficulty swallowing

_____ 6. Graying and thinning hair

_____ 7. Increases vulnerability to nosocomial infections

_____ 8. Increased risk of falls

_____ 9. Osteoporosis

_____ 10. Osteoarthritis

_____ 11. Dementia

_____ 12. Diverticulosis

_____ 13. Increased vulnerability to abrasions

_____ 14. Presbyopia

_____ 15. Atherosclerosis

_____ 16. Autoimmune diseases

_____ 17. Decreased elasticity of alveoli

_____ 18. Diabetes mellitus

Column B

a. Integumentary

b. Endocrine system

c. Gastrointestinal system

d. Immune system

e. Sensory system

f. Urinary system

g. Cardiovascular system

h. Nervous system

i. Musculoskeletal system

j. Respiratory system

k. Hematological system

9. Which of the following are reasons to educate the geriatric patient and their family about imaging procedures?
   1. Obtain their confidence
   2. Decreases patient stress
   3. Improve patient compliance
      a. 1 and 2 only
      b. 2 and 3 only
      c. 1 and 3 only
      d. 1, 2, and 3

10. How should the radiographer adjust his/her communication skills to accommodate an elderly patient who has a hearing loss?

11. Elimination of _____ will improve the listening environment for an elderly patient.

12. List three ways to increase the security for a geriatric patient when transporting them from the wheelchair to the examination table.

13. To reduce the risk of tearing the fragile skin of a geriatric patient, the use of _____ _____ for immobilization should be avoided.

14. The amount of contrast media administered to an elderly patient is varied because of:

15. Knowledge of age-related changes and disease processes _____ the radiographer's ability to meet the special care needs of the elderly patient.

    a. Improves
    b. Decreases
    c. Does not affect

Answer the following questions by selecting the best choice.

1. The branch of medicine dealing with the elderly and the problems of aging is termed:

    a. Pediatrics
    b. Geriatrics
    c. Psychiatry
    d. Endocrinology

2. To provide quality images and work well with the geriatric patient, the radiographer must be able to:

    a. Adapt procedures to accommodate disabilities and diseases unique to the geriatric population.
    b. Speak loudly and eliminate background noises.
    c. Adapt technical factors to ensure proper radiation protection.
    d. Calculate necessary contrast media adjustments.

3. It is important for the healthcare professional to not only know diseases and disorders common to specific age groups, but also to know:

    a. The associated economic status
    b. The resultant disabilities
    c. A particular ethnic group
    d. The effects on different genders

4. Which of the following are among the top ten chronic conditions for people over the age of 65 years?

    1. Visual impairment
    2. Cancer
    3. Diabetes
        a. 1 and 2 only
        b. 1 and 3 only
        c. 2 and 3 only
        d. 1, 2, and 3

5. A term used to describe the stereotyping of and discrimination against elderly persons is:

    a. Ageism
    b. Elderism
    c. Geriatricism
    d. Racism

6. What is one of the common psychological effects of aging?

    a. Gray hair
    b. Wrinkles
    c. Depression
    d. Alzheimer's disease

7. One of the most common health complaints of the elderly population is:

    a. Hair loss
    b. Depression
    c. Diabetes
    d. Fatigue

8. Which of the following can slow the progress of age-related joint stiffness, fatigue, weight gain, and bone mass loss?

    a. Vitamin supplements
    b. Nonsteroidal antiinflammatory drugs (NSAIDs)
    c. Mental games
    d. Low-impact exercise

9. Which of the following can cause cognitive impairment in elderly persons?

    1. Disuse
    2. Aging
    3. Disease
        a. 1 and 2 only
        b. 1 and 3 only
        c. 2 and 3 only
        d. 1, 2, and 3

10. Which of the following terms is defined as progressive cognitive impairment that eventually interferes with normal daily functioning?

    a. Dementia
    b. Senility
    c. Alzheimer's disease
    d. Depression

11. Alzheimer's disease is the most common form of:

    a. Depression
    b. Senility
    c. Dementia
    d. Ageism

12. Which body system is usually the first to show apparent signs of aging?

    a. Gastrointestinal system
    b. Integumentary system
    c. Cardiovascular system
    d. Musculoskeletal system

13. Which body system is responsible for most of the disabilities in persons over the age of 65 years?

    a. Integumentary system
    b. Nervous system
    c. Immune system
    d. Cardiovascular system

14. Hearing and visual impairments associated with aging are classified as disorders of the:

    a. Sensory system
    b. Integumentary system
    c. Nervous system
    d. Musculoskeletal system

15. What is the predominate age-related change in the blood vessels?

    a. Loss of elasticity
    b. Ulcerations
    c. Atherosclerosis
    d. Degeneration

16. The major hematological concern in geriatric patients is:

    a. Ischemia
    b. Atherosclerosis
    c. Diabetes
    d. Anemia

17. Which of the following is crucial to obtain an elderly patient's compliance and confidence?

    a. Education about imaging procedures
    b. Demonstration of empathy
    c. Knowledge of imaging procedures
    d. Demonstration of self-confidence and personal hygiene

18. Elimination of _____ will aid in listening and communications with geriatric patients.

    a. Extraneous words
    b. Body language
    c. Background noise
    d. Facial expressions

19. The elderly patient will often experience _____ when going from a recumbent position to a sitting position.

    a. Nausea
    b. Vertigo
    c. Fear
    d. Depression

20. The amount of contrast media used for imaging procedures is varied for elderly patients because of:

    a. Incontinence
    b. Anemia
    c. Age-related changes in cardiovascular system
    d. Age-related changes in liver and kidney functions

29 Mobile Radiography

EQUIPMENT, TECHNICAL CONSIDERATIONS, AND PATIENT CARE

There are many instances in which the technologist has to bring the imaging procedure to the patient, rather than the patient reporting to the radiology department. Mobile radiography is widely used to image those patients who are unable to come to the department for routine imaging examinations. Write the answer to each of the following questions regarding mobile equipment, technical considerations and patient care concerns.

1. List the common areas in which mobile radiography is performed.

2. When was mobile radiography first used, and by whom?

3. What other term is often used in place of "mobile"?

4. What technical controls are typically available on mobile equipment?

5. What is the typical range of milliampere-seconds (mAs) available on mobile x-ray machines?

6. What is the typical range of kilovolt peak (kVp) available on mobile x-ray machines?

7. What is the range of total power for most mobile units? How does this compare to stationary radiographic equipment?

8. What are the two categories of mobile x-ray machines?

261

9. What is the primary difference in the two categories of mobile x-ray machines?

10. What are the advantages of each type of mobile x-ray machine?

11. What three technical matters must be understood to be competent in mobile radiography?

12. For optimal mobile images, a grid must be:

    a. _____

    b. _____

    c. _____

13. Anode heel effect is more pronounced when using

    short _____, larger _____,

    and small _____.

14. Where should the cathode be positioned when performing a femur examination with a mobile x-ray machine?

    a. At the proximal femur
    b. At the distal femur

15. What is the preferred source–to–image-receptor distance (SID) for mobile examinations? Why?

16. True or False. Mobile radiography produces some of the highest occupational radiation exposures for radiographers.

17. Radiographers performing mobile examinations

    should wear a _____
    for proper radiation protection.

18. The single most effective means of radiation protection is:

    a. Shortest exposure time
    b. Maximum distance from the x-ray source
    c. Smaller field sizes
    d. Lower grid ratios

19. What is the recommended minimum distance between the radiographer and the x-ray tube?

20. Circle the five clinical situations in which gonadal shielding should be provided.

    a. Mobile exam on a child
    b. Mobile chest exam on a 28-year-old female in an intensive care unit
    c. Mobile pelvis and hip exam on a 75-year-old female in a surgical (post-op) recovery unit
    d. Emergency department (ED) patient requests shielding during a mobile knee exam
    e. Cross-table lateral lumbar spine image performed with a mobile unit on a 22-year-old male in the ED
    f. Routine hand exam on a 30-year-old patient
    g. Mobile KUB (kidney, ureter, and bladder) image in the ED on a 32-year-old female patient with blunt abdominal trauma

21. What two types of patients are often cared for in isolation units?

22. Because of the confidentiality of patient records, a radiographer may not know the specific disease of a patient in an isolation unit. Therefore all patients

should be handled using _____

_____.

23. Which of the following protective apparel should be worn when performing a mobile examination on a patient in strict isolation? Circle all that apply.
    a. Gown
    b. Gloves
    c. Mask
    d. Cap
    e. Shoe covers

24. What should be done to protect the image receptor (IR) when performing a mobile examination on a patient isolated with drainage secretion precautions?

25. What should be done to mobile equipment after performing an examination on a patient in an isolation unit?

MOBILE RADIOGRAPHIC EXAMINATIONS

The following exercises pertain to the performance of specific mobile radiographic procedures. Answer each question regarding the specific mobile examination.

1. Which of the following are preliminary steps for the radiographer before performing mobile radiography? Check all that apply.

   ____ a. Gather all necessary equipment.

   ____ b. Announce your presence to the nursing staff.

   ____ c. Confirm that you have the correct patient.

   ____ d. Introduce yourself to patient and family.

   ____ e. Explain the exam to the patient.

   ____ f. Process the images.

   ____ g. Observe medical equipment in room and move, if necessary.

   ____ h. Disconnect unnecessary medical equipment to remove artifacts.

Questions 2 through 6 pertain to the *AP projection of the chest, with the patient in an upright or supine position.*

2. Which position would be best to obtain a mobile AP chest radiograph on a conscious and alert patient?
   a. Sitting as upright as is tolerable by the patient
   b. Supine position
   c. Lateral decubitus position
   d. Trendelenburg's position

3. The IR should be placed about _____ above the shoulders for the AP projection of the chest performed with a mobile unit.

4. The central ray should be directed _____

   to the _____ on the mobile AP projection of the chest.

5. The central ray should enter the patient about

   _____ below the _____ on the mobile AP projection of the chest.

6. What device should be used if the kVp is above 90 for a mobile computed radiography AP projection of the chest?

Questions 7 through 10 pertain to the *AP projection of the chest with the patient in a right or left lateral decubitus position.*

7. When using the lateral decubitus position for a mobile chest examination, which position would be used if fluid were suspected in the left lung?

8. Describe the proper patient position to prevent rotation of the anatomy in an image of a lateral decubitus position.

9. What pathologic conditions would be demonstrated by the right lateral decubitus position?

10. True or False. Proper image ID should be demonstrated to indicate the decubitus position was used.

Questions 11 through 15 pertain to the *AP projection of the abdomen with the patient in a supine position.*

11. The grid IR should be centered at the level of the

    _____.

12. If the emphasis is on the upper abdomen, how does the grid IR center change?

13. What anatomy must be visualized on the radiograph if the lower abdomen is of primary interest?

14. The _____ must be seen at the top of the radiograph if the upper abdomen is of primary interest.

15. What error might occur if the patient is not in a true supine position, but the central ray is centered as if he/she is properly positioned?

Questions 16 through 18 pertain to the *AP projection of the abdomen with the patient in the left lateral decubitus position.*

16. How does one check for rotation on a radiograph of the abdomen taken in a left lateral decubitus position?

17. How long should the patient be in the left lateral decubitus position before exposure? Why?

18. The center of the grid IR should be centered

    _____ to include

    the _____ on the image.

Questions 19 through 21 pertain to the *AP projection of the pelvis.*

19. Where should the center of the grid IR be placed relative to the patient?

20. What possible contraindications prohibit proper positioning of the lower limbs for this examination?

21. What is the rationale for the position of the lower limbs for this examination?

Questions 22 through 25 pertain to the *AP and lateral projections of the femur.*

22. The grid IR should be placed _____ to the plane of the femoral condyles for the AP projection.

23. List the anatomy that must be included on a mobile femur examination.

24. When performing the mediolateral projection of the femur, the unaffected limb should be:

    a. Flexed at the knee for support
    b. Parallel to the grid IR
    c. Elevated and supported at a nearly vertical position
    d. Used to support the grid IR in a vertical position

25. When performing the lateromedial projection of the femur, the grid IR is placed:

    1. Perpendicular to the epicondylar plane
    2. Between the patient's legs
    3. Against the lateral aspect of the affected femur
       a. 1 and 2 only
       b. 2 and 3 only
       c. 1 and 3 only
       d. 1, 2, and 3

Questions 26 through 28 pertain to the *lateral projection of the cervical spine with the patient in the dorsal decubitus position.*

26. The top of the grid IR should be placed:

27. Proper alignment of the central ray with the grid IR

    will prevent _____.

28. What anatomic structures must be demonstrated on the image?

Questions 29 through 32 pertain to procedures performed with neonates, with the *AP projection of the chest and abdomen.*

29. Chest and abdomen combined projections are typically ordered on:

    a. Full-term infants
    b. Toddlers
    c. Adolescents
    d. Premature infants

30. Who should hold the infant during the radiographic examination?

31. True or False. A covering should be placed over the IR if it is placed directly under the infant.

32. Explain the risks of straightening the head of a neonate with an endotracheal tube.

Questions 33 through 35 pertain to procedures performed with neonates, with the *lateral projection of a patient in the dorsal decubitus position.*

33. True or False. The infant does not need to be elevated for the dorsal decubitus position.

34. What anatomy is of special interest in this position?

35. What pathology, if present, can be demonstrated in this position?

Answer the following questions by selecting the best choice.

1. Mobile radiography is defined as:

    a. Using digital equipment to transmit images to remote sites
    b. Using transportable radiographic equipment to bring imaging services to the patient
    c. Using radiographic imaging to increase patient mobility
    d. Using PACSs (picture archiving and communication systems) to transmit images to patients in their homes

2. Which of the following are common sites in which mobile radiography is performed?

    1. Intensive care units
    2. Patient hospital rooms
    3. Surgery
        a. 1 and 2 only
        b. 2 and 3 only
        c. 1 and 3 only
        d. 1, 2, and 3

3. The typical mAs range on a mobile unit is:

    a. 0.04 to 320 mAs
    b. 1 to 10 mAs
    c. 1 to 100 mAs
    d. 0.5 to 500 mAs

4. The typical kVp range on a mobile unit is:

    a. 1 to 100 kVp
    b. 10 to 500 kVp
    c. 40 to 130 kVp
    d. 50 to 150 kVp

5. What is a "deadman's" brake?

    a. A brake that allows the operator to remotely engage it
    b. A brake that does not require maintenance
    c. A brake that requires minimal force to engage it
    d. A brake that instantly stops the machine when the push-handle is released

6. What are the primary advantages of a battery-powered mobile unit?

    a. They are lightweight and easy to maneuver.
    b. They are cordless and provide constant kVp and mAs levels.
    c. They do not require much time to charge before the exposure.
    d. They are inexpensive and low-maintenance.

7. What is the primary advantage of a capacitor discharge mobile unit?

    a. They are cordless and provide constant kVp and mAs levels.
    b. They are lightweight and easy to maneuver.
    c. They do not require much time to charge before the exposure.
    d. They are inexpensive and low-maintenance.

8. When performing a mobile examination of the abdomen, where should the cathode be placed for the AP projection?

    a. The down side of the abdomen
    b. Over the symphysis pubis
    c. Over the diaphragm
    d. No designation for cathode placement

9. The anode heel effect is more pronounced with:

    1. Larger field sizes
    2. Larger anode angles
    3. Shorter SID
        a. 1 and 2 only
        b. 1 and 3 only
        c. 2 and 3 only
        d. 1, 2, and 3

10. If the SID is increased, what risk is also increased?

    a. Imaging of patient motion
    b. Tube overload
    c. Imaging of patient artifacts
    d. Grid cut-off

11. For optimum radiation safety, the radiographer should stand:

    a. At a right angle to the patient
    b. At a right angle to the x-ray tube
    c. Anywhere, as long as a lead apron is worn
    d. At least 6 feet away from the patient and x-ray tube

12. At what kVp level should a grid be employed for mobile chest examinations?

    a. Above 60 kVp
    b. Above 75 kVp
    c. Above 90 kVp
    d. Above 100 kVp

13. Which of the following evaluation criteria for the mobile AP chest is used to evaluate adequate density and contrast?

    a. Medial portion of clavicles equidistant from the vertebral column
    b. Ribs and thoracic intervertebral disc spaces faintly visible through the heart shadow
    c. Psoas muscles, lower margin of liver, and kidney margins demonstrated
    d. Symmetric appearance of the vertebral column and iliac wings

267

14. Which of the following evaluation criteria for the mobile AP chest is used to evaluate patient rotation?

   a. Medial portion of clavicles equidistant from the vertebral column
   b. Ribs and thoracic intervertebral disc spaces faintly visible through the heart shadow
   c. Psoas muscles, lower margin of liver, and kidney margins demonstrated
   d. Symmetric appearance of the vertebral column and iliac wings

15. What is the proper position of the median coronal plane for the right lateral decubitus position of the chest?

   a. Horizontal
   b. Perpendicular to the IR
   c. Vertical
   d. Aligned to the center of the IR

16. When performing a mobile lateral decubitus chest examination, how long should the patient be in position prior to exposure?

   a. 1 minute
   b. 5 minutes
   c. 8 minutes
   d. 20 minutes

17. What is the danger of straightening the head and neck of a neonate during a mobile AP projection of the chest and abdomen?

   a. Risk of physical injury to the underdeveloped vertebra
   b. Risk of transmission of infectious organisms
   c. Risk of increased occupational exposure
   d. Risk of advancing the endotracheal tube too far into the trachea

18. Which position would be used to demonstrate fluid in the right lung of a patient in an intensive care unit?

   a. Right lateral decubitus
   b. Left lateral decubitus
   c. Supine
   d. Prone

19. Which position would be used to demonstrate free air or fluid levels in a neonate?

   a. Right lateral decubitus
   b. Left lateral decubitus
   c. Dorsal decubitus
   d. Supine

20. Which of the following are contraindications to positioning the feet of a trauma patient during a mobile AP projection of the pelvis?

   a. Decreased level of consciousness
   b. Suspicion of hip fracture
   c. No one available to hold the patient
   d. Increased risk of occupational exposure

30 Surgical Radiography

Exercise 1

Listed below are personnel who may be found working within an operating room during surgical procedures. In the space provided, write S if that person is a sterile team member or N if that person is a nonsterile team member.

_____ 1. Surgeon

_____ 2. Circulator

_____ 3. Radiographer

_____ 4. Anesthesiologist

_____ 5. Surgical assistant

_____ 6. Physician's assistant

_____ 7. Monitoring technician

_____ 8. Biomedical technician

_____ 9. Certified surgical technologist

_____ 10. Certified registered nurse anesthetist

Exercise 2

Answer each statement as either true or false. Explain any statement you believe is false.

1. True or False. A certified surgical technologist is a sterile team member within the operating room (OR).

2. True or False. The anesthesia provider is a sterile team member within the OR.

3. True or False. Street clothes should never be worn within semirestricted areas of the surgical suite.

4. True or False. It takes two people—a radiographer and a sterile team member—to place an image receptor (IR) into a sterile IR cover.

5. True or False. The floor of the OR is always considered contaminated before a surgical procedure begins.

6. True or False. Only sterile items can be used within the sterile field.

7. True or False. A radiographer may touch only non-sterile items within the OR.

8. True or False. Items of doubtful sterility must be considered nonsterile.

9. True or False. Sterile gowns are considered sterile in front from shoulder to the level of the knees.

10. True or False. The sleeves of gowns are considered to be sterile from the cuff to the shoulder.

11. True or False. Lifting sterile drapes on a table above table level compromises the sterile field.

12. True or False. The radiographer should place sterile drapes over both ends of the C-arm before entering the OR.

13. True or False. When a mobile x-ray unit becomes contaminated, it should never be cleaned while still inside the OR.

14. True or False. When positioning the C-arm during an operative cholangiogram, it is not necessary to cover the C-arm's image intensifier with a sterile drape if the patient's abdomen is already covered with a sterile drape.

15. True or False. The radiographer should be the person who places sterile drapes over both ends of the C-arm.

16. True or False. For the AP projection image of the lumbar spine, the spine should be centered in the vertical axis of the monitor.

17. True or False. When lining up the screw holes in the nail during a retrograde femoral nailing procedure, the hole should be imaged perfectly round and centered on the monitor.

18. True or False. When lining up the screw holes in the nail during a retrograde femoral nailing procedure, it may be necessary for the radiographer to manipulate the patient's leg.

19. True or False. To prevent overheating of the C-arm, a sterile drape should not be placed over the image intensifier.

20. True or False. When positioning the C-arm for imaging a tibial nail insertion, the C-arm should be tilted to match the angle of the affected leg.

21. True or False. When positioning the C-arm for use during a transsphenoidal resection of a pituitary tumor, the C-arm should be positioned for a lateral image.

22. True or False. *Road mapping* is a procedure that often is used during femoral arteriography.

23. True or False. The femur and the tibia should be seen in the image after subtraction technique is performed during femoral and tibial arteriography.

24. True or False. When performing a radiograph of an extremity during surgical procedures to install reduction hardware, the radiographer should remove sterile draping from the affected extremity to ensure proper centering.

25. True or False. *Strike-through* refers to moisture from a nonsterile surface soaking through to a sterile surface and causing bacteria to reach a sterile area.

270

Chapter **30** **Surgical Radiography**   Workbook for Merrill's Atlas of Radiographic Positioning and Procedures • Volume 2

Answer the following questions by selecting the best choice.

1. Which of the following personnel is a member of the sterile team during a surgical procedure?

   a. Circulator
   b. Radiographer
   c. Anesthesia provider
   d. Physician's assistant

2. Which of the following personnel is *not* a member of the sterile team during a surgical procedure?

   a. Surgeon
   b. Radiographer
   c. Surgical assistant
   d. Certified surgical technologist

3. What is the accepted protocol for the wearing of street clothes within the semirestricted and restricted areas of a surgical suite?

   a. They should never be worn in either area.
   b. They can be worn only in the semirestricted areas.
   c. They can be worn in either area only before the surgical procedure begins.
   d. They can be worn in either area only after the surgical procedure is completed.

4. What is the accepted protocol for the wearing of surgical caps within the semirestricted and restricted areas of a surgical suite?

   a. They should always be worn in either area.
   b. They should be worn only in the restricted areas.
   c. They should be worn in either area only after the surgical procedure begins.
   d. They should be worn in either area only before the surgical procedure begins.

5. What should a radiographer do with shoe covers after radiography services are no longer needed in the surgical suite?

   a. Remove them and hand them to the circulator.
   b. Remove and dispose of them before leaving the surgical area.
   c. They should be saved for use during the next visit to the surgical suite.
   d. Wear them until after returning to the radiology department, and then properly dispose of them.

6. What procedure should be followed if the radiographer who routinely performs surgical radiography has either an acute infection or a sore throat, and radiography services are requested within the OR?

   a. Send a different radiographer to the surgical suite.
   b. Ensure that the sick radiographer changes into proper operating room attire.
   c. Send another radiographer to assist the sick radiographer inside the operating room.
   d. Ensure that the sick radiographer wears gloves and a facemask when inside restricted areas of the surgical suite.

7. What procedure should a radiographer do if the sterile field is accidentally compromised?

   a. Immediately notify a member of the OR staff.
   b. Wipe down the mobile unit and repeat the procedure.
   c. Quickly finish the procedure and leave the operating room.
   d. Change into clean operating room attire and finish the procedure.

8. What is the proper procedure for placing an IR into a sterile IR cover?

   a. A radiographer should hand the IR to the surgeon so he or she can put it into a sterile IR cover.
   b. A radiographer should open the sterile IR cover and place the IR into it.
   c. A surgical technologist should open the sterile IR cover and hold it open for the radiographer to insert the IR into it.
   d. A radiographer should open the sterile IR cover and hold it open for the surgical technologist to insert the IR into it.

9. Which article of his/her operating room attire should a radiographer remove before handling the IR after performing a surgical radiography procedure?

   a. Cap
   b. Mask
   c. Gloves
   d. Shoe covers

10. What procedure should a radiographer perform if an exposed IR becomes contaminated in the operating room?

   a. Leave the contaminated IR in the OR.
   b. Repeat the examination with a clean IR.
   c. Wrap the contaminated IR in a sterile drape.
   d. Clean the IR with a hospital-approved disinfectant before leaving the OR.

11. When cleaning contaminated x-ray equipment within the OR suite, why is it preferred that cleaning solutions be poured instead of sprayed onto a rag?

    a. To conserve cleaning solutions
    b. To prevent possible contamination from the spray
    c. To reduce the amount of time it takes to clean the equipment
    d. To enable the cleaning of x-ray equipment while using only one hand

12. When using a C-arm to image a pregnant patient during an operative cholangiogram, where should a lead shield be placed to protect the patient?

    a. On top of the sterile field
    b. Under the patient and under the pelvic region
    c. On top of the patient and over the right upper quadrant
    d. Under the patient and under the right upper quadrant

13. Where should the C-arm be centered for an operative cholangiogram?

    a. Over the left side of the abdomen and superior to the rib line
    b. Over the left side of the abdomen and inferior to the rib line
    c. Over the right side of the abdomen and superior to the rib line
    d. Over the right side of the abdomen and inferior to the rib line

14. Why is it necessary to demonstrate a catheter from its insertion point to its terminal end with a C-arm unit when performing a line placement examination?

    a. To ensure there are no kinks in the catheter and to ensure that it is in the proper position
    b. To ensure there are no kinks in the catheter and to accurately measure the length of the catheter
    c. To accurately measure the depth of penetration and to ensure that it is in the proper position
    d. To accurately measure the depth of penetration and to accurately measure the length of the catheter

15. How many degrees and in which direction should the C-arm be tilted for the AP projection of the cervical spine during an ACDF procedure?

    a. 15 degrees caudad
    b. 15 degrees cephalad
    c. 25 degrees caudad
    d. 25 degrees cephalad

16. When using a C-arm unit to perform the lateral projection of the cervical spine, what procedure should be accomplished to place the spine into the center of the monitor?

    a. Raise or lower the C-arm.
    b. Remove padding from under the patient.
    c. Raise or lower the surgery table and patient.
    d. Place radiolucent cushions under the patient.

17. After obtaining a PA projection when using the C-arm during a hip pinning procedure, what procedure should be done to obtain a lateral image?

    a. Rotate the image intensifier 90 degrees.
    b. Rotate the C-arm under the leg and table.
    c. Rotate the patient's leg to the lateral position.
    d. Rotate the patient into a lateral recumbent position.

18. Where should a radiographer position the C-arm for use during a hip pinning procedure?

    a. Alongside the upper torso
    b. Between the patient's legs
    c. At right angles to the patient on the affected side
    d. At right angles to the patient on the unaffected side

19. When using the C-arm during a hip pinning procedure, what structures should be visualized to determine a starting point and to ensure no hardware enters the joint?

    a. Distal end of the femur and acetabular rim
    b. Distal end of the femur and intercondylar fossa
    c. Lateral side of the femur and acetabular rim
    d. Lateral side of the femur and intercondylar fossa

20. When using the C-arm during a tibial nailing procedure, how is it determined that the C-arm is correctly positioned over the patient's affected leg?

    a. Tilt the tube and image intensifier to match the angle of the leg.
    b. Tilt the tube and image intensifier to match the angle of the femur.
    c. Turn the wheels of the machine parallel with the patient to move the machine longitudinally.
    d. Turn the wheels of the machine perpendicular to the patient to move the machine towards the patient.

21. When using the C-arm during a tibial nailing procedure, what is the purpose for turning the wheels of the C-arm parallel with the long axis of the affected tibia?

    a. To prevent the C-arm from tilting during the procedure
    b. To prevent the C-arm from moving during the procedure
    c. To enable the C-arm to move towards the midline of the patient
    d. To enable the C-arm to move longitudinally alongside the patient

22. Why should a sterile drape not be allowed to remain on the C-arm's tube for a long time?

    a. The tube may overheat.
    b. The drape may become contaminated.
    c. The drape may cause artifacts on the image.
    d. The drape may contaminate the sterile field.

23. When imaging the patient during a transsphenoidal resection of a pituitary tumor, how should the C-arm be positioned relative to the patient?

    a. AP
    b. Lateral
    c. AP axial with 30 degrees caudal angulation
    d. AP axial with 30 degrees cephalad angulation

24. Which surgical procedure will most likely require subtraction technique with C-arm-arm imaging?

    a. Hip pinning
    b. Femoral nailing
    c. Chest line placement
    d. Femoral arteriography

25. What are two reasons for performing a lateral projection of thoracic or lumbar spine inside the OR?

    a. To identify specific vertebrae and to show the position of hardware
    b. To identify specific vertebrae and to perform an operational check of the portable unit
    c. To demonstrate intervertebral foramina and to show the position of hardware
    d. To demonstrate intervertebral foramina and to perform an operational check of the portable unit

31 Computed Tomography

Computed tomography (CT) is used so extensively that an understanding of this modality is becoming essential information for all radiographers. The following questions provide a brief review of CT. Answer each of the fill-in-the-blank, short answer, true/false, and multiple choice questions below.

1. Define *computed tomography*.

2. Fill in the blanks to describe the basic scanning steps in CT.

   The x-ray tube _____ around the patient or part.

   A _____ measures the radiation exiting the patient and feeds the data to a computer. The computer compiles and calculates the data according to a preselected

   _____ and assembles it into a _____. The image is then displayed on a

   _____.

3. List the three major components of a CT scanner.

   a. _____

   b. _____

   c. _____

4. Match the terms in Column A to the definition in Column B.

   Column A

   ____ 1. Detector assembly

   ____ 2. Matrix

   ____ 3. Hounsfield unit

   ____ 4. Data acquisition system (DAS)

   ____ 5. Field of view (FOV)

   ____ 6. Voxel

   ____ 7. Window level

   ____ 8. Gantry

   ____ 9. Window width

   ____ 10. Pixel

   Column B

   a. Number used to describe average density of tissue

   b. Area of anatomy displayed by the cathode ray tube (CRT)

   c. Volume element; determined by slice thickness

   d. Part of detector assembly that converts analog signals to digital signals

   e. Determines the midpoint of the range of gray levels displayed

   f. The range of CT numbers used to map signals into shades of gray

   g. Part of scanner that houses the x-ray tube, cooling system, detector assembly, and DAS

   h. One individual cell surface within an image matrix used for CRT image display; picture element

   i. Electronic component of scanner that measures remnant radiation exiting the patient and converts it to a proportional analog signal

   j. The array of numbers arranged in a grid; comprises the digital image

275

5. What is multiplanar reconstruction?

6. What are the most commonly used filming devices?

   a. _____

   b. _____

7. What are the three most commonly requested CT procedures?

8. By what three routes is contrast introduced for CT procedures?

9. The four main factors that affect CT image quality are:

   a. _____

   b. _____

   c. _____

   d. _____

10. The amount of blurring in a CT image is described as

    _____.

11. The ability to differentiate between small differences

    in density within the image is termed _____

    _____.

12. The most common cause of noise in a CT image arises from the random variation in photon detection,

    or _____.

13. Why would it be best to schedule a CT abdomen on a patient several days after the patient's gastrointestinal (GI) fluoroscopy procedure?

14. Indicate the image quality factor(s) affected by the scan parameter or item listed by writing *S* for spatial resolution, *C* for contrast resolution, *N* for noise, and *A* for artifacts.

    _____ 1. FOV

    _____ 2. Matrix size

    _____ 3. Slice thickness

    _____ 4. Dental fillings

    _____ 5. X-ray beam energy

    _____ 6. Focal spot size

    _____ 7. Residual barium

    _____ 8. Reconstruction algorithm

    _____ 9. Patient size

15. List four image quality factors that are under the technologist's control.

16. Which new CT data acquisition method involves the continuous rotation of the gantry as the table moves through the gantry?

17. Which new CT data acquisition technology has detectors arrays containing multiple rows of elements along the z-axis, instead of a single row of detectors?

18. List three advantages of CT angiography (CTA) over conventional angiography.

19. The three common techniques used for creating three-dimensional (3D) images from CT data are:

20. Which 3D-imaging technique is commonly used for CTA?

21. 3D reconstructions are particularly useful in

_____.

22. Indicate the preferred or more useful imaging modality by writing *CT* or *MRI* in the blank beside each item listed below.

_____ 1. Bony structures

_____ 2. Less scan time

_____ 3. Soft tissue

_____ 4. Claustrophobic patients

_____ 5. Better low-contrast resolution

_____ 6. Less costly

23. Most CT systems require _____ or

_____ preventative maintenance to ensure proper operation.

24. What method was first used to describe CT dose as a result of multiple scan locations?

25. List the factors that directly influence the CT radiation dose to the patient.

a. _____

b. _____

c. _____

d. _____

e. _____

f. _____

g. _____

h. _____

Radiographers are expected to recognize CT images from other modalities, identify basic anatomic structures, and identify the imaging plane. Answer each question related to the images provided to aid in your ability to analyze CT images.

1. Which image in Fig. 31-1—A or B—is the CT image?

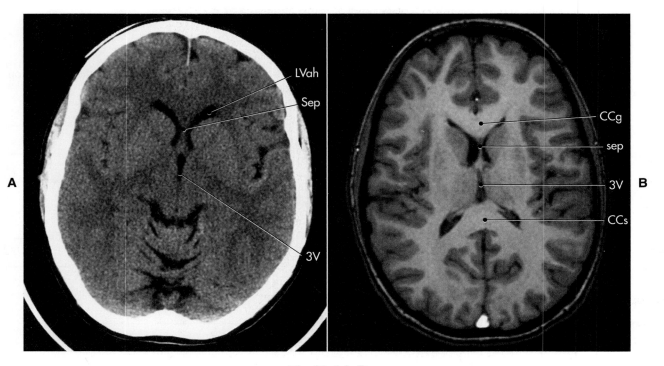

Fig. 31-1 A, B

2. Identify each lettered structure shown in Fig. 31-2.

A. _____

B. _____

C. _____

D. _____

E. _____

F. _____

G. _____

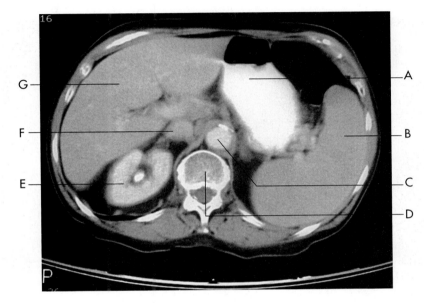

Fig. 31-2 Axial CT image of abdomen.

3. Label each image in Fig. 31-3 as a soft tissue window or a bone window.

A: _____

B: _____

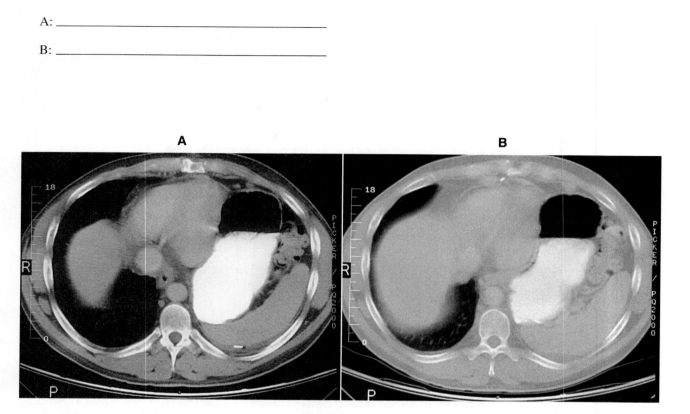

Fig. 31-3 A, B

Indicate the imaging plane, coronal or axial for Figs. 31-4 to 31-7.

4. Fig. 31-4: _____ plane

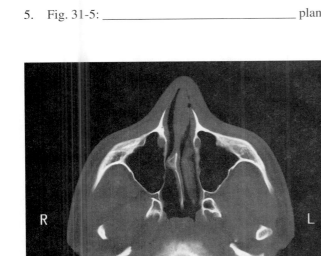

Fig. 31-4

5. Fig. 31-5: _____ plane

Fig. 31-5

6. Fig. 31-6: _____ plane

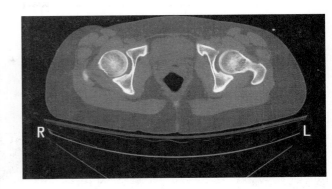

Fig. 31-6

7. Fig. 31-7: _____ plane

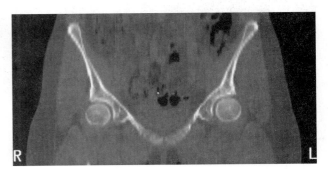

Fig. 31-7

Which of the images below demonstrate contrast media administration? Indicate by circling your answer provided below each image.

8. Fig. 31-8:

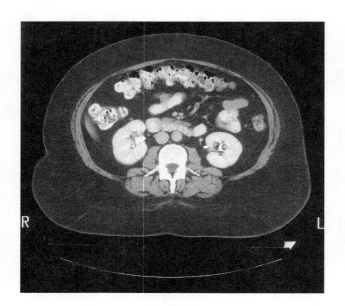

Fig. 31-8

Contrast   Noncontrast

9. Fig. 31-9:

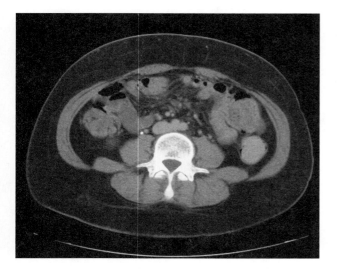

Fig. 31-9

Contrast   Noncontrast

10. Fig. 31-10:

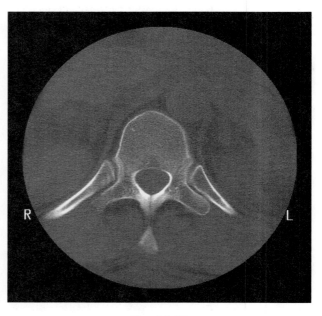

Fig. 31-10

Contrast   Noncontrast

Answer the following questions by selecting the best choice.

1. What term is applied to a single square, or picture element, in the image display matrix?

   a. CT number
   b. Hounsfield unit
   c. Pixel
   d. Raw data

2. What determines the amount of data displayed on the monitor?

   a. Number of volume elements
   b. Pixel size
   c. Tissue density
   d. FOV

3. A volume element is called a:

   a. Pixel
   b. Voxel
   c. Matrix
   d. CT number

4. A relative comparison of x-ray attenuation of a voxel of tissue to an equal volume of water is a(n):

   a. CT number
   b. Matrix
   c. FOV
   d. Scan profile

5. What is the CT number of water?

   a. −1000
   b. −500
   c. 0
   d. 1000

6. Which of the following are the major system components of a CT scanner?

   a. Gantry, computer and operator's console, and patient table
   b. CRT, gantry, and aperture
   c. Computer and operator's console, patient table, and DAS
   d. Patient table, computer, and 3D-reconstruction algorithms

7. A circular device that houses the x-ray tube, DAS, and detector array is called the:

   a. Gantry
   b. Computer
   c. Aperture
   d. Algorithm

8. X-ray tubes used in advanced CT scanners can tolerate:

   a. 0.5 to 1.5 million heat units (MHU)
   b. 2 to 3 MHU
   c. 4 to 5 MHU
   d. 6 to 10 MHU

9. Which of the following can be selected at the operator's console?

   1. Slice thickness
   2. Table index
   3. Radiographic technique factors
      a. 1 and 2 only
      b. 1 and 3 only
      c. 2 and 3 only
      d. 1, 2, and 3

10. The range of CT numbers that are used to map signals into shades of gray is called the:

    a. Window level
    b. Window width
    c. Image registration
    d. Matrix display

11. The midpoint of the range of gray levels to be displayed on the monitor is the:

    a. Window level
    b. Window width
    c. Hounsfield center
    d. Algorithm point

12. A narrow window width would display:

    a. A long gray scale
    b. Many shades of gray
    c. Low contrast
    d. High contrast

13. The window level should be set to:

    a. One half of the algorithm point
    b. The Hounsfield center
    c. One fourth of the window width
    d. The CT number of the tissue of interest

14. The preferred device for producing hard copies of CT images is the:

    a. Matrix camera
    b. Laser printer
    c. Xerox dry printer
    d. Conventional x-ray processor

15. CT is the examination of choice for:

    a. Limb fractures
    b. Head trauma
    c. The GI tract
    d. The genitourinary system

16. The amount of blurring in a CT image is termed:
    a. Noise
    b. Artifact
    c. Spatial resolution
    d. Contrast resolution

17. The ability to differentiate between small differences in density within the CT image is called:
    a. Spatial resolution
    b. Contrast resolution
    c. Windowing
    d. Gray level mapping

18. Which of the following is the most significant geometric factor that contributes to spatial resolution?
    a. Detector aperture width
    b. Focal spot size
    c. Slice thickness
    d. Detector array

19. Random variation in photon detection results in:
    a. Quantum noise
    b. Streak artifacts
    c. Beam hardening
    d. Image misregistration

20. Which of the following contribute to image noise in CT?
    1. Detector aperture width
    2. Matrix size
    3. Patient size
    a. 1 and 2 only
    b. 1 and 3 only
    c. 2 and 3 only
    d. 1, 2, and 3

21. Metallic objects, such as dental fillings, can cause:
    a. Image misregistration
    b. Quantum noise
    c. Windowing gauss
    d. Artifacts

22. High-resolution CT scans are made using:
    a. Shorter scan times
    b. Thinner sections or slices
    c. Wider window widths
    d. Volume rendering algorithms

23. Which of the following quality factors is affected by x-ray beam energy?
    1. Contrast resolution
    2. Spatial resolution
    3. Noise
    a. 1 and 2 only
    b. 1 and 3 only
    c. 2 and 3 only
    d. 1, 2, and 3

24. Which image quality factor is affected by focal spot size?
    a. Noise
    b. Artifacts
    c. Spatial resolution
    d. Contrast resolution

25. Tissue density differences of less than _____ can be distinguished by CT.
    a. 0.01%
    b. 0.1%
    c. 0.5%
    d. 1.0%

26. Reconstruction algorithm affects all of the image quality factors *except* for:
    a. Artifacts
    b. Contrast resolution
    c. Spatial resolution
    d. Noise

27. The image that appears on the CRT depends on the:
    a. Focal spot size
    b. Detector array
    c. Detector aperture width
    d. Scan diameter

28. What is based on the principle that different structures enhance at different rates after contrast administration?
    a. Dynamic scanning
    b. 3D imaging
    c. Spiral CT
    d. Image misregistration

29. What new CT data acquisition method involves continuous gantry rotations combined with constant table movement through the aperture?
    a. Dynamic scanning
    b. Maximun intensity projection
    c. Volume rendering
    d. Spiral or helical CT

30. Which 3D-imaging technique is commonly used for CTA?
    a. Dynamic scanning
    b. Maximum intensity projection
    c. Shaded surface display
    d. Volume rendering

284

Appendix: Supplemental Exercises for Skull Positioning

SKULL POSITIONING REVIEW

Note to Students: The exercises in this appendix pertain to information referenced from Chapters 20 through 22 and should be completed after you have completed the review exercises for those chapters.

Exercise 1

Match each projection in Column A with the number of degrees and direction of central ray angulation in Column B. Choices from Column B may be used once, more than once, or not at all.

Column A

_____ 1. AP axial (cranium)

_____ 2. AP axial (cranium; Towne method)

_____ 3. AP axial (temporomandibular articulations)

_____ 4. AP axial (zygomatic arches; modified Towne method)

_____ 5. PA axial (mandibular rami)

_____ 6. PA axial (cranium; Haas method)

_____ 7. PA axial (sinuses; Caldwell method)

_____ 8. PA axial (cranium; Caldwell method)

_____ 9. Axiolateral oblique (mandible)

_____ 10. Axiolateral oblique (temporomandibular articulations)

_____ 11. Axiolateral oblique (petromastoid portion; Arcelin method [anterior profile])

_____ 12. Axiolateral oblique (petromastoid portion; Stenvers method [posterior profile])

_____ 13. Parietoacanthial (sinuses; Waters method)

_____ 14. Parietoorbital oblique (optic foramen; Rhese method)

_____ 15. Axiolateral oblique (mastoids; modified Law method [single-tube angulation method])

Column B

a. Perpendicular

b. 10 degrees caudad

c. 10 degrees cephalad

d. 12 degrees caudad

e. 12 degrees cephalad

f. 15 degrees caudad

g. 15 degrees cephalad

h. 20 degrees caudad

i. 20 degrees cephalad

j. 23 degrees caudad

k. 23 degrees cephalad

l. 25 degrees caudad

m. 25 degrees cephalad

n. 30 degrees caudad

o. 30 degrees cephalad

p. 35 degrees caudad

q. 35 degrees cephalad

r. 37 degrees cephalad

Exercise 2

Match the projections in Column A with the locations in Column B. Each location in Column B is either a centering point for the body part or a point where the central ray should enter or exit the patient. Not all locations in Column B may apply to the projections listed in Column A.

Column A

_____ 1. Lateral (cranium)

_____ 2. Lateral (nasal bones)

_____ 3. Lateral (facial bones)

_____ 4. Submentovertical (cranium; Schüller)

_____ 5. Lateral (paranasal sinuses)

_____ 6. Tangential (zygomatic arch)

_____ 7. PA axial (cranium; Haas method)

_____ 8. PA axial (cranium; Caldwell method)

_____ 9. Parietoacanthial (sinuses; Waters method)

_____ 10. AP axial (zygomatic arches; modified Towne method)

_____ 11. AP axial (temporomandibular articulations)

_____ 12. Axiolateral oblique (temporomandibular articulations)

_____ 13. Axiolateral oblique (petromastoid portion; Arcelin method [anterior profile])

_____ 14. Axiolateral oblique (petromastoid portion; Stenvers method [posterior profile])

_____ 15. Axiolateral oblique (mastoids; modified Law method [single-tube angulation method])

Column B

a. Nasion

b. Glabella

c. Acanthion

d. Zygomatic bone

e. External acoustic meatus (EAM)

f. ½ inch (1.2 cm) distal to the nasion

g. 1½ inches (3.8 cm) above the nasion

h. 3 inches (7.6 cm) above the nasion

i. ½ to 1 inch (1.2 to 2.5 cm) posterior to the outer canthus

j. 1 inch (2.5 cm) posterior to the outer canthus

k. ½ inch (1.2 cm) anterior to the EAM

l. 1 inch (2.5 cm) anterior to the EAM

m. 1 inch (2.5 cm) posterior to the EAM

n. 2 inches (5 cm) superior to the EAM

o. ¾ inch (1.9 cm) anterior to the level of the EAM

p. 1 inch (2.5 cm) anterior and ¾ inch (1.9 cm) superior to the EAM

Examine the following diagrams of various projections of the skull (e.g., cranium, facial bones, sinuses). Listed after the diagrams are the names and characteristics of skull projections. In the space provided, write the letter of the diagram that corresponds to each name or characteristic. Not all diagrams may apply to the listed names and characteristics, and some diagrams may be used more than once.

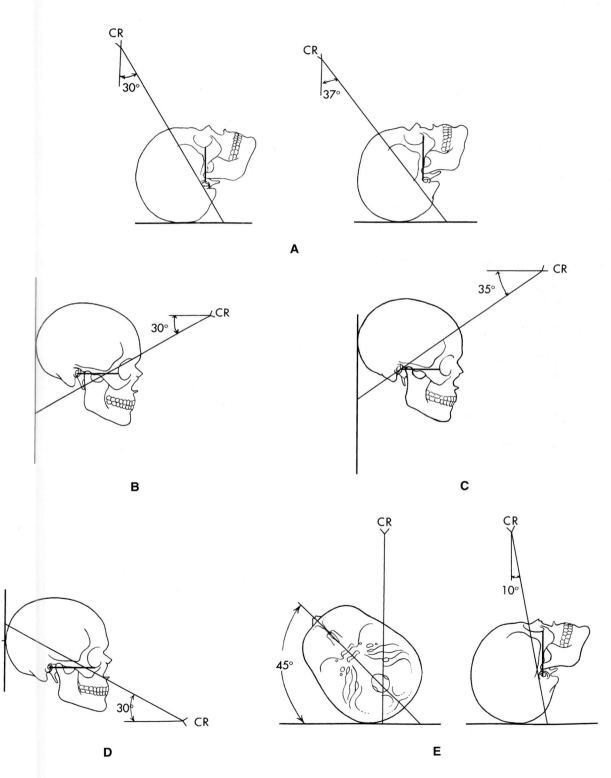

287

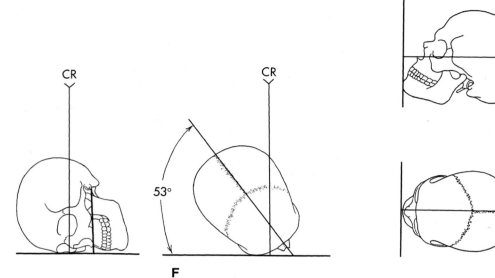

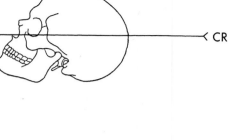

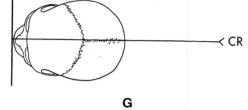

F

G

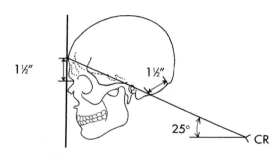

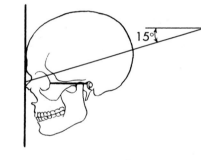

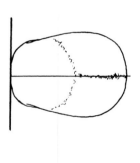

H

I

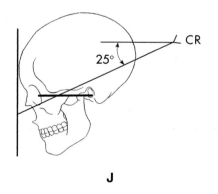

J

288

Appendix: Supplemental Exercises for Skull Positioning   Workbook for Merrill's Atlas of Radiographic Positioning and Procedures • Volume 2

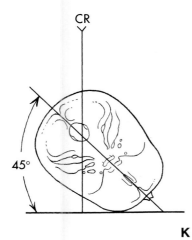

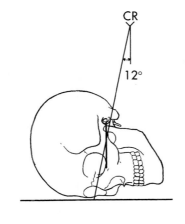

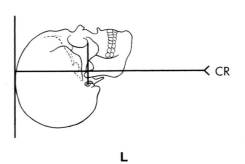

K

L

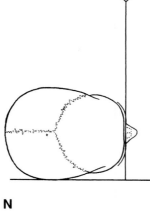

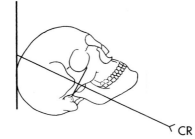

M

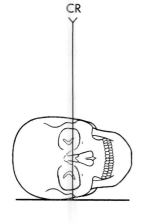

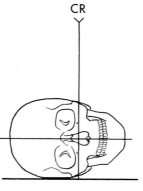

N

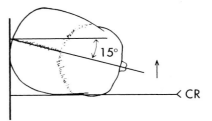

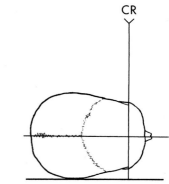

O

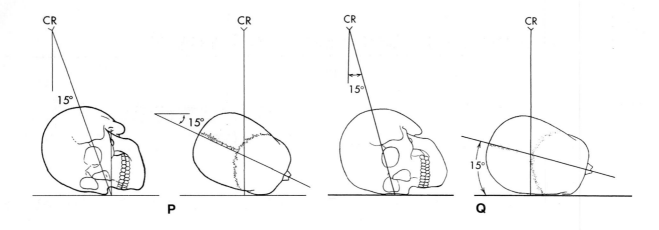

P   Q

1. Parietoacanthial projection (Waters method)

2. Full basal projection of the cranium

3. AP axial projection (cranium, Towne method)

4. AP axial projection demonstrating temporomandibular joints (TMJs)

5. PA axial projection (cranium, Haas method)

6. PA axial projection (cranium, Caldwell method)

7. Parietoorbital oblique projection (Rhese method)

8. Demonstrates one TMJ

9. Best projection for demonstrating the maxillary sinuses

10. Tangential projection for demonstrating an individual zygomatic arch

11. Petrous ridges should be projected immediately below the maxillae.

12. Demonstrates the mastoid air cells of the side closest to the cassette

13. Lateral projection and central ray alignment for demonstrating the nasal bones

14. Lateral projection and central ray alignment for demonstrating the facial bones

15. Orbitomeatal line (OML) should form an angle of 37 degrees with the cassette.

16. Petrous ridges should be projected into the lower one third of the orbits.

17. Shows a profile image of the part of the petromastoid closest to the cassette

18. Axiolateral oblique projection (petromastoid portion, Arcelin method [anterior profile])

19. Axiolateral oblique projection (petromastoid portion, Stenvers method [posterior profile])

20. AP axial projection and central ray alignment for demonstrating bilateral zygomatic arches

21. AP axial projection and central ray alignment for demonstrating TMJs

22. Produces a slightly oblique tangential image of one zygomatic arch free from superimposed shadows

23. Central ray should enter 2 inches (5 cm) posterior to and 2 inches (5 cm) superior to the upside EAM.

Answers to Exercises: Volume 2

CHAPTER 13: TRAUMA RADIOGRAPHY

Review

1. A sudden, unexpected, dramatic, forceful, or violent event
2. Level I trauma centers provide the most comprehensive medical and emergency care, whereas level IV trauma centers provide care for basic injuries and can assess and stabilize patients for transfer to a larger trauma center.
3. 6 feet
4. Cool, clammy skin; excessive sweating; increased drowsiness; loss of consciousness; and patient complains of thirst
5. Document the alterations for the referring physician and radiologist.
6. Lateral projection, dorsal decubitus position
7. When the entire cervical spine and the interspace between C7 and T1 is not well demonstrated with the lateral projection
8. Permission is granted from the attending physician after review of the lateral projection.
9. When the patient cannot depress the tube-side shoulder
10. To blur rib shadows
11. The attending physician
12. The compound central ray angle will cause grid cutoff.
13. At a compound angle of 15 to 20 degrees cephalad and 45 degrees lateromedially
14. Slightly lateral to the midsagittal plane at the level of the thyroid cartilage, and passing through C4
15. Lateral projection, dorsal decubitus position
16. Horizontal and perpendicular to the center of the IR
17. Permission from the attending physician to transfer the patient to the radiographic table
18. Immediately inform the attending physician.
19. To prevent grid cutoff and image distortion
20. To allow any free air to rise and be visualized
21. Internal hemorrhaging and hemorrhagic shock
22. Immediately alert the attending physician.
23. Approximately perpendicular
24. Always include both joints.
25. Do not remove unless directed to do so by the attending physician.
26. Cardiopulmonary resuscitation
27. Motor vehicle accident
28. Gunshot wound
29. Cerebrovascular accident
30. Emergency department
31. Orbitomeatal line
32. Infraorbitomeatal line
33. Mentomeatal line
34. Intravenous urography
35. External acoustic meatus

Self-Test: Trauma Radiography

1. d	5. a	9. a	13. d	17. c
2. b	6. d	10. c	14. b	18. d
3. c	7. d	11. b	15. d	19. c
4. a	8. c	12. b	16. c	20. a

CHAPTER 14: MOUTH AND SALIVARY GLANDS

Review

1. A. Posterior arch
   B. Anterior arch
   C. Tonsil
   D. Hard palate
   E. Uvula
   F. Soft palate
   G. Tongue
2. A. Orifice of the submandibular duct
   B. Tongue
   C. Frenulum of the tongue
   D. Sublingual fold
3. A. Parotid duct
   B. Sublingual ducts
   C. Submandibular duct
   D. Sublingual gland
   E. Parotid gland
   F. Submandibular gland
4. A. Muscle tissue
   B. Ramus of mandible
   C. Parotid gland
   D. Tongue
   E. Dens
   F. Atlas
   G. Spinal cord
5. A. Mandible
   B. Oropharynx
   C. Cervical vertebral body
   D. Sublingual gland
   E. Submandibular gland
   F. Tip of parotid gland
6. Mouth
7. The process of chewing and grinding food into small pieces
8. Teeth
9. To soften food, keep the mouth moist, and contribute digestive enzymes
10. Parotid, sublingual, and submandibular
11. Radiographic examination of the salivary glands and ducts with the use of a contrast medium
12. Water-soluble, iodinated medium
13. Salivary gland pairs are in close proximity.
14. To detect any condition demonstrable without the use of a contrast medium, and to establish the optimal exposure factors

291

15. Tangential and lateral projections
16. b
17. Perpendicular to the image receptor along the lateral surface of the mandibular ramus
18. True
19. True
20. False (Only one parotid gland can be demonstrated with each tangential projection.)
21. a. Tangential projection
    b. Parotid
    c. The patient can fill the mouth with air and then puff the cheeks out as much as possible.
22. a. Lateral projection
    b. Parotid
    c. Parotid
23. a. Lateral projection
    b. Submandibular
    c. Submandibular

Self-Test: Mouth and Salivary Glands

1. a	5. a	9. a	13. a
2. a	6. b	10. c	14. c
3. b	7. d	11. a	15. b
4. a	8. b	12. a	

CHAPTER 15: ANTERIOR PART OF THE NECK

Review

1. A. Nasal septum
   B. Nasopharynx
   C. Uvula
   D. Epiglottis
   E. Vocal folds
   F. Larynx
   G. Laryngeal pharynx
   H. Soft palate
   I. Piriform recess
   J. Rima glottidis
2. A. Soft palate
   B. Nasopharynx
   C. Uvula
   D. Oropharynx
   E. Epiglottis
   F. Vocal cords
   G. Larynx
   H. Hard palate
   I. Hyoid bone
   J. Laryngeal pharynx
   K. Trachea
   L. Thyroid cartilage
   M. Esophagus
3. A. Superior parathyroid gland
   B. Thyroid gland
   C. Inferior parathyroid gland
   D. Esophagus
   E. Thyroid cartilage
   F. Isthmus of the thyroid
   G. Trachea
4. A. Hyoid bone
   B. Thyroid cartilage
   C. Trachea

5. A. Base of the tongue
   B. Epiglottis
   C. Vestibular fold (false vocal cord)
   D. Rima glottidis (open)
   E. Rima glottidis (closed)
   F. Vocal fold (true vocal cord)
6. Posterior; anterior
7. Trachea
8. Esophagus
9. Thyroid; parathyroid
10. Pharynx
11. Nasopharynx
12. Oropharynx
13. Larynx
14. Glottis
15. AP projection; lateral projection
16. Breathing, phonation, stress maneuvers, and swallowing
17. a. Supine
    b. Upright
18. Laryngeal prominence
19. a. Level of the external acoustic meatuses
    b. Level of the mandibular angles
    c. Level of the laryngeal prominence
20. A. Air-filled pharynx
    B. Hyoid bone
    C. Laryngeal structures
    D. Trachea

Self-Test: Anterior Part of the Neck

1. c	6. d
2. a	7. b
3. d	8. b
4. b	9. b
5. c	10. b

CHAPTER 16: DIGESTIVE SYSTEM: ABDOMEN AND BILIARY TRACT

SECTION 1: ANATOMY OF THE DIGESTIVE SYSTEM: ABDOMEN AND BILIARY TRACT

Exercise 1

1. A. Left lobe of the liver
   B. Falciform ligament
   C. Right lobe of the liver
   D. Gallbladder
   E. Ascending colon
   F. Ileum
   G. Appendix
   H. Diaphragm
   I. Esophagus
   J. Stomach
   K. Spleen
   L. Pancreas
   M. Descending colon
   N. Transverse colon
   O. Small intestine
   P. Urinary bladder
2. A. Tongue
   B. Sublingual gland
   C. Submandibular gland

292

D. Gallbladder
E. Biliary ducts
F. Visceral surface of the liver
G. Vermiform appendix
H. Parotid gland
I. Pharynx
J. Esophagus
K. Stomach
L. Spleen
M. Pancreas
N. Large intestine
O. Small intestine

3. A. Hepatopancreatic ampulla
B. Cystic duct
C. Right lobe of the liver
D. Gallbladder
E. Liver
F. Falciform ligament
G. Quadrate lobe of the liver
H. Left lobe of the liver
I. Left hepatic duct
J. Caudate lobe of the liver
K. Common hepatic duct
L. Common bile duct
M. Pancreatic duct
N. Pancreas
O. Duodenum

4. A. Cut surface of the liver
B. Gallbladder
C. Cystic duct
D. Right kidney
E. Common hepatic duct
F. Common bile duct
G. Spleen
H. Left kidney
I. Pancreas
J. Duodenum

5. A. Liver
B. Duodenum
C. Stomach
D. Inferior vena cava
E. Right kidney
F. Aorta
G. Pancreas
H. Left kidney
I. Spleen

Exercise 2

1. b
2. e
3. i
4. a
5. c
6. k
7. d
8. f
9. g
10. h

Exercise 3

1. Peritoneum
2. Parietal; visceral
3. Parietal
4. Visceral
5. Liver
6. Liver

7. Bile
8. Common hepatic duct
9. Gallbladder
10. Liver
11. Common bile duct
12. Pancreatic duct
13. Cholecystokinin
14. Hepatopancreatic ampulla
15. Pancreas
16. True
17. False (The gallbladder is located on the inferior surface of the right lobe of the liver, within the abdominal cavity.)
18. True
19. True
20. True

SECTION 2: POSITIONING OF THE ABDOMEN AND BILIARY TRACT

Exercise 1: Positioning for the Abdomen

1. Supine KUB, AP upright abdomen, and PA chest
2. To demonstrate abdominal free air that may accumulate under the diaphragm
3. Left lateral decubitus
4. Gonadal shielding is desirable if the gonads lie within close proximity (2 inches [5 cm]) to the primary x-ray field; gonadal shielding should be used if the clinical objectives of the examination will not be compromised; and gonadal shielding should be used if the patient has a reasonable reproductive potential.
5. Psoas
6. KUB
7. Midsagittal
8. Iliac crests
9. 2 inches (5 cm) above the iliac crests (high enough to include the diaphragm) and to the level of the iliac crests (to include the bladder)
10. Diaphragm (to demonstrate any free air within the abdominal cavity that may rise and become trapped under the diaphragm)
11. Suspend respiration at the end of expiration.
12. So that abdominal organs are not compressed
13. A right or left marker and an appropriate marker indicating the patient is upright
14. A reduction in the radiation exposure to the gonads
15. b, d, e
16. Demonstration of air-fluid levels
17. To enable rising free air to be seen through the homogeneous background density of the liver instead of becoming superimposed with air in the stomach
18. The patient should be recumbent in a lateral position with the left side down (left lateral recumbent), both arms raised above the diaphragm, and the knees slightly flexed.
19. To allow any air to rise to its highest level within the abdomen
20. A vertically placed IR should be centered against the patient's posterior side of the abdomen at the level of the iliac crests.
21. Suspend respiration after expiration.

22. Perpendicular (horizontally) to the midpoint of the IR, entering at the level of the iliac crests
23. The dependent "down" side
24. The "up" side
25. Diaphragm
26. Markers indicating the side of the patient and which side is up
27. True
28. False (The midcoronal plane should be perpendicular and centered to the IR.)
29. False (Make the exposure after the patient suspends respiration after expiration.)
30. The iliac crests, or 2 inches above the iliac crests to include the diaphragm
31. Across the pelvis
32. To a point on the midcoronal plane at the level of the iliac crests
33. Pelvis and lumbar vertebrae
34. Dorsal decubitus
35. To relieve strain on the patient's back by reducing the lordotic curvature
36. Midcoronal plane
37. 2 inches (5 cm)
38. False (Make the exposure after the suspension of expiration.)
39. True
40. b, c, d

Exercise 2: Contrast Studies for the Biliary Tract

1. Cholecystography
2. Biliary ducts
3. Sonography
4. CT and MRI
5. Percutaneous transhepatic cholangiography
6. Obstructive jaundice
7. a
8. True
9. False (A local anesthetic is used.)
10. False (Retrieval baskets can be used once the drainage catheter has been in place for a while.)
11. 1. Demonstrate patency and caliber of biliary ducts
    2. Demonstrate the status of the sphincter of the hepatopancreatic ampulla
    3. Demonstrate the presence of residual or previously undetected stones or other pathologic conditions in the biliary ducts
12. c
13. To allow the tube to fill with bile to minimize the possibility of air bubbles entering the ducts. Air bubbles can mimic cholesterol (radiolucent) stones.
14. Water-soluble, iodinated
15. RPO; RUQ
16. Endoscopic retrograde cholangiopancreatography
17. When the biliary ducts are not dilated and when the ampulla is not obstructed
18. Sonography; pancreatic pseudocysts
19. The duodenum
20. No food or drink for at least 1 hour after the procedure to allow time for the effects of the local anesthetic to subside

1. a	8. d	15. d	22. a	29. a
2. d	9. a	16. b	23. c	30. d
3. d	10. d	17. a	24. a	31. d
4. b	11. d	18. a	25. a	32. d
5. d	12. b	19. d	26. b	33. b
6. c	13. a	20. c	27. b	34. b
7. b	14. a	21. a	28. a	35. a

CHAPTER 17: DIGESTIVE SYSTEM: ALIMENTARY CANAL

SECTION 1: ANATOMY OF THE ALIMENTARY CANAL

Exercise 1

1. A. Tongue
   B. Sublingual gland
   C. Submandibular gland
   D. Gallbladder
   E. Biliary ducts
   F. Vermiform appendix
   G. Rectum
   H. Parotid gland
   I. Pharynx
   J. Esophagus
   K. Stomach
   L. Spleen
   M. Pancreas
   N. Large intestine
   O. Small intestine
2. A. Cardiac antrum
   B. Cardia
   C. Lesser curvature
   D. Angular notch
   E. Pyloric sphincter
   F. Duodenum
   G. Pyloric canal
   H. Pyloric antrum
   I. Greater curvature
   J. Cardiac notch
   K. Fundus
   L. Body
3. A. Cardiac sphincter
   B. Pyloric sphincter
   C. Duodenum
   D. Pyloric canal
   E. Rugae
4. A. Major duodenal papilla (orifice of biliary and pancreatic ducts)
   B. Hepatopancreatic ampulla
   C. Gallbladder
   D. Cystic duct
   E. Common hepatic duct
   F. Common bile duct
   G. Pylorus
   H. Stomach
   I. Pancreatic duct
   J. Pancreas
   K. Duodenum

5. A. Ileum
   B. Vermiform appendix
   C. Cecum
   D. Ascending colon
   E. Right colic flexure
   F. Transverse colon
   G. Left colic flexure
   H. Descending colon
   I. Sigmoid colon
   J. Rectum
6. A. Sacrum
   B. Anal canal
   C. Rectum
   D. Rectal ampulla

Exercise 2

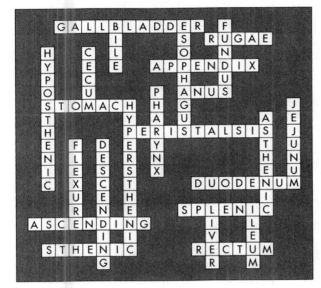

Exercise 3

1. b	6. c	11. b	16. a
2. a	7. a	12. c	17. b
3. a	8. a	13. c	18. a
4. b	9. c	14. c	19. c
5. c	10. b	15. a	20. c

Exercise 4

1. f	6. b
2. e	7. k
3. g	8. h
4. a	9. i
5. d	10. c

Exercise 5

1. Esophagus
2. Cardiac antrum
3. Cardiac orifice
4. Stomach
5. Rugae
6. Right (medial)

7. Pylorus
8. Greater curvature
9. a. Hypersthenic
   b. Sthenic
   c. Hyposthenic
   d. Asthenic
10. Cardia, fundus, body, and pylorus
11. Cardia
12. Fundus
13. Pyloric
14. Pyloric orifice
15. Duodenum; jejunum; ileum
16. Duodenum
17. Duodenal bulb
18. Ileocecal valve
19. Duodenum
20. Jejunum
21. Ileum
22. Duodenum; ileum
23. Small
24. Ileocecal valve
25. Cecum
26. Cecum
27. Right colic
28. Ascending
29. Transverse
30. Left colic
31. Descending
32. Descending colon; rectum
33. Rectum
34. Anal canal
35. Anus

SECTION 2: POSITIONING OF THE ALIMENTARY CANAL

Exercise 1: Positioning for the Esophagus

1. AP or PA projection, AP or PA oblique projection (RAO or LPO position), and lateral projection
2. A high-density barium product and carbon dioxide crystals
3. The LAO position may superimpose vertebral shadows with the distal esophagus.
4. T5-T6 (top of IR should be at the level of the mouth)
5. RAO and LPO
6. It allows more complete contrast filling of the esophagus.
7. The esophagus should be adequately demonstrated through the superimposed thoracic vertebrae.
8. To the left of the vertebral column, between the thoracic vertebrae and the heart
9. Partially obscured by thoracic vertebrae
10. Posterior ribs; they should be superimposed.
11. 35; 40
12. Cardiac orifice
13. True
14. True

15. False (A 30% to 50% weight per volume suspension is acceptable. The most important criterion for the barium is that the flow must be sufficient to coat esophageal walls.)

Exercise 2: The Gastrointestinal Series

1. UGI
2. To reduce the production of intestinal gas and fecal material
3. The coating ability of the barium could be diminished because the secretion of gastric juices may be stimulated.
4. A barium sulfate product of 30% to 50% weight per volume concentration
5. Single-contrast examination and double-contrast examination
6. 30% to 50%
7. Small lesions are readily demonstrated, and the mucosal lining of the stomach can be more clearly visualized.
8. High-density barium sulfate suspension and gas-producing substance
9. False (The examination should begin with the patient upright.)
10. False (Most radiographs are obtained with the patient in the recumbent position to provide better coating of the mucosal surface.)
11. True
12. To coat the mucosal lining of the stomach
13. The patient should be instructed not to belch.
14. To relax the gastric tract, enabling gastric structures to expand and thus be better demonstrated
15. A biphasic GI examination is a UGI examination in which the patient is first examined with a double-contrast procedure, after which a low weight per volume barium sulfate suspension is administered, and the patient is examined with a single-contrast procedure.
16. Double-contrast
17. With intubation and without intubation
18. True
19. True
20. True
21. False (The patient should be in the recumbent position.)
22. True
23. True
24. False (A compression band should not be used to immobilize the patient, because its use can cause filling defects and interfere with the filling and emptying of the duodenal bulb.)
25. The patient's weight should be supported by cushions placed under the thorax and pelvis.
26. Center over the midline of the grid a sagittal plane passing halfway between the vertebral column and the left lateral border of the abdomen.
27. Centered about 1 to 2 inches above the lower rib margin, at the level of Ll-L2
28. Center the IR 3 to 6 inches (7.5 to 15 cm) lower.
29. Asthenic
30. Suspend respiration after expiration.
31. Perpendicular to the center of the IR

32. Instruct the patient to turn toward the left, elevating the left side away from the x-ray table and to support the raised left side with the left forearm and flexed left knee.
33. Perpendicular to the center of the IR
34. c
35. c
36. True
37. False (The patient should suspend respiration after expiration.)
38. Supine
39. Right
40. 45
41. Midway between the xiphoid process and the lower lateral margin of the ribs
42. To a point midway between the midsagittal plane and the left lateral margin of the abdomen and centered to a level midway between the xiphoid process and the lower lateral margin of the ribs
43. True
44. False (An air-contrast image, not a barium-filled image, of the pyloric canal and duodenal bulb is produced with the LPO position.)
45. A. Distal esophagus
    B. Fundus
    C. Body
    D. Pylorus
    E. Duodenum
46. d
47. b
48. a
49. c
50. b
51. Perpendicular to the center of the IR and midway between the midcoronal plane and the anterior surface of the abdomen
52. a. Gas-filled
    b. Barium-filled
    c. Barium-filled
53. A. Fundus
    B. Body
    C. Duodenum
    D. Duodenal bulb
    E. Pyloric portion
54. b
55. c
56. Center the midsagittal plane to the midline of the grid.
57. Center a sagittal plane passing midway between the midsagittal plane and the lateral margin of the left ribs to the midline of the grid.
58. Midway between the tip of the xiphoid process and the lower margin of the ribs
59. a. Gas-filled (double-contrast)
    b. Barium-filled
    c. Gas-filled (double-contrast)
    d. Gas-filled (double-contrast)
60. A. Fundus
    B. Body
    C. Pyloric portion
    D. Duodenal loop

296

Exercise 3: Small Intestine Examination

1. Orally, reflux filling, and intubation (direct injection)
2. a
3. a, b, f, g
4. c
5. a
6. b
7. b
8. a
9. c
10. b
11. b
12. c
13. b
14. b
15. b
16. c
17. a
18. a
19. a
20. a, b, d, e, f, g, i

Exercise 4: Large Intestine Examination

1. c
2. Barium sulfate
3. To obtain better coating of the lumen
4. Air and carbon dioxide
5. When the patient cannot tolerate retrograde filling of the colon
6. Although it may vary, typical preparation includes a restrictive diet, laxatives, and a cleansing enema.
7. The entire colon should be as clean as possible; no fecal material should be present.
8. Approximately 85° to 90° F
9. Barium that is too warm may be unpleasant and debilitating to the patient, may injure internal tissues, and may produce irritation that makes it difficult for the patient to retain the barium for as long as required.
10. Approximately 41° F
11. Cold barium causes less irritation to the colon, relaxes the colon, and stimulates tonal contraction of the anal sphincter to increase patient comfort, facilitate better toleration of the examination, and improve retention of the barium.
12. Maintain tight contraction of the anal sphincter around the enema tip, relax the abdominal muscles, and concentrate on deep oral breathing.
13. 24 inches (61 cm)
14. About 3½ to 4 inches (8.9 to 10 cm)
15. Postevacuation (or postevac) image
16. a
17. c
18. a

19. A. Left colic flexure
    B. Right colic flexure
    C. Transverse colon
    D. Descending colon
    E. Ascending colon
    F. Cecum
    G. Sigmoid
    H. Rectum
20. b
21. c
22. b
23. c
24. False (Superior colic structures [transverse colon and both flexures] need not be demonstrated.)
25. A. Left colic flexure
    B. Transverse colon
    C. Sigmoid
    D. Rectum
26. True
27. False (The central ray should be directed perpendicular to the center of the IR.)
28. True
29. True
30. A. Left colic flexure
    B. Right colic flexure
    C. Descending colon
    D. Ascending colon
    E. Sigmoid
31. c
32. b
33. A. Left colic flexure
    B. Right colic flexure
    C. Transverse colon
    D. Descending colon
    E. Ascending colon
    F. Vermiform appendix
    G. Sigmoid
34. To the level of the anterior superior iliac spines
35. Hips and femurs should be superimposed.
36. a
37. c
38. A. Sigmoid
    B. Sacrum
    C. Rectum
    D. Pubic symphysis
39. Midsagittal
40. Iliac crests
41. True
42. True
43. A. Left colic flexure
    B. Transverse colon
    C. Right colic flexure
    D. Descending colon
    E. Ascending colon
    F. Sigmoid
44. b
45. d
46. 2 inches (5 cm) below the level of the anterior superior iliac spines
47. The inferior margin of the pubic symphysis

297

48. A. Descending colon
    B. Sigmoid
    C. Rectum
49. PA oblique; RAO
50. 35; 45
51. Right
52. Right colic
53. A. Left colic flexure
    B. Right colic flexure
    C. Descending colon
    D. Ascending colon
    E. Sigmoid
    F. Rectum
54. LAO
55. Left colic
56. 35 to 45 degrees
57. A. Left colic flexure
    B. Transverse colon
    C. Right colic flexure
    D. Descending colon
    E. Ascending colon
    F. Sigmoid
58. d
59. Support the patient on a radiolucent pad.
60. Area from the flexures to the rectum
61. a. Right lateral decubitus
    b. Left lateral decubitus
62. a. Fig. 17-38
    b. Fig. 17-37
    c. Fig. 17-37
    d. Fig. 17-38
    e. Fig. 17-38
    f. Fig. 17-37
63. It is lower—generally 2 to 3 inches (5 to 7.5 cm)—because of the gravitational effect.
64. a. Upright
    b. Liquid barium can be seen settling to the lower levels of the colon.
65. 1. g
    2. c
    3. e
    4. d
    5. a
    6. b
    7. f
    8. h

CHAPTER 18: URINARY SYSTEM

SECTION 1: ANATOMY OF THE URINARY SYSTEM

Exercise 1

1. A. Right kidney
   B. Inferior vena cava
   C. Aorta
   D. Left kidney
   E. Left ureter
   F. Urinary bladder
2. A. Right kidney
   B. Right ureter
   C. Urinary bladder
   D. Rectum
   E. Prostate
   F. Anal canal
3. A. Hilum
   B. Renal papilla
   C. Renal pelvis
   D. Renal cortex
   E. Renal sinus
   F. Renal medulla
   G. Renal pyramid
   H. Minor calyx
   I. Major calyx
4. A. Cortex
   B. Medulla
   C. Afferent arteriole
   D. Efferent arteriole
   E. Glomerulus
   F. Distal convoluted tubule
   G. Glomerular capsule
   H. Proximal convoluted tubule
   I. Descending limb of Henle's loop
   J. Ascending limb of Henle's loop
   K. Collecting duct

5. A. Ovary
   B. Uterine tube
   C. Uterus
   D. Bladder
   E. Pubic symphysis
   F. Urethra
   G. Vagina
   H. Rectum
6. A. Bladder
   B. Pubic symphysis
   C. Urethra
   D. Sacrum
   E. Rectum
   F. Prostate

Exercise 2

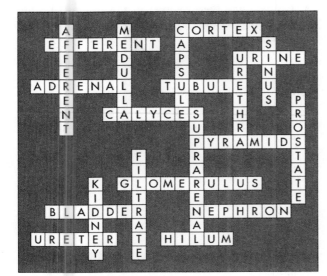

Exercise 3

1. l	6. g	11. o
2. p	7. j	12. e
3. a	8. f	13. m
4. d	9. h	14. c
5. k	10. n	15. i

Exercise 4

1. Urinary
2. Kidney
3. Suprarenal
4. Hilum
5. Medial
6. T12
7. Nephron
8. Cortex
9. Glomerular
10. Glomerulus
11. Renal
12. Afferent; efferent
13. Glomerular filtrate
14. Calyces
15. Calyces

16. Pelvis
17. Ureters
18. Urinary bladder
19. Urethra
20. Prostate

Exercise 5: Abbreviations

1. Voiding cystourethrogram
2. Blood urea nitrogen
3. Intravenous
4. American College of Radiology
5. Benign prostatic hyperplasia

Exercise 6: Venipuncture and IV Contrast Media Administration

1. b
2. a
3. b
4. c
5. c
6. a
7. b
8. a.
9. b, d, g, h
10. Using tincture of iodine 1% to 2% or isopropyl alcohol 70%, wipe the skin with a circular motion, covering an area that is approximately 2 inches in diameter, without lifting the swab from the skin until the process is completed.
11. 6 to 8 inches
12. Bevel up
13. 45 degrees
14. The vein has been successfully penetrated by the needle.
15. Remove the needle and apply direct pressure to the puncture site.
16. c
17. c
18. b
19. a, b, c, d
20. a, b, c, e, f

SECTION 2: POSITIONING OF THE URINARY SYSTEM

Exercise 1: Excretory Urography

1. Urography
2. d
3. a, b, c, e
4. a, c, e, f, j, k
5. a
6. a, c, e, g
7. To distend the stomach with gas, thus providing a negative background density that better demonstrates renal structures
8. Inappropriate abdominal pressure might retard the excretion of fluid from the kidneys and might cause distortion of ureteral structures.

299

9. To retard the flow of opacified urine into the bladder, allowing renal structures to be better filled and demonstrated
10. The anterior surface of the lower abdomen, about 2 inches (5 cm) above the pubic symphysis
11. Rapid releasing of the ureteral compression device might rupture some of the viscera within the pelvis.
12. Increased doses of contrast agents and the use of contrast media of higher concentrations produce better demonstration of ureters.
13. To demonstrate the mobility of the kidneys
14. Patient data, side marker, time interval, and position indicator
15. Elastic waistbands in the underwear can produce unwanted densities in the image because of soft tissue skin folds.
16. c
17. b, c, d, e, h
18. d
19. a
20. b
21. c
22. b
23. True
24. True
25. False (Postinjection radiographs are most often obtained with the patient supine.)
26. d
27. c
28. a
29. c
30. c
31. b
32. A. Renal calyces
    B. Renal pelvis
    C. Abdominal ureter
    D. Pelvic ureter
    E. Urinary bladder
33. b
34. a
35. c
36. c
37. b
38. a
39. Midcoronal
40. Arms extended in front of the patient, elbows flexed, and hands placed under the head
41. Pelvis and lumbar vertebrae
42. Expiration
43. Short
44. Supine
45. Midcoronal
46. a
47. b
48. True
49. False (The exposure should be made at the end of expiration.)
50. True

Exercise 2: Retrograde Urography

1. False (Contrast agents are injected into a selected renal pelvis by means of catheters that pass through the urethra, the bladder, and the ureter to the selected kidney.)
2. False (Special cystoscopic-radiographic tables are used for retrograde studies.)
3. c
4. c
5. a
6. The urologist intravenously injects a color dye, and the function of each kidney is determined by the time required for the dye substance to appear in the urine as it passes through the respective catheter.
7. A preliminary radiograph showing catheter insertion, a pyelogram, and a ureterogram
8. By retarding the excretion of the contrast medium from the kidney, the filling of the renal pelvis is enhanced.
9. b
10. a

Exercise 3: Retrograde Cystography

1. By means of a catheter passed through the urethra into the bladder
2. d
3. b
4. c
5. b
6. c
7. b
8. a
9. b
10. b
11. c
12. b
13. c
14. c
15. a, b
16. a
17. b
18. d
19. b
20. c

Exercise 4: Male Cystourethrography

1. The radiographic examination of the urinary bladder and urethra after the introduction of a contrast medium by means of a catheter inserted into the bladder
2. A catheter is inserted through the urethral canal into the bladder.
3. d
4. c
5. d
6. True
7. True
8. True

9. False (Only the bladder and urethra need to be demonstrated in their entirety.)
10. A. Bladder
    B. Prostatic urethra
    C. Membranous urethra
    D. Spongy (cavernous) urethra

Exercise 5: Identifying Urinary System Radiographs

1. d	6. b
2. a	7. a
3. b	8. a
4. b	9. b
5. a	10. d

Self-Test: Anatomy and Positioning of the Urinary System

1. a	10. d	19. d
2. b	11. a	20. a
3. c	12. b	21. c
4. b	13. a	22. a
5. d	14. b	23. c
6. c	15. d	24. d
7. c	16. b	25. d
8. b	17. b	
9. c	18. c	

CHAPTER 19: REPRODUCTIVE SYSTEM

SECTION 1: ANATOMY OF THE REPRODUCTIVE SYSTEM

Exercise 1

1. A. Fundus
   B. Round ligament
   C. Ovarian ligament
   D. Uterine tube
   E. Ovary
2. A. Uterine tube (cut)
   B. Cervix
   C. Uterine ostium
   D. Rectum
   E. Ovary
   F. Uterine tube
   G. Uterus
   H. Round ligament (cut)
   I. Urinary bladder
   J. Pubic symphysis
   K. Urethral orifice
   L. Vaginal orifice
3. Ovaries
4. Ova
5. Uterine (or fallopian)
6. Two
7. Uterus
8. Fundus, body, isthmus, and cervix
9. Cervix

10.
    1. e
    2. a
    3. b
    4. d
    5. c

Exercise 2

1. A. Testicular artery
   B. Ductus deferens
   C. Epididymis
   D. Head of the epididymis
   E. Testis
2. A. Sacrum
   B. Rectum
   C. Prostate
   D. Testes
   E. Bladder
   F. Pubis
   G. Urethra
3. A. Ureter
   B. Ductus deferens
   C. Bladder
   D. Seminal vesicle
   E. Ampulla
   F. Prostate
   G. Epididymis
   H. Testis
4. Testes (or testicles)
5. Spermatozoa
6. Epididymis
7. Ductus deferens
8. Ejaculatory
9. Prostate
10. Urethra

SECTION 2: RADIOGRAPHY OF THE REPRODUCTIVE SYSTEM

Exercise 1: Radiography of the Female Reproductive System

1.
   1. a
   2. a
   3. b
   4. a
   5. b
   6. b
2.
   1. b
   2. b
   3. d
   4. e
   5. c, e, f
   6. c, f
   7. f
   8. a, b, d, e
   9. a, b
   10. c
   11. f
   12. e
   13. c, e, f
   14. f
   15. c

3. i. d
   ii. c
   iii. b
   iv. b
   v. a

Exercise 2: Radiography of the Male Reproductive System

1. Water-soluble, iodinated
2. To improve radiographic contrast of examined structures
3. Prostate
4. Level of superior border of pubic symphysis
5. Ultrasound

Self-Test: Reproductive System

1. a	6. c	11. d
2. c	7. c	12. b
3. b	8. a	13. b
4. a	9. d	14. c
5. b	10. d	15. d

CHAPTER 20: SKULL

SECTION 1: OSTEOLOGY OF THE SKULL

Exercise 1

1. A. Parietal bone
   B. Glabella
   C. Greater wing of the sphenoid
   D. Nasal bone
   E. Temporal bone
   F. Zygomatic bone
   G. Perpendicular plate of the ethmoid
   H. Vomer
   I. Maxilla
   J. Frontal bone
   K. Sphenoid bone
   L. Lacrimal bone
   M. Ethmoid bone
   N. Middle nasal concha
   O. Infraorbital foramen
   P. Inferior nasal concha
   Q. Anterior nasal spine
   R. Mandible
2. A. Frontal bone
   B. Sphenoid bone
   C. Glabella
   D. Nasal bone
   E. Lacrimal bone
   F. Ethmoid bone
   G. Anterior nasal spine (acanthion)
   H. Zygomatic bone (zygoma)
   I. Temporal process
   J. Maxilla
   K. Mental foramen
   L. Mandible
   M. Bregma
   N. Coronal suture

O. Parietal bone
P. Squamosal suture
Q. Lambda
R. Lambdoidal suture
S. Occipital bone
T. External occipital protuberance (inion)
U. Mastoid process
V. Temporal bone
W. External acoustic meatus
X. Styloid process

3. A. Orbital plate
   B. Lesser wing
   C. Greater wing
   D. Optic groove
   E. Foramen ovale
   F. Foramen spinosum
   G. Temporal bone
   H. Petrous portion
   I. Clivus
   J. Occipital bone
   K. Crista galli
   L. Cribriform plate
   M. Optic canal and foramen
   N. Tuberculum sellae
   O. Anterior clinoid process
   P. Sella turcica
   Q. Posterior clinoid process
   R. Foramen lacerum
   S. Dorsum sellae
   T. Jugular foramen
   U. Hypoglossal canal
   V. Foramen magnum
4. A. Frontal bone
   B. Frontal sinus
   C. Crista galli
   D. Nasal bone
   E. Ethmoid bone
   F. Vomer
   G. Maxilla
   H. Parietal bone
   I. Sphenoidal sinus
   J. Petrous portion
   K. Internal acoustic meatus
   L. Occipital bone
   M. Squamous portion of the temporal bone
   N. Clivus
   O. Pterygoid hamulus
   P. Palatine bone
5. A. Frontal squama
   B. Supraorbital foramen
   C. Supraorbital margin
   D. Glabella
   E. Nasal spine
   F. Superciliary arch
   G. Frontal eminence

6. A. Superior nasal concha
   B. Middle nasal concha
   C. Perpendicular plate
   D. Crista galli
   E. Ethmoidal sinus
   F. Air cells in the labyrinth
   G. Cribriform plate
7. A. Parietal
   B. Frontal
   C. Frontal
   D. Sphenoid
   E. Occipital
   F. Occipital
   G. Mastoid
   H. Temporal
8. A. Anterior clinoid processes
   B. Posterior clinoid processes
   C. Dorsum sellae
   D. Lateral pterygoid lamina
   E. Pterygoid hamulus
   F. Optic canal and foramen
   G. Lesser wing
   H. Superior orbital fissure
   I. Greater wing
9. A. Squama
   B. Foramen magnum
   C. Basilar portion
   D. Occipital condyle
   E. External occipital protuberance (inion)
10. A. Squamous portion
    B. Mastoid portion
    C. External acoustic meatus
    D. Tympanic portion
    E. Styloid process
    F. Mandibular fossa
    G. Articular tubercle
    H. Zygomatic process
    I. Petrous portion
11. A. External acoustic meatus
    B. Cartilage
    C. Tympanic membrane
    D. Auditory ossicles
    E. Semicircular canals
    F. Stapes (in oval window)
    G. Internal acoustic meatus
    H. Cochlear nerve
    I. Cochlea
    J. Round window
    K. Auditory (eustachian) tube
    L. Nasopharynx
    M. External acoustic meatus
    N. Auditory tube
12. A. Neck
    B. Condyle
    C. Alveolar process
    D. Mental foramen
    E. Symphysis
    F. Coronoid process
    G. Ramus

H. Body
I. Mental protuberance
J. Angle
K. Gonion
13. A. Body
    B. Greater cornu
    C. Lesser cornu

Exercise 2

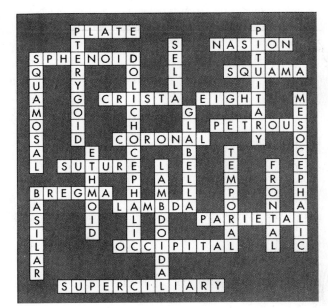

Exercise 3

1. a	6. f	11. e	16. a
2. a	7. b	12. f	17. b
3. c	8. d	13. e	18. d
4. d	9. f	14. d	19. d
5. d	10. b	15. e	20. d

Exercise 4

1. m	6. n	11. g
2. q	7. r	12. j
3. i	8. l	13. f
4. c	9. k	14. b
5. a	10. p	15. s

Exercise 5

1. i	6. o	11. a
2. g	7. f	12. j
3. a	8. b	13. l
4. d	9. n	14. k
5. c	10. m	15. p

Exercise 6

1. Cranial; facial
2. Frontal (1); ethmoid (1); parietal (2); sphenoid (1); temporal (2); and occipital (1)
3. Nasal (2); lacrimal (2); maxillae (2); zygomatic (2); palatine (2); inferior nasal conchae (2); vomer (1); and mandible (1)
4. Mesocephalic (47 degrees); brachycephalic (54 degrees); and dolichocephalic (40 degrees)
5. Flat
6. Diploë
7. Bregma; lambda
8. Bregma
9. Lambda
10. Frontal
11. Ethmoid
12. Parietal
13. Eminence
14. Sagittal
15. Coronal
16. Occipital
17. Lambdoidal
18. Sphenoid
19. Occipital
20. Basilar
21. Foramen magnum
22. Sphenoid
23. C1 vertebra (atlas)
24. Sphenoid
25. Temporal
26. Tympanic
27. Mastoid
28. Petrous portion (pars petrosa, petrous pyramid)
29. Temporal
30. Auricle
31. Malleus (hammer); incus (anvil); stapes (stirrup)
32. Temporal
33. Temporal
34. Nasal
35. Lacrimal
36. Maxilla
37. Maxillary sinus
38. Alveolar process
39. Maxillae
40. Acanthion
41. Zygomatic
42. Zygomatic
43. Palatine
44. Inferior nasal conchae
45. Vomer
46. Mandible
47. Ramus
48. Hyoid
49. Condyle; coronoid
50. Condyle

Exercise 7: Abbreviations

1. Acanthiomeatal line
2. Top of ear attachment
3. Internal acoustic meatus
4. Interpupillary line
5. Glabellomeatal line

SECTION 2: RADIOGRAPHY OF THE SKULL

Exercise 1: Skull Topography

1. A. Angle of the mandible (gonion)
   B. Infraorbitomeatal margin
   C. Outer canthus
   D. Midsagittal plane
   E. Glabella
   F. Interpupillary line
   G. Inner canthus
   H. Nasion
   I. Acanthion
   J. Mental point
2. A. External acoustic meatus
   B. Angle of the mandible (gonion)
   C. Glabellomeatal line
   D. Orbitomeatal line
   E. Infraorbitomeatal line
   F. Acanthiomeatal line
   G. Glabelloalveolar line
   H. Glabella
   I. Nasion
   J. Acanthion
   K. Mental point
3. 1. c
   2. f
   3. a
   4. e
   5. h
   6. d
   7. b
   8. i
   9. g
4. 1. e
   2. b
   3. h
   4. d
   5. i
   6. g
   7. f
5. a. 7
   b. 8

Exercise 2: Positioning for the Cranium

1. c
2. a. Parallel
   b. Perpendicular
3. c
4. d
5. 2 inches (5 cm) above the EAM
6. Perpendicular to a point approximately 2 inches (5 cm) above the EAM
7. a
8. False (The central ray should enter at a point 2 inches [5 cm] superior to the EAM.)
9. True
10. b, c, d, e, f, g, h, j

11. a. A support should be placed under the thorax to raise the inferior aspect of the head and to place the midsagittal plane parallel with the IR.

   b. A radiolucent sponge should be placed under the head to make the midsagittal plane parallel with the IR.

12. A. Orbital roof
   B. Sella turcica
   C. Sphenoidal sinus
   D. Petrous portion of the temporal bone
   E. Temporomandibular joint
   F. EAM
   G. Mandibular rami

13. a. Perpendicular
   b. Perpendicular

14. c

15. 1. a
    2. b
    3. d
    4. c

16. Nasion

17. Nasion

18. Stop breathing.

19. a, c, g, h, i

20. A. Dorsum sellae
   B. Superior orbital margin
   C. Sphenoid plane
   D. Petrous ridge
   E. Ethmoidal sinus
   F. Inferior orbital margin
   G. Crista galli

21. a. Perpendicular
   b. Perpendicular

22. Perpendicularly

23. Cephalically

24. a

25. c

26. a, c, g, h, j

27. a. 15 degrees cephalad (The petrous ridges lie in the lower third of the orbits.)
   b. Perpendicularly (The petrous ridges fill the orbits.)

28. d

29. c

30. Orbitomeatal; infraorbitomeatal

31. a

32. d

33. c

34. b, f, g, i

35. A. Parietal bone
   B. Occipital bone
   C. Foramen magnum
   D. Petrous ridge
   E. Posterior clinoid process
   F. Dorsum sellae

36. True

37. False (Hypersthenic patients must be either prone or upright.)

38. c

39. a

40. b

41. c

42. a, c, g, i

43. A. Occipital bone
   B. Foramen magnum
   C. Petrous ridge
   D. Posterior clinoid process
   E. Dorsum sellae

44. a. Perpendicular
   b. Parallel

45. Infraorbitomeatal

46. On the midsagittal plane of the throat between the angles of the mandible, passing through a point ¾ inch (1.9 cm) anterior to the level of the EAM

47. a

48. b, e

49. a, d, f, h, i

50. A. Maxillary sinus
   B. Ethmoidal air cells
   C. Mandible
   D. Sphenoidal sinus
   E. Foramen spinosum
   F. Mandibular condyle
   G. Dens (odontoid process)
   H. Petrosa
   I. Mastoid process

Exercise 3: Positioning for the Temporal Bone

1. From true lateral, with the affected mastoid centered to the IR, rotate the head until the midsagittal plane forms a 15-degree angle with the IR.

2. a

3. c

4. d

5. 15 degrees caudad

6. Approximately 2 inches (5 cm) posterior and 2 inches (5 cm) above the uppermost EAM

7. False (The head should be rotated 15 degrees from true lateral, moving the face closer to the IR.)

8. False (The head should be rotated 15 degrees from true lateral.)

9. True

10. a, b, f, g, i, j

11. A. Internal and external acoustic meatus
    B. Mastoid air cells
    C. Mastoid process
    D. Mandibular condyle

12. Forehead, nose, and cheek

13. 12 degrees cephalad

14. d

15. d

16. d

17. c

18. A. Internal acoustic canal
    B. Arcuate eminence
    C. Mastoid air cells
    D. EAM and canal
    E. Mandibular condyle
    F. Mastoid process

19. True
20. False (The midsagittal plane should form an angle of 45 degrees with the IR.)
21. True
22. 10 degrees caudad
23. On the zygomatic bone approximately 1 inch (2.5 cm) anterior to and ¾ inch (1.9 cm) above the EAM
24. d
25. b, e, f, g, h, j

Exercise 4: Positioning for the Optic Canal and Foramen

1. b
2. b
3. a
4. True
5. True
6. False (The central ray should be directed perpendicularly through the affected orbit closer to the IR.)
7. True
8. False (Incorrect angulation of the acanthiomeatal line causes longitudinal deviation from the preferred location of the optic canal and foramen. Any lateral deviation from the preferred location for the optic canal and foramen is caused by incorrect rotation of the head.)
9. b, e, f, g
10. A. Superior orbital margin
    B. Lateral orbital margin
    C. Optic canal and foramen
    D. Medial orbital margin
    E. Lesser wing of the sphenoid
    F. Ethmoidal sinus
    G. Inferior orbital margin

Exercise 5: Evaluating Radiographs of the Skull

1. a. Fig. 20-40 (Certain structures of the skull are superimposed with their opposite side [orbital roofs, mandibular rami, mastoid regions, EAMs, and temporomandibular joints], and no rotation is visible.)
   b. Fig. 20-39 (Cranial structures [orbital roofs, temporomandibular joints, and EAMs] are longitudinally separated.)
   c. Fig. 20-38 (Cranial structures [orbital roofs, temporomandibular joints, and EAMs] are laterally separated.)
   d. Fig. 20-39
2. a. Caudally 15 degrees
   b. In the lower third of the orbits
   c. The distance from the lateral border of the skull to the lateral border of the orbit is not equal on both sides.
   d. The head is rotated, moving the occipital bone closer to the left shoulder. The midsagittal plane is not perpendicular to the IR.
3. a. Perpendicular to the nasion
   b. The petrous ridges should fill the orbits.
   c. Yes

d. The distance from the lateral border of the skull to the lateral border of the orbit is not equal on both sides.
   e. The head is rotated, moving the occipital bone closer to the right shoulder. The midsagittal plane is not perpendicular to the IR.
4. a. Acceptable
   b. Unacceptable
   c. The head is rotated, moving the occipital bone closer to the left shoulder. The midsagittal plane is not perpendicular to the IR.
   d. Perpendicularly
5. The mandibular symphysis does not superimpose the anterior frontal bone.
6. a. Fig. 20-47 (The optic foramen is demonstrated in the inferior and lateral quadrant of the orbit.)
   b. Fig. 20-46 (The position of the optic foramen is posterior to the lateral orbital margin.)
   c. Fig. 20-48 (The position of the optic foramen is too much toward the medial aspect of the orbit.)

Self-Test: Osteology and Radiography of the Skull

1. a	15. a	29. b	43. b	57. c
2. d	16. b	30. d	44. c	58. d
3. a	17. a	31. b	45. b	59. c
4. b	18. c	32. d	46. c	60. d
5. c	19. b	33. b	47. a	61. a
6. d	20. c	34. c	48. a	62. b
7. d	21. d	35. c	49. c	63. d
8. d	22. b	36. c	50. c	64. d
9. b	23. a	37. a	51. a	65. c
10. a	24. b	38. d	52. c	66. b
11. c	25. a	39. c	53. d	67. c
12. d	26. c	40. b	54. a	68. a
13. a	27. d	41. d	55. d	69. a
14. c	28. c	42. d	56. d	70. a

CHAPTER 21: FACIAL BONES

Radiography of the Facial Bones

Exercise 1: Positioning for Facial Bones and Nasal Bones

1. Lengthwise
2. Midsagittal
3. b
4. d
5. d
6. Perpendicularly
7. Halfway between the outer canthus and the external acoustic meatus.
8. a, b, d, g
9. A. Frontal sinus
   B. Nasal bone
   C. Sella turcica
   D. Maxillary sinus
   E. External acoustic meatus
   F. Maxilla
   G. Mandible

10. a. 37-degree angulation
    b. Perpendicular
11. b
12. a
13. a. Too far below maxillae (The maxillae will appear foreshortened.)
    b. Immediately below the maxillae
    c. Superimpose maxillary sinuses
14. d, e
15. A. Orbit
    B. Zygomatic arch
    C. Maxillary sinus
    D. Maxilla
    E. Mandibular angle
16. Supine
17. Parietoacanthial; Waters
18. b
19. c
20. a
21. a
22. c
23. d, e
24. A. Orbit
    B. Zygomatic bone
    C. Maxillary sinus
25. a. Perpendicular
    b. Parallel
26. Two
27. Nasion
28. Perpendicular to the bridge of the nose at a point ½ inch (1.2 cm) distal to the nasion
29. c, d
30. A. Frontonasal (nasofrontal)
    B. Nasal bone
    C. Anterior nasal spine of the maxilla

Exercise 2: Positioning for Zygomatic Arches

1. True
2. False (The zygomatic arches should be free from overlying structures.)
3. False (The posterior cranium need not be included in the image.)
4. False (The midsagittal plane should be perpendicular to the IR.)
5. c
6. c
7. c
8. a
9. a, b, d
10. True
11. True
12. Infraorbitomeatal
13. Perpendicularly to the infraorbitomeatal line and centered to the zygomatic arch at a point approximately 1 inch (2.5 cm) posterior to the outer canthus
14. b
15. a. Perpendicular
    b. Perpendicular

16. a. 30 degrees caudad
    b. 37 degrees caudad
17. Nasion
18. True
19. False (Close beam restriction to zygomatic arches and adjacent structures may exclude the vertex.)
20. A. Occipital bone
    B. Mandible
    C. Zygomatic arch

Exercise 3: Positioning for the Mandible

1. b
2. a
3. Perpendicular
4. Stop breathing for the exposure.
5. b
6. b
7. True
8. False (The central portion of the mandible is superimposed with the cervical vertebrae.)
9. a, c
10. A. Condyle
    B. Mastoid process
    C. Fracture of the mandibular ramus
    D. Body
11. b
12. c
13. a
14. c
15. d
16. a
17. a, c, d
18. Fig. 21-18
19. Fig. 21-16
20. Fig. 21-18
21. Fig. 21-17
22. Fig. 21-16
23. Fig. 21-17
24. Fig. 21-17
25. NA
26. Figs. 21-16, 21-17, and 21-18
27. NA
28. NA
29. Figs. 21-16, 21-17, and 21-18
30. Fig. 21-18
31. Fig. 21-16
32. True
33. False (The neck should be extended to place the mandibular body parallel with the transverse axis of the IR.)
34. True
35. A. Coronoid process
    B. Ramus
    C. Body
    D. Hyoid bone
    E. Angle

Exercise 4: Positioning for the Temporomandibular Joints (TMJs)

1. True
2. False (The head should be positioned the same way as for an AP projection, with the midsagittal plane perpendicular to the plane of the IR.)
3. Occlusion of the incisors places the mandible in a position of protrusion in which the condyles are carried out of the mandibular fossae.
4. Any trauma to the mandible where the mandible is suspected to be fractured; because of the danger of fracture displacement
5. c
6. c
7. c
8. c
9. a, c
10. a, d
11. c
12. c
13. c
14. 15 degrees caudad
15. The TMJ closer to the IR
16. In the mandibular fossa
17. False (To exit through the EAM closest to the IR, the caudally directed central ray should enter about 1½ inches [4 cm] superior to the upside EAM.)
18. True
19. False (Close beam restriction should surround the affected TMJ.)
20. A. Mandibular fossa
    B. Articular tubercle
    C. Condyle

Exercise 5: Evaluating Radiographs of Facial Bones

1. The mandibular rami are not superimposed, and the orbital roofs are not superimposed.
2. a. Fig. 21-26
   b. Fig. 21-24
   c. Fig. 21-25
3. a. The zygomatic arches are not symmetric, and the left zygomatic arch is superimposed with cranial structures.
   b. The midsagittal plane was not perpendicular to the IR because the patient's head was slightly tilted.
4. a. The base of the occipital partially superimposes the mandible, and the mandibular rami are not seen without superimposition from surrounding structures.
   b. Reposition the head, ensuring that the forehead is in contact with the vertical grid device or x-ray table surface, to image the mandible without cranial superimposition.
5. a. The opposite side of the mandible superimposes the mandibular body.
   b. Position the head so that the uppermost side of the mandible will be projected above the mandibular body closer to the IR.

Self-Test: Radiography of the Facial Bones

1. a.	6. d	11. b	16. d
2. a	7. a	12. c	17. d
3. d	8. d	13. d	18. a
4. a	9. a	14. b	19. d
5. d	10. b	15. b	20. b

CHAPTER 22: PARANASAL SINUSES

Review

1. Frontal, sphenoidal, ethmoidal, and maxillary
2. A. Sphenoidal
   B. Maxillary
   C. Frontal
   D. Ethmoidal
3. a
4. b
5. d
6. d
7. c
8. c
9. To demonstrate the presence or absence of fluid and to differentiate between shadows caused by fluid and those caused by other pathologic conditions
10. Underpenetration produces shadows simulating pathologic conditions that do not exist.
11. a. Parallel
    b. Perpendicular
12. d
13. a
14. d
15. d
16. a, b, c, d, e, f
17. A. Frontal sinus
    B. Sella turcica
    C. Sphenoidal sinus
    D. Ethmoidal sinuses
    E. Maxillary sinus
    F. Superimposed mandibular rami
18. c
19. c
20. c
21. a
22. a
23. b
24. c, d, e, g, h, k, 1, m
25. A. Frontal sinus
    B. Ethmoidal sinuses
    C. Petrous ridge
    D. Sphenoidal sinuses
    E. Maxillary sinus
26. Maxillary
27. Superimposed with the maxillary sinuses
28. Foreshortened
29. Orbitomeatal
30. Mentomeatal
31. Acanthion
32. Immediately below the maxillary sinuses

33. One on each side, just inferior to the medial aspect of the orbital floor and superior to the roof of the maxillary sinuses
34. False (Only the chin should touch the vertical grid device.)
35. True
36. c, e, g, j, k
37. A. Frontal sinus
    B. Ethmoidal sinuses
    C. Foramen rotundum
    D. Maxillary sinus
    E. Petrous pyramid
    F. Mastoid air cells
38. Acanthion
39. Chin
40. Orbitomeatal
41. Sphenoidal
42. c, e, g, h, j, k
43. False (The head should rest on its vertex.)
44. False (The IOML should be as close to parallel with the IR as possible.)
45. True
46. True
47. True
48. False (To demonstrate the paranasal sinuses, close restriction of the beam to the sinus area may exclude the occipital bone.)
49. Sphenoidal and ethmoidal
50. The mandibular symphysis should superimpose the anterior frontal bone.
51. Anterior to the petrous ridges
52. The IOML was not parallel with the IR because the neck was not extended far enough (assuming the central ray was correctly directed).
53. The IOML was not parallel with the IR because the neck was extended too far or the vertical IR holder was tilted too far toward the patient (assuming the central ray was correctly directed).
54. d, e, f
55. A. Maxillary sinus
    B. Ethmoidal sinus
    C. Mandible
    D. Vomer
    E. Sphenoidal sinus
    F. Mandibular condyle
    G. Petrosa

Self-Test: Radiography of the Paranasal Sinuses

1. d	6. a	11. d	16. c	21. b
2. d	7. b	12. c	17. d	22. c
3. d	8. a	13. d	18. c	23. d
4. d	9. a	14. d	19. a	24. c
5. b	10. b	15. b	20. a	25. b

CHAPTER 23: MAMMOGRAPHY

SECTION 1: ANATOMY AND PHYSIOLOGY OF THE BREAST

Exercise 1

1. A. Axillary prolongation (tail) of the breast
   B. Serratus anterior
   C. Pectoralis minor
   D. Pectoralis major (cut)
2. A. Fat
   B. Nipple
   C. Lactiferous tubules
   D. Fat
   E. Inframammary crease
   F. Pectoralis major
   G. Retromammary fat

Exercise 2

1. Mammary
2. Milk
3. Tail
4. Base
5. Nipple
6. Areola
7. 15; 20
8. Acini
9. Smaller
10. Involution
11. Fat
12. Lactiferous
13. Cooper's
14. Axilla
15. Sternum

Exercise 3

1. h
2. g
3. b
4. e
5. i
6. f
7. d
8. c

SECTION 2: RADIOGRAPHY OF THE BREAST

Exercise 1

1. Because the mammogram will record the slightest wrinkle in any cloth covering
2. These substances will resemble calcifications on the resultant image.
3. Craniocaudal and mediolateral oblique projections
4. To locate a nipple that is not in profile
5. Compress the breast with an approved mammographic compression device.
6. Place a radiopaque marker such as a BB on the breast overlying the mass.
7. To evaluate whether or not sufficient breast tissue is demonstrated

309

8. Nipple and chest wall, or edge of the image, whichever comes first
9. 1 cm
10. Clean the IR surface and face guard with a disinfectant.

Exercise 2

1. a
2. d
3. c
4. b

Exercise 3

1. b
2. a, b, c, d
3. b, d
4. a, b, c
5. d
6. a, b, c, d
7. a
8. b
9. c
10. a

Exercise 4

1. a
2. a
3. b
4. c
5. b
6. a
7. d
8. d

Self-Test: Mammography

1. a	6. d	11. b
2. c	7. a	12. a
3. d	8. c	13. c
4. d	9. c	14. c
5. b	10. c	15. a

CHAPTER 24: CENTRAL NERVOUS SYSTEM

SECTION 1: ANATOMY OF THE CENTRAL NERVOUS SYSTEM

1. A. Cerebrum
   B. Corpus callosum
   C. Cerebrum
   D. Cerebellum
   E. Pituitary gland
   F. Medulla oblongata
   G. Cerebellum
   H. Pons
2. A. Gray substance
   B. White substance
   C. Posterior nerve root
   D. Anterior nerve root

3. A. Pons
   B. Medulla oblongata
   C. Spinal cord
   D. Dural sac for the cauda equina
4. A. Fourth ventricle
   B. Inferior horn
   C. Interventricular foramen
   D. Anterior horn
   E. Body of the lateral ventricle
   F. Third ventricle
   G. Posterior horn
   H. Cerebral aqueduct
5. A. Body of the lateral ventricle
   B. Anterior horn
   C. Inferior horn
6. A. Fourth ventricle
   B. Body of the lateral ventricle
   C. Third ventricle
   D. Anterior horn
   E. Inferior horn
   F. Lateral recess
   G. Posterior horn
7. Brain and spinal cord
8. Cerebrum, cerebellum, and brain stem
9. Diencephalon, midbrain (mesencephalon), pons, and medulla oblongata
10. Cerebellum, pons, and medulla oblongata
11. Cerebrum (forebrain)
12. Forebrain
13. Midbrain (mesencephalon)
14. Longitudinal fissure
15. Pituitary gland
16. Cerebellum
17. Medulla oblongata
18. Meninges
19. Pia mater
20. Dura mater
21. Lateral
22. Cerebrum (forebrain)
23. Interventricular
24. Monro
25. Cerebral aqueduct and aqueduct of Sylvius

SECTION 2: RADIOGRAPHY OF THE CENTRAL NERVOUS SYSTEM

1. Radiographic examination of the spinal cord after the injection of a contrast medium into the subarachnoid space
2. L2-L3, L3-L4, and cisterna cerebellomedullaris (cisterna magna)
3. Extrinsic spinal cord compression
4. Nonionic, water-soluble (They provide good visualization of nerve roots and good enhancement for follow-up computerized tomography, and they are readily absorbed by the body.)
5. To prevent it from accidentally contacting the spinal needle
6. Explain details of the examination to the patient before beginning the procedure.

7. Prone and lateral recumbent with the spine flexed
8. Varying the angulation of the table
9. To compress the cisterna cerebellomedullaris, preventing the contrast medium from entering cranial structures
10. Cross-table lateral of the cervical spine

Self-Test: Central Nervous System

1. b	6. a	11. b
2. b	7. c	12. a
3. c	8. d	13. b
4. b	9. c	14. d
5. b	10. d	15. c

CHAPTER 25: CIRCULATORY SYSTEM

SECTION 1: ANATOMY OF THE CIRCULATORY SYSTEM

Exercise 1

1. A. Superior sagittal sinus
   B. Transverse sinus
   C. Internal jugular vein
   D. Right subclavian artery and vein
   E. Superior vena cava
   F. Brachial artery and basilic vein
   G. Celiac axis (artery)
   H. Portal vein
   I. Renal artery and vein
   J. Superior mesenteric artery and vein
   K. Common iliac artery and vein
   L. Common femoral artery and vein
   M. Popliteal artery
   N. Anterior tibial artery
   O. Posterior tibial artery
   P. Anterior facial artery and vein
   Q. Common carotid artery
   R. Aortic arch
   S. Pulmonary artery and vein
   T. Aorta
   U. Inferior vena cava
   V. Inferior mesenteric vein
   W. Radial artery and cephalic vein
   X. Ulnar artery and basilic vein
   Y. Deep femoral artery
   Z. Superficial femoral artery
   AA. Popliteal vein
   BB. Large saphenous vein
2. A. Aortic arch
   B. Superior vena cava
   C. Right pulmonary artery
   D. Right pulmonary veins
   E. Right atrium
   F. Right atrioventricular (tricuspid) valve
   G. Right ventricle
   H. Inferior vena cava
   I. Descending aorta
   J. Left ventricle
   K. Left atrioventricular (bicuspid or mitral) valve
   L. Left lung
   M. Left atrium

3. A. Right coronary artery
   B. Left coronary artery
4. A. Coronary sinus
   B. Great cardiac vein
5. A. Capillaries
   B. Lungs
   C. Right atrium
   D. Right ventricle
   E. Liver
   F. Intestine
   G. Aorta
   H. Left atrium
   I. Left ventricle
   J. Stomach
   K. Spleen
   L. Pancreas
6. A. External carotid artery
   B. Internal carotid artery
   C. Right common carotid artery
   D. Right vertebral artery
   E. Right subclavian artery
   F. Brachiocephalic artery
   G. Brachial artery
   H. Radial artery
   I. Ulnar artery
   J. Left subclavian artery
   K. Left vertebral artery
   L. Left common carotid artery
   M. Thyroid
7. A. Anterior communicating cerebral artery
   B. Posterior communicating artery
   C. Anterior cerebral artery
   D. Middle cerebral artery
   E. Internal carotid artery
   F. Posterior cerebral artery
   G. Basilar artery
   H. Vertebral artery
8. A. Inferior vena cava
   B. Common iliac artery
   C. External iliac artery
   D. Deep femoral artery
   E. Popliteal artery
   F. Anterior tibial artery
   G. Abdominal aorta
   H. Internal iliac artery
   I. Femoral artery
   J. Dorsalis pedis artery
9. A. Axillary nodes
   B. Common iliac nodes
   C. Deep inguinal nodes
   D. Cervical nodes
   E. Thoracic duct
   F. Lumbar nodes
   G. Superior inguinal nodes

Exercise 2

1. Blood-vascular; lymphatic
2. Pulmonary; systemic
3. Pulmonary
4. Arteries

5. Veins
6. Arterioles
7. Capillaries
8. Venules
9. Venules
10. Pulmonary
11. Superior vena cava
12. Inferior vena cava
13. Myocardium
14. Endocardium
15. Epicardium
16. Left ventricle
17. Pericardial cavity
18. Atria
19. Ventricles
20. Atria
21. Ventricles
22. Tricuspid
23. Mitral; bicuspid
24. Right
25. Left
26. Left ventricle
27. Coronary
28. Cardiac
29. Right
30. Aorta
31. Iliac
32. Femoral
33. Popliteal
34. Tibial
35. Portal
36. Hepatic
37. Inferior vena cava
38. Pulmonary
39. Pulmonary
40. Pulmonary
41. Systole
42. Diastole
43. Common carotid; vertebral
44. Left common carotid
45. Subclavian
46. Basilar
47. Internal; external
48. Cerebral
49. Posterior cerebral
50. Jugular
51. Brachiocephalic
52. Subclavian
53. Brachial
54. Radial; ulnar
55. Forearm
56. Aorta (abdominal)
57. Brain
58. Heart
59. Thoracic
60. Subclavian; jugular

SECTION 2: RADIOGRAPHY OF THE CIRCULATORY SYSTEM

1. The risk of extravasation is reduced; most body parts can be reached for selective injection; the patient can be positioned as needed; and the catheter can be safely left in the body while the radiographs are being examined.
2. Seldinger
3. Femoral
4. b
5. b, c, g
6. b, d, e
7. The patient's legs should be elevated, and intravenous fluids may be administered.
8. To reduce the possibility of the aspiration of vomitus
9. To saturate the kidneys and minimize kidney damage from iodinated contrast media
10. T6
11. A. Brachiocephalic artery
    B. Ascending aorta
    C. Right coronary artery
    D. Intercostal arteries
    E. Left common carotid artery
    F. Left subclavian artery
    G. Left coronary artery
    H. Descending thoracic aorta
12. From the diaphragm to the aortic bifurcation
13. Lateral
14. A. Hepatic artery
    B. Right renal artery
    C. Right common iliac artery
    D. Splenic artery
    E. Left renal artery
    F. Abdominal aorta
15. A. Celiac axis
    B. Superior mesenteric artery
    C. Abdominal aorta
16. AP
17. Expiration
18. A. Left gastric artery
    B. Hepatic artery
    C. Gastroduodenal artery
    D. Splenic artery
    E. Celiac axis
19. To ensure exact positioning of the tube-part-film alignment and close collimation of the x-ray tube
20. Splenic
21. Proximally
22. Upper
23. a
24. b
25. b
26. A. Ulnar artery
    B. Posterior interosseous artery
    C. Brachial artery
    D. Right subclavian artery
27. In the superficial vein at the wrist (when demonstrating the entire upper limb) or at the elbow (when demonstrating the upper arm)

28. A. Cephalic vein
    B. Basilic vein
    C. Subclavian vein
29. Extended and internally rotated 30 degrees
30. A. Common iliac artery
    B. External iliac artery
    C. Profunda femoris artery
    D. Femoral artery
    E. Popliteal artery
    F. Anterior tibial artery
    G. Peroneal artery
    H. Posterior tibial artery
31. c
32. c
33. a
34. c
35. a
36. a. Capillary
    b. Arterial
    c. Venous
37. Infraorbitomeatal
38. Away from the injected side
39. a
40. b

Self-Test: Anatomy and Radiography of the Circulatory System

1. c	6. b	11. c	16. d
2. d	7. a	12. b	17. b
3. c	8. a	13. c	18. a
4. a	9. a	14. c	19. b
5. d	10. b	15. c	20. d

CHAPTER 26: SECTIONAL ANATOMY FOR RADIOGRAPHERS

Review

1. A. Frontal bone
   B. Superior sagittal sinus
   C. Parietal bone
   D. White matter
   E. Falx cerebri
2. A. Genu of corpus callosum
   B. Caudate nucleus
   C. Thalamus
   D. Posterior horn of lateral ventricle
   E. Straight sinus
   F. Frontal lobe
   G. Anterior horn of lateral ventricle
   H. Lentiform nucleus
   I. Splenium of corpus callosum
   J. Choroid plexus
   K. Occipital lobe
3. A. Frontal sinus
   B. Crista galli of ethmoid bone
   C. Anterior cerebral artery
   D. Posterior cerebral artery
   E. Cerebellum
   F. Middle cerebral artery
   G. Pons

   H. Tentorium cerebelli
   I. Internal occipital protuberance
4. A. Ethmoid sinuses
   B. Sphenoid sinuses
   C. Basilar artery
   D. Pons
   E. Fourth ventricle
   F. Globe of eye
   G. Pituitary gland
   H. Temporal lobe
   I. Transverse sinus
   J. Cerebellum
5. A. Lateral ventricle
   B. Third ventricle
   C. Optic chiasm
   D. Pituitary gland
   E. Sphenoidal sinus
   F. Clivus
   G. Nasopharynx
   H. Maxilla
   I. Tongue
   J. Corpus callosum
   K. Superior sagittal sinus
   L. Corpora quadrigemina
   M. Cerebral aqueduct
   N. Straight sinus
   O. Cerebellum
   P. Fourth ventricle
   Q. Pons
   R. Basilar artery
   S. Cervical spinal cord
   T. C2 vertebral body
6. A. Superior sagittal sinus
   B. Falx cerebri
   C. Lateral ventricle
   D. Caudate nucleus
   E. Insula
   F. Lateral fissure
   G. Sphenoid sinus
   H. Parotid gland
   I. Corpus callosum
   J. Septum pallucidum
   K. Third ventricle
   L. Optic chiasm
   M. Pituitary gland
7. A. Lateral ventricle
   B. Third ventricle
   C. Temporal bone (petrous portion)
   D. Lateral mass of C1
   E. C2 body
   F. Thalamus
   G. External acoustic meatus
   H. Dens (odontoid process) of C2
   I. Parotid gland
8. A. Corpus callosum
   B. Fourth ventricle
   C. Cerebellum
   D. Lateral ventricle
   E. Superior cistern
   F. Transverse sinus

9. A. Trachea
   B. Clavicle
   C. Pectoralis major and minor
   D. Subclavian vein
   E. Axillary artery and vein
   F. Humeral head
   G. Glenoid
   H. Acromion
   I. Lung
   J. Esophagus
   K. Trapezius muscles
   L. Supraspinatus muscle
   M. Scapular spine
   N. Infraspinatus muscle
   O. Subscapularis muscle
   P. Subclavian artery
   Q. Rib
   R. Brachiocephalic vein
   S. Common carotid artery
10. A. Sternum
    B. Ascending aorta
    C. Pectoralis muscles
    D. Superior vena cava
    E. Right main bronchus
    F. Esophagus
    G. Descending aorta
    H. Left main bronchus
    I. Left pulmonary artery
    J. Pulmonary trunk
11. A. Sternum
    B. Root of aorta
    C. Right atrium
    D. Superior lobe of lung
    E. Middle lobe of lung
    F. Right pulmonary vein
    G. Inferior lobe of lung
    H. Esophagus
    I. Descending aorta
    J. Left atrium
    K. Scapula
    L. Latissimus dorsi muscle
    M. Left ventricle
    N. Interventricular septum
    O. Right ventricle
12. A. Pharynx
    B. Tongue
    C. Epiglottis
    D. Trachea
    E. Left brachiocephalic vein
    F. Manubrium
    G. C2 vertebra
    H. Spinal cord
    I. Intervertebral disk
    J. Brachiocephalic artery
    K. Aortic arch
    L. Right pulmonary artery
13. A. Spinal cord
    B. Sternocleidomastoid muscle
    C. Right lung
    D. Tracheal bifurcation

   E. Heart
   F. Left subclavian artery
   G. Clavicle
   H. Acromion
   I. Humeral head
   J. Aortic arch
   K. Pulmonary trunk
14. A. Caudate lobe of liver
    B. Inferior vena cava
    C. Crus of diaphragm
    D. Aorta
    E. Lung
    F. Spleen
    G. Stomach
    H. Greater omentum
    I. Diaphragm
    J. Left lobe of liver
15. A. Rectus abdominis muscle
    B. External oblique muscle
    C. Portal vein
    D. Right lobe of liver
    E. Latissimus dorsi muscle
    F. Inferior vena cava
    G. Caudate lobe of liver
    H. Aorta
    I. Left crus of diaphragm
    J. Spleen
    K. Greater omentum
    L. Splenic flexure
    M. Stomach
    N. Left lobe of liver
16. A. Head of pancreas
    B. Duodenum
    C. Hepatic flexure
    D. Right lobe of liver
    E. Inferior vena cava
    F. Left renal vein
    G. Aorta
    H. Left kidney
    I. Spleen
    J. Descending colon
    K. Origin of superior mesenteric artery
    L. Transverse colon
    M. Superior mesenteric vein
17. A. Right common iliac artery
    B. Ileum
    C. Ascending colon
    D. Ilium
    E. Common iliac veins
    F. Left common iliac artery
    G. Psoas muscle
    H. Descending colon
    I. Small bowel
    J. Ureter
18. A. Bladder
    B. Gluteus maximum muscle
    C. Ischium
    D. Rectum
    E. Cervix
    F. Sciatic nerve

314

G. Greater trochanter
H. Femoral head
I. Femoral nerve
J. Femoral artery
K. Femoral vein
L. Pubis

19. A. Spermatic cord
    B. Prostate
    C. Ischium
    D. Seminal vesicle
    E. Rectum
    F. Coccyx
    G. Urethra
    H. Sciatic nerve
    I. Gluteus maximus muscle
    J. Greater trochanter
    K. Femoral head
    L. Femoral artery
    M. Femoral vein
    N. Pubis

20. A. Rectus abdominis muscle
    B. Bladder
    C. Pubis
    D. Coccyx
    E. Uterus
    F. Uterine cavity
    G. Rectum
    H. Sacrum
    I. Cauda equina
    J. L4-L5 intervertebral disk

21. A. Aorta
    B. Rectus abdominis muscle
    C. Bladder
    D. Pubic bone
    E. Corpora cavernosa
    F. Cauda equina
    G. L4 vertebra
    H. Sacrum
    I. Rectum
    J. Coccyx
    K. Prostatic urethra (within the prostate)
    L. Corpous spongiosum
    M. Testicles (testes)

22. A. Sigmoid colon
    B. Bladder
    C. Ductus deferens
    D. Prostate
    E. Gracilis muscle
    F. Psoas muscle
    G. Iliacus (iliac) muscle
    H. Ilium
    I. Gluteus medius muscle
    J. Gluteus minimus muscle
    K. Acetabulum
    L. Pubic ramus
    M. Corpous spongiosum
    N. Scrotum

CHAPTER 27: PEDIATRIC IMAGING

Review

1. Communication skills and immobilization techniques
2. a, b, e, f
3. School-age children, 6 to 8 years old
4. Premature infants
5. Gastroschisis
6. b
7. Osteogenesis imperfecta
8. Consult a radiologist or other attending physician.
9. Pigg-O-Stat
10. "Bunny" wrap
11. True
12. a
13. Octagonal infant immobilizer
14. a, b, e, f
15. Contralateral (uninjured); comparison
16. Salter-Harris fractures
17. It is less comfortable and more traumatic.
18. a. PA projection of chest on inspiration
    b. PA projection chest on expiration
    c. Lateral projection of chest
19. d
20. General anesthesia; risk

Self-Test: Pediatric Imaging

1. b	6. b	11. d	16. a	21. a
2. a	7. b	12. a	17. b	22. d
3. d	8. d	13. b	18. a	23. d
4. a	9. c	14. d	19. b	24. c
5. c	10. c	15. c	20. c	25. a

CHAPTER 28: GERIATRIC RADIOGRAPHY

Review

1. Geriatrics is defined as the branch of medicine dealing with the elderly and the problems of aging.
2. b
3. Arthritis, hypertension, hearing impairment, heart disease, cataracts, deformity or orthopedic impairment, chronic sinusitis, diabetes, visual impairment, and varicose veins.
4. Weight gain, fatigue, loss of bone mass, joint stiffness, loneliness.
5. Dementia
6. False (Although the incidence of dementia increases with age, not all elderly persons will develop dementia.)
7. Alzheimer's disease
8. 1. k
   2. f
   3. e
   4. g
   5. c
   6. a
   7. d
   8. h
   9. i

10. i
11. h
12. c
13. a
14. e
15. g
16. d
17. j
18. b
9. d
10. Speak lower and closer; speak slowly, directly, and distinctly.
11. Background noise
12. 1. Providing assistance when there is a step up or step down
    2. Allowing time for rest between position changes
    3. Use of table handgrips and proper RT assistance
13. Adhesive tape
14. Age-related changes in liver and kidney function
15. a

Self-Test: Geriatric Radiography

1. b	6. c	11. c	16. d
2. a	7. d	12. b	17. a
3. c	8. d	13. b	18. c
4. b	9. d	14. a	19. b
5. a	10. a	15. c	20. d

CHAPTER 29: MOBILE RADIOGRAPHY

SECTION 1: EQUIPMENT, TECHNICAL CONSIDERATIONS, AND PATIENT CARE

1. Mobile radiography is commonly performed in patient rooms, emergency rooms, intensive care units, surgery and recovery rooms, as well as nursery and neonatal units.
2. Mobile radiography was first used in World War I by the military for treating battlefield injuries.
3. Portable, because the first units were carried
4. kVp and mAs
5. Typical range is 0.04 to 320 mAs
6. Typical range is 40 to 130 kVp
7. The total power range for mobile units is 15 to 25 kilowatts (kW), which is much lower than stationary units, which can have as much as 150 kW.
8. Mobile x-ray machines are classified into two categories—*battery operated* and *capacitor discharge*—depending on the power source.
9. The power source
10. Battery operated: cordless and provide constant kVp and mAs; capacitor discharge: smaller size and ease of movement
11. The grid, anode heel effect, and source–to–image-receptor distance (SID)
12. a. Level
    b. Centered to the central ray
    c. Used at the recommended focal distance or radius
13. SID; field sizes; anode angles

14. a
15. 40 inches (102 cm); the mA limitations of a mobile unit necessitate longer exposure times when the SID exceeds 40 inches (102 cm).
16. True
17. Lead apron
18. b
19. 6 feet
20. a, b, d, e, f
21. 1. Patients who have infectious microorganisms that could be spread to health care workers and visitors
    2. Patients who need protection from potentially lethal microorganisms that may be carried by health care workers and visitors
22. Universal precautions
23. Mask, gown, and gloves
24. The IR should be placed in a clear, impermeable cover.
25. All equipment that touched the patient or the patient's bed must be wiped with a disinfectant according to appropriate aseptic technique.

SECTION 2: MOBILE RADIOGRAPHIC EXAMINATIONS

1. a, b, c, d, e, g
2. a
3. 2 inches (5 cm)
4. Perpendicular; long axis of the sternum
5. 3 inches; jugular notch
6. A grid
7. Left lateral decubitus position
8. The coronal plane passing through the shoulders and hips should be vertical.
9. A pneumothorax (free air levels) in the left lung or fluid in the right lung
10. True
11. Iliac crests
12. 2 inches (5 cm) above the iliac crest, or high enough to include the diaphragm on the image
13. Symphysis pubis
14. Diaphragm
15. Grid cut-off
16. Look for symmetric appearance of the vertebral column and iliac wings.
17. 5 minutes; to allow air to rise and fluid levels to settle
18. 2 inches (5 cm) above the iliac crests; diaphragm
19. Midway between the anterior superior iliac spine (ASIS) and the pubic symphysis, or about 2 inches (5 cm) inferior to the ASIS and 2 inches (5 cm) superior to the pubic symphysis
20. Fractured hip or pelvis
21. To place the greater trochanters in profile and eliminate foreshortening of the femoral necks
22. Parallel
23. Distal ⅔ of femur and the knee joint
24. c
25. a
26. 1 inch (2.5 cm) above the external acoustic meatus
27. Grid cut-off

28. Seven cervical vertebrae, including the base of the skull and the soft tissues surrounding the neck
29. d
30. A nurse wearing a lead apron
31. True
32. Straightening the head and neck of a neonatal infant may advance the endotracheal tube too far into the trachea.
33. False (The infant must be elevated on a radiolucent support to include all pertinent anatomy on the image.)
34. The costophrenic angles of the lungs
35. Air-fluid levels

Self-Test: Mobile Radiography

1. b	6. b	11. d	16. b
2. d	7. b	12. c	17. d
3. a	8. c	13. b	18. a
4. c	9. b	14. a	19. c
5. d	10. a	15. c	20. b

CHAPTER 30: SURGICAL RADIOGRAPHY

Exercise 1

1. S
2. N
3. N
4. N
5. S
6. S
7. N
8. N
9. S
10. N

Exercise 2

1. True
2. False (The anesthesia provider is a nonsterile team member.)
3. True
4. True
5. True
6. True
7. True
8. True
9. False (Sterile gowns are considered sterile in front from the shoulder to the level of the sterile field.)
10. False (The sleeves of gowns are considered to be sterile from the cuff to the elbow.)
11. True
12. False (The C-arm should be covered with sterile drapes only after it is inside an OR.)
13. False (Cleaning within the OR helps reduce the possibility of cross contamination.)
14. False (The image intensifier must be covered with a sterile drape because it is positioned over the sterile field.)
15. False (Only a member of the sterile team can touch sterile supplies; the radiographer is not a member of the sterile team.)

16. True
17. True
18. False (Only a member of the sterile team—most likely the surgeon—can manipulate the patient's limb.)
19. False (To prevent overheating, the tube should not be covered for too long.)
20. True
21. True
22. True
23. False (The tibia and the femur should not be seen after subtraction is performed.)
24. False (The radiographer should never touch sterile draping overlying the surgical area.)
25. True

Self-Test: Surgical Radiography

1. d	6. a	11. b	16. a	21. d
2. b	7. a	12. b	17. b	22. a
3. a	8. c	13. c	18. b	23. b
4. a	9. c	14. a	19. c	24. d
5. b	10. d	15. b	20. a	25. a

CHAPTER 31: COMPUTED TOMOGRAPHY

Review

1. Computed tomography is the process of creating a cross-sectional tomographic plane of any part of the body.
2. Rotates; detector assembly; algorithm; matrix; liquid crystal display (LCD) or cathode ray tube (CRT)
3. a. Gantry
   b. Computer and operator console
   c. Patient table
4. 1. i
   2. j
   3. a
   4. d
   5. b
   6. c
   7. e
   8. g
   9. f
   10. h
5. A digital postprocessing technique that has the ability to reconstruct CT axial images into other planes without additional radiation to the patient.
6. a. Matrix camera
   b. Laser printer
7. Head, chest, and abdomen
8. IV, orally, or rectally
9. a. Spatial resolution
   b. Contrast resolution
   c. Noise
   d. Artifacts
10. Spatial resolution
11. Contrast resolution
12. Quantum noise
13. To reduce the chance of residual barium in the GI tract causing artifacts on the CT

317

14. 1. S
    2. N, S
    3. S, C, N
    4. A
    5. N, C
    6. S
    7. A
    8. S, C, N
    9. C, N
15. Slice thickness, scan time, scan diameter, and patient instructions
16. Spiral CT
17. Multi-slice spiral/helical CT (MSHCT)
18. a. Less invasive—does not require arterial puncture
    b. Postprocessing capable of eliminating overlying structures so that only the vascular anatomy is reconstructed
    c. Any image made with CT can be reconstructed without additional radiation exposure or IV contrast administration.
19. Maximum intensity projection (MIP), shaded surface display (SSD), and volume rendering (VR)
20. MIP
21. Surgical procedures or presurgical planning
22. 1. CT
    2. CT
    3. MRI
    4. CT
    5. MRI
    6. CT
23. Weekly; biweekly
24. Multiple Scan Average Dose (MSAD)
25. a. Beam energy (kVp)
    b. Tube current (mA)
    c. Rotation or exposure time (seconds)
    d. Section or slice thickness (collimation)
    e. Object thickness and attenuation (size of patient)
    f. Pitch and/or section spacing (table distance traveled in one rotation)
    g. Dose reduction techniques (mA modulation)
    h. Distance from the tube to the isocenter

CT Image Analysis

1. A
2. A. Stomach
   B. Spleen
   C. Abdominal aorta
   D. Vertebral body (thoracic)
   E. Right kidney
   F. Inferior vena cava
   G. Liver

3. A. Soft tissue window
   B. Bone window
4. Coronal
5. Axial
6. Axial
7. Coronal
8. Contrast
9. Noncontrast
10. Noncontrast

Self-Test: Computed Tomography

1. c	7. a	13. d	19. a	25. c
2. d	8. c	14. b	20. d	26. a
3. b	9. d	15. b	21. d	27. d
4. a	10. b	16. c	22. b	28. a
5. c	11. a	17. b	23. b	29. d
6. a	12. d	18. a	24. c	30. b

APPENDIX: SUPPLEMENTAL EXERCISES FOR SKULL POSITIONING

Skull Positioning Review
Exercise 1

1. g	6. m	11. b
2. n	7. a	12. e
3. p	8. f	13. a
4. n	9. m	14. a
5. m	10. f	15. f

Exercise 2

1. n	6. j	11. h
2. f	7. g	12. k
3. d	8. a	13. p
4. o	9. c	14. l
5. i	10. b	15. m

Exercise 3

1. G	7. F	13. N	19. K
2. L	8. P	14. O	20. B
3. A	9. G	15. G	21. C
4. C	10. M	16. I	22. M
5. H	11. G	17. K	23. Q
6. I	12. Q	18. E	